汉英对照

Chinese—English Edition

针灸组合穴图解

编著　刘炎
Compiler　Liu Yan

翻译　王静
Translator　Wang Jing

Illustration of Composed Acupoints in Acupuncture-Moxibustion Use

上海科学技术出版社
SHANGHAI SCIENTIFIC & TECHNICAL PUBLISHERS

图书在版编目(CIP)数据

汉英对照针灸组合穴图解/刘炎编著;王静译.—上
海:上海科学技术出版社,2004.6
ISBN 7—5323—7136—0

Ⅰ.汉...　Ⅱ.①刘...②王...　Ⅲ.针灸疗法—图解
Ⅳ.R245—64

中国版本图书馆 CIP 数据核字(2003)第 053301·号

世 纪 出 版 集 团
上海科学技术出版社　出版、发行
(上海瑞金二路 450 号　邮政编码 200020)
苏州望电印刷有限公司印刷
新华书店上海发行所经销
开本 787×1092　1/16　印张 26.75　字数 450 千字
2004 年 6 月第 1 版　2004 年 6 月第 1 次印刷
印数:1—3 500
定价:85.00 元

本书如有缺页、错装或坏损等严重质量问题,
请向本社出版科联系调换

　　针灸组合穴指由二个或二个以上的腧穴或穴点组合而成的穴组，是目前腧穴组合发展的一个新组成、新形式。全书共介绍了临床常用组合穴553个，分成四章，其中头面颈项部71个，躯干部141个，四肢部172个，全身性组合穴169个。均为临床常用有效的组合穴。由于大多数穴位组合并不复杂，读者阅后即可运用，并可获得较为理想的效果。

　　全书内容易学易懂，并采取汉英对照、图文并茂方式，更便于国内外医务人员和针灸爱好者学习和应用。

　　Composed acupoints is the group of acupoints composed of two points or more, it's a new combination and new form in the development of acupoints. There are 553 composed acupoints in common use in clinic introduced in this book, which is divided into four chapters: 71 on the head, face, neck and nape regions, 141 on the trunk, 172 on the four limbs and 169 composed points located on the whole body. They are all the effective composed acupoints commonly used in clinic. Most of the acupoints are not complicated, so after reading the book, the readers can use them and obtain preferable effects.

　　The content of this book is easy to learn and easy to comprehend, and it takes the form of Chinese-English description and illustration, which is more convenient for the doctors and lovers of acupuncture and moxibustion at home and abroad.

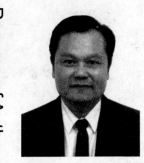

刘炎，男，出生于1941年6月，汉族，上海松江人。大学本科(6年制)毕业。上海中医药大学教授，针灸推拿学院首任院长，中华全国高等中医院校针灸教育研究会前任会长，上海市中医药学会中医综合疗法研究会会长，中国针灸学会刺灸分会副理事长。

主要贡献：擅长中医针灸各科。1965年毕业后一直从事医疗教学工作，中年起参加科研，近年则致力于著书立说和总结工作，有着丰富的临床和教学经验，其医疗作风正派，针法娴熟，下手如飞，堪称针家一绝，被誉为"飞针"专家，深受医患欢迎。曾被评为上海中医学院、龙华医院先进工作者，1993年受到《解放日报》、《工人日报》及《冶金报》等报的表彰。负责并完成了"针刺手法测定仪"、"不同针法灸法的生理病理效应"等科研课题4项，并获得了3项奖。教学经验丰富，1983年曾去美国加州讲学，受到美方的欢迎和该州考试委员会的表彰，教学录像《毫针刺法》、《灸法》曾先后在全国中西医院校有声读物评展中获得2项优秀教材奖，以及优秀片奖、教学奖等。《古典针法》一书别具一格，新颖别致，集科学艺术于一体，获得了全国比赛一等奖，此为全国中医院校在历届比赛中所取得的最高奖，受到了国际国内同道的一致好评。先后发表了《谈高校的针灸教学》、《练针前后针刺手法测定》、《脐海探秘》等医疗教学科研文章40篇。出版专著有《中华自然疗法》、《中华特种针疗法》、《中华脐疗大成》、《中华古今食疗荟萃》、《中华古今药膳荟萃》、《中华奇穴大成》、《中华组合穴集成》、《江浙沪名医秘方精粹》、《腧穴刺灸法》等近20本。此外，还以副主编、编委身份参加了《新编针灸大辞典》等10余部著作的撰写工作；近还积极参与"针药结合戒毒的临床和机制研究"、"丹芪益心贴透皮吸收方法学实验研究"等7项国家部局级课题的研究工作,在全国针灸界影响颇深,其业绩已被载入《中国当代名人录》、《中国名医列传·当代卷》、《中国当代教育名人大辞典》、《中国教育专家名典》、《中华英才大典》、《中华兴国大典》、《世界名人录》、《世界优秀人才大典》、《中华人民共和国人物辞典》等50余种书中。

Liu Yan, male, born in June of 1941, Han nationality and a native of Songjiang County, Shanghai, and graduated from the undergraduate program (6—year program) in 1965, a professor and first director of Acu-Moxi and Tuina College of Shanghai University of TCM, a former director of Acupuncture Education Society of All-China Higher TCM Institution, a director of TCM Comprehensive Therapy Association of Shanghai Society of Chinese Medicine and Pharmacy and a deputy board chairman of Needling and Moxibustion Technique Association of China Acupunctures Society.

Main contributions: Professor Liu is a professional specialist in various aspects in acupuncture therapy of Chinese medicine. After he graduated in 1965, he has been engaged in the medical service and educational work and in the scientific research since his middle age. In recent years, he has been contributing his efforts in book complication of his previous professional expertise. By his rich experience in clinical treatment and education, his ethical style in medical service and proficient needling techniques, he is honoured as a specialist of "Flying Needling Technique" and has been deeply appreciated by the patients. He used to be awarded model medical worker of Shanghai College of Traditional Chinese Medicine and Long Hua Hospital. He was awarded by *Jiefang Daily*, *Workers'*

Daily and *Metallurgical Newspaper* in 1993. He organized and completed 4 research projects of "Determination Apparatus of Needling Techniques" and "Physiopathological Efficacy of Different Needling Techniques" etc. and was awarded 3 prizes. In 1983 he was invited by US as a visiting scholar to give lectures in California, US and was highly appreciated by US partners and Acupuncture Licensing Committee of the state. His educational videotapes on "Needling Techniques of Filiform Needles" and "Moxibustion Methods" were honored two prizes of Outstanding Teaching Materials Award, and Excellent Tape Award and Education Award in audio-video publication exhibition of national medical institutions of western and Chinese medicine. His book on *Classic Needling Techniques*, compiled with a unique style and in combination of science and art was awarded a first prize in competition in whole China, also a highest prize in the successive competitions of the national institutions of Chinese medicine, and was highly evaluated and appreciated by international and domestic colleagues. He has published over 40 pieces of these on his achievements in medical service and education, such as "On Acupuncture Education in Universities", "Determination of Needling Techniques before and after Practice" and "Exploration of Naval Therapy", and has also published around 20 books, such as *Natural Therapies in China*, *Special Needle Therapies in China*, *Compendium of Chinese Naval Therapies*, *Collection of Chinese Ancient and Current Dietetic Therapy*, *Collection of Chinese Ancient and Current Medicated Meals*, *Compendium of Chinese Extraordinary Points*, *Collection of Chinese Combined Points*, *Secret Formulas Selected From Famous Doctors in Jiangsu and Zhejiang Province and Shanghai* and *Needling and Moxibustion Methods of*

Acupoints. In addition, he also participated the compilation and edition of over 10 books, such as *New Edition of Acupuncture and moxibustion Dictionary*, as a deputy editor-in-chief and editing member. Recently, he also takes part in seven research projects of ministry and bureau level, such as "Clinical and Mechanism Study on Drug Abuse Treated by Acupuncture and Herbal Preparation" and "Experimental Study on Methodology of Transdermal Absorption of Salvia and Astragalus Heart-Benefiting Plaster." He is impressive in the circle of TCM acupuncture in the whole country and his achievements have been recorded in over 50 books of *Chinese Famous Professionals of Contemporary Times*, Volume of *Contemporary Times-Biographies of Chinese Famous Doctors*, *Dictionary of Chinese Famous Professionals of Contemporary Education*, *Dictionary of Chinese Educational Specialists*, *Dictionary of Chinese Talents*, *Dictionary of Chinese Flourish*, *Biography of World Famous Persons*, *Dictionary of World Outstanding Talents* and *Personage Dictionary of P.R. China*.

　　针灸是中医学一颗璀璨的明珠，也是它的一个重要组成部分。而腧穴又是学好针灸的基础，是历代针灸医家所十分重视和研究的内容。

　　组合穴是由二个或二个以上的腧穴或穴点组合而成的穴组。它大体上可分为如下几种：一为经穴的组合，即由二个或二个以上的经穴与经穴组合而成，如三里二穴是由手、足三里二穴组合而成，还如合谷与太冲组合成的"四关"穴等，似这般组合的还包括特定穴的组合如心募巨阙与心俞组合成的心募俞穴，肺经原穴太渊与大肠经络穴偏历组合的肺原络穴等；二为奇穴组合，如大、小骨空，手三关穴等，以及本身由多个点组合而成的奇穴组合如十宣、四缝等；三为经穴与奇穴或阿是穴的组合，如腹下三针是由中极与子宫穴组合而成，极泉中心由极泉和其上下左右四个阿是穴组合而成等。总之，只要形成一个穴组，各穴或点均有明确的定位，具有共同的主治，冠以一个总的名称，并经临床验证确有疗效的，均可成为一个组合穴。

　　在临床实践中，有些组合穴本身就是一个小型的配方，如胁肋疼痛取阳陵泉和支沟，胃脘疼痛取中脘、内关、足三里，肩痛取肩髃、肩前、肩后等。这些小配方在临床上用之卓有成就，因而渐渐地把它固定下来，也便成了组合穴。在众多组合穴中，类似这种例子颇多，并充分体现了原来配穴处方中的本经配穴法，前后配穴法，表里配穴法，上下配穴法，左右配穴法等法。而今组合穴的出现，对于针灸腧穴学分类来说无疑是一种突破、一种创新，它的产生实际上是腧穴学的一个新发展，也是针灸学发展的一个方向，必将有其广阔的前景。

Acumoxi (Acupuncture and Moxibustion), a bright pearl in the treasure house of Traditional Chinese Medicine, is an important component part of Traditional Chinese Medicine. Acupoints is the base of Acumoxi as well as the content that Acumoxi doctors through the ages have paid much attention to and made researches on.

Composed points is the acupoints composed of two points or more. It has several forms as follows: First, the combination of the meridian acupoints, i.e. the group is composed of two meridian acupoints or more, such as Siguan, which is composed of Hegu and Taichong. Such combination also includes the specific points, such as Xinshumuxue which is composed of Juque, the Front—Mu Point of Heart and Xinshu, the Back-Shu Point of Heart, Feiyuanluo which is composed of Taiyuan, the Yuan-Primary Point of the Lung Meridian and Pianli, the Luo—Connecting Point of the Large Intestine Meridian, etc.. Second, the combination of extraordinary acupoints, such as Daxiaogukong, Shousanguanxue, etc., and the extraordinary acupoints which are composed of multi—point themselves such as Shixuan, Sifeng, etc., and Jiquanzhongxin, which is composed of Jiquan and four Ashi points superior, inferior and lateral to it, etc.. Third, the combination of the meridian acupoints and extraordinary acupoints or Ashi points, such as Fuxiasanzhen, which is composed of Zhongji and Zigong. In a word, so long as there is a group of acupoints which is entitled a name, each acupoint of the group has its specific location, common indications, and the group has certain curative effect proved by clinical use, then the group can be called a composed acupoints.

In the clinical use, some composed acupoints are abbreviated prescriptions themselves. For example, Yanglingquan and Zhigou can be used to treat the pain in the hypochondriac region, Zhongwan, Neiguan and Zusanli can be used to treat the gastric pain, Jianyu, Jianqian and Jianhou can be used to treat the pain in the shoulder, etc.. These small prescriptions have great effect in the clinical use, therefore they have a fixed form gradually, thus the composed acupoints take shape. There are many such examples in so many composed acupoints, and they embody the methods of combination of the same meridian, combination of the anterior and the posterior, combination of the exterior and the interior, combination of the above and the subjacent and combination of the left and the right of the original selection of acupoints and prescription. Composed acupoints is a kind of breakthrough as well as a kind of innovation for the classification of the acupoints of Acumoxi. It's a new development of the study of acupoints and a direction of the development of Acumoxi, it will surely have great prospect.

第一章 头面颈项部组合穴

CHAPTER 1 COMPOSED ACUPOINTS ON THE HEAD, FACE, NECK AND NAPE

Contents

目录

第二章 躯干部组合穴

CHAPTER 2 COMPOSED ACUPOINTS ON THE TRUNK

目录

Contents

Contents

Contents

第三章 四肢部组合穴

CHAPTER 3 COMPOSED ACUPOINTS ON THE FOUR LIMBS

目录

Contents

Contents

Contents

第四章 全身性组合穴

CHAPTER 4 COMPOSED ACUPOINTS ON THE WHOLE BODY

 261

Contents

Contents

Contents

Contents

第一章　头面颈项部组合穴

CHAPTER 1 COMPOSED ACUPOINTS ON THE HEAD, FACE, NECK AND NAPE

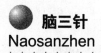

脑三针
Naosanzhen

组成　本穴组由脑户、脑空二穴组合而成。

位置　脑户：风府穴直上1.5寸。

脑空：风池穴直上1.5寸。

主治　帕金森综合征，智力低下，运动功能障碍，共济失调脑性瘫痪等。

操作　将针尖顺着头皮向下刺入，第一针脑户向后发际正中方向捻进1.5寸；然后分别向双侧风池方向取左、右侧脑空穴，深度1.5寸。采用缓慢捻进法，得气后少提插，多捻转，以针感向脑后放散为度，留针30分钟，间隔5~10分钟行捻转1次。

Composition　This group of acupoints is composed of Naohu (GV17) and Naokong(GB19).

Location　Naohu：1.5 cun directly above Fengfu (GV16).

Naokong：1.5 cun directly above Fengchi(GB20).

Indications　Parkinson's disease, feeble-mindedness, dyskinesia, ataxic cerebral paralysis, etc..

Method　The needle is inserted downwards along the scalp. The first needle is rotated into Naohu in the direction of the median posterior hairline and then Naokong on left and right sides are needled in the direction of Fengchi on each side respectively, the depth is 1.5 cun. Slow rotation-inserting method is selected, more rotation, less lifting and thrusting after the acu-esthesia is obtained and radiates to the posterior side of the head. The needles are retained for 30 minutes, and rotated once every 5-10 minutes.

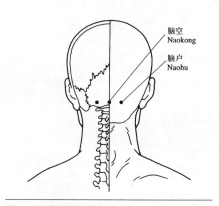

图1-1　脑三针
Fig. 1-1　Naosanzhen

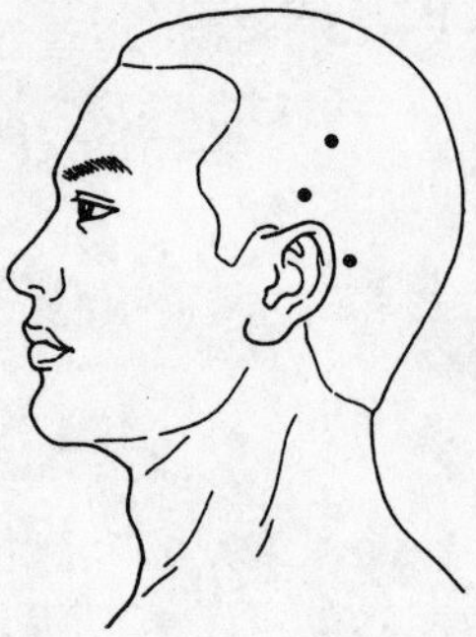

颞三
Niesan

组成　本穴组由颞部的三个点组合而成。

位置　三个点分别位于顶骨节下缘前1厘米处，耳尖上1.5厘米处，耳尖下后2厘米处。

主治　儿童脑性麻痹。

操作　向后平刺3厘米，不捻转，不强刺激，留2小时，2日1次，10次为1疗程。

按注　本穴有书称颞三针。

Composition　This group of acupoints is composed of three points in the temporal part of the head.

Location　The point 1 cm anterior to the lower border of the parietal tubercle. The point 1.5 cm above the ear apex. The point 2 cm posterior to the point 2 cm below the ear apex.

Indication　Infantile cerebral palsy.

Method　The needle is inserted horizontally backwards without rotation or strong stimulation. Retain the needles for 2 hours. Treat once every other day, ten times as one course of treatment.

Note　This group of acupoints is also called Niesanzhen in some books.

智三针
Zhisanzhen

组成　本穴组由神庭、本神二穴组合而成。

位置　神庭：前发际正中直上0.5寸。

本神：神庭穴（督脉）旁3寸，当神庭穴与头维穴连线的内2/3与外1/3连接点处。

主治　儿童智力低下，脑发育不全，小儿多动综合征，老年性痴呆等。

操作　进针方向有两种：一为向头顶百会方向平刺，二为沿前额皮肤向下平刺。儿童多采用后者，青壮年及老人多采用前者。进针深度在儿童为1寸，成年人为1.5～2寸。

弱智儿童以快速进针法或"飞针"法进针，也可以快速捻进法，进针后捻转补泻；成年人以缓慢捻进法为主，进针后以

图1-2　颞三
Fig. 1-2　Niesan

捻转结合小幅度提插，务使针感向额部前后左右放散。得气后均留针30分钟，间隔10分钟行针1次，视阴阳的偏胜偏衰而补泻。

Composition　This group of acupoints is composed of Shenting (GV24) and Benshen(GB13).

Location　Shenting：0.5 cun directly above the midpoint of the anterior hairline.

Benshen：3 cun lateral to Shenting (Du Meridian), at the junction of the medial two thirds and lateral third of the line connecting Shenting and Touwei(ST8).

Indications　Children's feeble-mindedness, encephalic hypoplasia, hyperkinetic syndrome of childhood, senile dementia.

Method　There're two inserting directions, one is to insert the needle horizontally towards Baihui on the vertex of the head, the other is to needle horizontally downwards along the forehead skin. The latter is used more in the children while the former more in the young people, adults and old people. The inserting depth is 1 cun for the children, 1.5—2 cun for the adults.

Quick-inserting method,needle-flying method or quick rotation-inserting method can be used for retarded children, the reducing or reinforcing techniques by rotation are applied after the needle is inserted. For adults, slow rotation-inserting method is mainly used, after the needle is inserted, the reducing or reinforcing techniques by rotation are applied in combination with light inserting and lifting, be sure to make the acu-esthesia distribute over the forehead. The needles are retained for 30 minutes after the acu-esthesia is obtained, manipulated once every 10 minutes.The reinforcing or reducing method is applied according to the excess or deficiency of yin or yang.

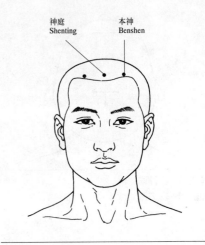

神庭　Shenting　本神　Benshen

图1-3　智三针
Fig. 1—3　Zhisanzhen

四神聪
Sishencong

组成　本穴组由百会前、后、左、右各1寸处的四个点组合而成。

位置　百会前、后、左、右各1寸。

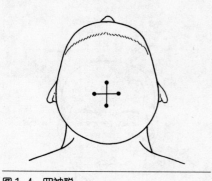

图1-4 四神聪
Fig. 1-4 Sishencong

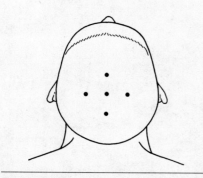

图1-5 四神针
Fig. 1-5 Sishenzhen

主治 头痛，眩晕，失眠，健忘，癫痫，低智，痴呆。

操作 平刺0.5～1寸。

Composition This group of acupoints is composed of the four points respectively 1 cun anterior, posterior and bilateral to Baihui (GV20).

Location Four points respectively 1 cun anterior, posterior and lateral to Baihui.

Indications Headache, vertigo, insomnia, poor memory, epilepsy, feeble-mindedness, dementia.

Method Needle horizontally 0.5-1 cun.

● 四神针
Sishenzhen

组成 本穴组由百会穴左右前后各旁开1.5寸的四穴点组合而成。

位置 百会穴前后左右旁开1.5寸。

主治 智力低下，巅顶头痛，眩晕。

操作 针尖向外方向平刺,或针尖向内即百会方向平刺1～1.2寸，行捻转手法。

Composition This group of acupoints is composed of the four points respectively 1.5 cun anterior, posterior and bilateral to Baihui(GV20).

Location 1.5 cun anterior, posterior and lateral to Baihui.

Indication Feeble-mindedness, parietal headache, vertigo.

Method The needles are inserted 1-1.2 cun outwards, or inwards, i.e. towards Baihui horizontally. The rotating method is applied.

● 治脑四穴
Zhinaosixue

组成 本穴组由治脑、强脑、益脑、一光四穴组合而成。

位置 治脑：颈部正中线、第二、第三颈椎棘突之间点。

强脑：颈部正中线、第三、第四颈椎棘突之间点。

益脑：颈部正中线、第四、第五颈椎棘突之间点。

一光：颈部正中线、第五、第六颈椎棘突之间点。

主治　大脑发育不良，癫、狂、痫。

操作　针0.3～0.5寸，局部酸胀感。

Composition　This group of acupoints is composed of Zhinao, Qiangnao, Yinao and Yiguang.

Location　Zhinao：On the midline of the nape, at the midpoint of the spinous processes of the 2nd and 3rd cervical vertebrae.

Qiangnao：On the midline of the nape, at the midpoint of the spinous processes of the 3rd and 4th cervical vertebrae.

Yinao：On the midline of the nape, at the midpoint of the spinous processes of the 4th and 5th cervical vertebrae.

Yiguang：On the midline of the nape, at the midpoint of the spinous processes of the 5th and 6th cervical vertebrae.

Indications　Encephalic hypogenesis, mania, epilepsy.

Method　The needle is inserted 0.3－0.5 cun, the acu-esthesia of soreness and distension should be obtained.

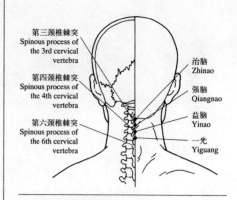

图1-6　治脑四穴

Fig. 1-6　Zhinaosixue

 治脑纵线要穴

Zhinaozongxianyaoxue

组成　本穴组由第一颈椎至第二胸椎棘突间的八个点组合而成。

位置　项背部正中线，入后发际0.5寸处一穴，第二、第三颈椎棘突之间点一穴，第三、第四、第四、第五、第六、第六、第七颈椎棘突之间点各一穴，第七颈椎与第一胸椎棘突之间点一穴，第一、第二胸椎棘突之间点一穴。

主治　大脑发育不良。

操作　针0.3～0.8寸，针感局部酸、胀。

Composition　This group of acupoints is composed of the eight points locating in the area from the spinous process of the 1st cervical vertebra to the spinous process of the 2nd thoracic vertebra.

Location　On the midline of the nape and the back, 8 points in all. They are：the point 0.5 cun above the posterior hairline, the points between the spinous pro-

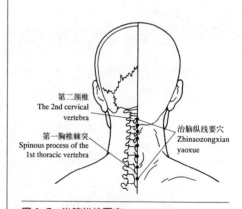

图1-7　治脑纵线要穴

Fig. 1-7　Zhinaozongxianyaoxue

cesses of the 2nd and 3rd, 3rd and 4th, 4th and 5th, 5th and 6th, 6th and 7th cervical vertebrae, the point between the spinous processes of the 7th cervical vertebra and the 1st thoracic vertebra and the point between the spinous processes of the 1st and 2nd thoracic vertebrae.

Indication　Encephalic hypogenesis.

Method　The needle is inserted 0.3−0.8 cun, the acu-esthesia of soreness and distension should be obtained.

四中
Sizhong

组成　本穴组由百会左、右、前、后各2~3寸的四个点组合而成。

位置　位于百会穴前、后、左、右各2~3寸处。

主治　脑积水。

操作　平刺1~2寸。

按注　注意囟门突出者应避开斜刺。

Composition　This group of acupoints is composed of the 4 points respectively 2−3 cun anterior, posterior and bilateral to Baihui(GV20).

Location　2−3 cun anterior, posterior and lateral to Baihui.

Indication　Hydrocephalus.

Method　The needle is inserted 1−2 cun horizontally.

Note　The protuberant fontanel should be avoided when the needle is inserted.

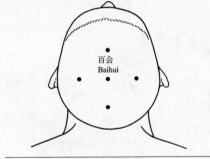

图1-8　四中
Fig. 1−8　Sizhong

百囟
Baixin

组成　本穴组由百会、囟会二穴组合而成。

位置　百会：后发际正中直上7寸。

囟会：前发际正中直上2寸。

主治　卒中。

操作　一针从百会向囟会透刺进针3寸，一针从囟会向百会透刺3寸用泻法。留针20分钟。

Composition　This group of acupoints is composed of

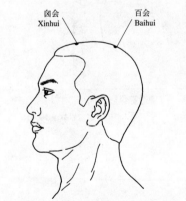

图1-9　百囟
Fig. 1−9　Baixin

Baihui (GV20) and Xinhui (GV22).

Location Baihui：7 cun directly above the midpoint of the posterior hairline.

Xinhui：2 cun directly above the midpoint of the anterior hairline.

Indication Apoplexy.

Method One needle is penetrated 3 cun from Baihui to Xinhui, another needle is penetrated 3 cun from Xinhui to Baihui. The reducing method is used. Retain the needles for 20 minutes.

颈中二穴
Jingzhongerxue

组成 本穴组由颈中、翳明下二穴组合而成。

位置 颈中：位于颈后部、颈肌隆起外缘入后发际1寸的凹陷中与胸锁乳突肌停止处乳突下凹连线之中点直下2寸处，当风池穴与翳明穴连线之中点直下2寸处。

翳明下(又名颈中2)：位于颈部、乳突下凹直下2寸，胸锁乳突肌后缘，当翳明穴下2寸处。

主治 半身不遂。

操作 直刺0.5～1.5寸，针感酸麻沉重。

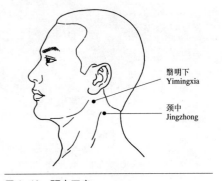

图1-10 颈中二穴
Fig. 1-10 Jingzhongerxue

Composition This group of acupoints is composed of Jingzhong and Yimingxia.

Location Jingzhong：on the nape, 2 cun directly below the midpoint of the line connecting the depression 1 cun above the posterior hairline to the lateral border of the neck muscle with the depression below the mastoid process where the sternocleidomastoid muscles end, i.e. the point 2 cun below the midpoint of the line connecting Fengchi(GB20) with Yiming(EX-HN14).

Yimingxia (Jingzhong2)：on the neck, 2 cun directly under the depression below mastoid process, to the posterior border of the sternocleidomastoid muscles, i.e. 2 cun below Yiming.

Indication Hemiplegia.

Method The needle is inserted perpendicularly. The acu-esthesia of soreness, numbness and heaviness should be obtained.

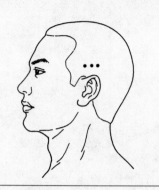

图 1-11　颞三针
Fig. 1-11　Niesanzhen

● 颞三针
Niesanzhen

组成　本穴组由颞部的三个点组合而成。

位置　于偏瘫对侧颞部，耳尖直上 2 寸处为第一针，然后以第一针为中点、同一水平前后各旁开 1 寸分别为第二针，第三针。

主治　中风后遗症偏瘫，智力低下儿童运动功能障碍，帕金森综合病征，小儿多动综合征，扭体痉挛综合征。

操作　于偏瘫对侧颞部耳尖直上 2 寸处，呈 30°角朝下刺入，针刺深度 1~1.2 寸，局部有麻胀感或放射至整个头部为度，用同样方法针第二针，第三针（一般不灸）。

多采用提插捻转手法。中风偏瘫患者进针后每间隔 5 分钟行针 1 次，半小时后出针，可在针刺过程中令患者配合活动患侧肢体。

Composition　This group of acupoints is composed of the three points on the temporal part of the head.

Location　On the temporal part of the head contralateral to the hemiplegic side. The first point is 2 cun directly above the ear apex. The 2nd and 3rd points are 1 cun horizontally lateral to the first point.

Indications　Apoplectic sequelae, hemiplegia, feeble-mindedness, infantile dyskinesia, Parkinson's disease, MBD, torsion spasm.

Methods　The needle is inserted downwards at the point 2 cun directly above the ear apex on the temporal part of the head contralateral to the hemiplegic side, the angle is 30°, the depth 1-1.2 cun. Manipulate the needle till the acu-esthesia of numbness or distension is obtained in this part or distributes over the whole head. The 2nd and 3rd needles are inserted with the same method (Usually moxibustion is not applied).

The techniques of thrusting, lifting and rotating are used more. For the patients with apoplexy and hemiplegia, manipulate the needles every 5 minutes after the needles are inserted, and withdraw the needles after half an hour. The patient can be instructed to exercise the affected limbs during the treatment.

前后神聪
Qianhoushencong

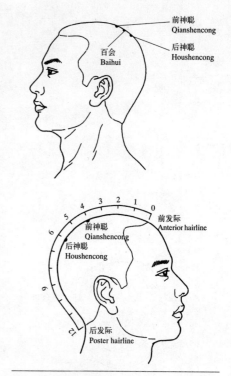

组成　本穴组由前、后神聪二穴组合而成。

位置　前神聪：位于头项正中线，前发际后4寸处。

后神聪：位于头项正中线，前后发际之中点处。

主治　中风，癫痫，头痛，眩晕，失眠，健忘，弱智。

操作　沿皮向后、向前针0.5～1寸，局部抽痛胀感。

Composition　This group of acupoints is composed of Qianshencong and Houshencong.

Location　Qianshencong：on the midline of the head, 4 cun above the anterior hairline.

Houshencong：on the midline of the head, midpoint of the anterior and posterior hairline.

Indications　Apoplexy, epilepsy, headache, vertigo, insomnia, poor memory, feeble-mindedness.

Method　The needles are inserted 0.5–1 cun backwards or forwards. The acu-esthesia of pain and distension should be obtained in this part.

图1-12　前后神聪
Fig. 1-12　Qianhoushencong

舌三针
Shesanzhen

组成　本穴组由颌下的三个点组合而成。

位置　以拇指第一、第二指骨间横纹平贴于下颌前缘，拇指尖处为第一针，其左右各旁开1寸为第二针，第三针。

主治　中风语言謇涩，弱智儿童流涎，语言发育迟缓，语不连贯，发音不清。

操作　头稍仰，针尖向舌根方向呈60°～45°针刺，儿童进针深度约0.8寸，成人1～1.2寸。

Composition　This group of acupoints is composed of the three points on the jaw.

Location　Align the transverse crease between the 1st and 2nd phalanges of the thumb with the anterior border of the jaw, the first point is at the end of the tip of the thumb, the 2nd and 3rd points are 1 cun lateral to the first point.

Indications　Apoplectic stuttering speech, feeble-minded

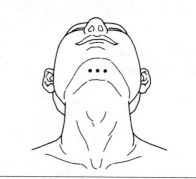

图1-13　舌三针
Fig. 1-13　Shesanzhen

children's salivation, retarded development of speech, disconnected speech, alalia.

Method The head is bent upwards a bit, the needle is inserted at the angle of 60° −45° toward the tongue root. For children, the depth is about 0.8 cun, and 1−1.2 cun for adults.

难言
Nanyan

组成 本穴组由金津、玉液、廉泉、风府四穴组合而成。

位置 金津、玉液：舌系带两侧静脉上，左为金津，右为玉液。

廉泉：舌骨体上缘的中点处。

风府：后发际正中直上1寸。

主治 中风舌强难言。

操作 金津、玉液用三棱针点刺出血，廉泉、风府针刺3厘米左右，皆用泻法，留针30分钟。

Composition This group of acupoints is composed of Jinjin(EX-HN12), Yuye(EX-HN13), Lianquan (CV23) and Fengfu(GV16).

Location Jinjin, Yuye：on the veins lateral to the frenulum of the tongue, Jinjin is on the left vein, Yuye on the right one.

Lianquan：at the midpoint of the upper border of the hyoid bone.

Fengfu：1 cun directly above the midpoint of the posterior hairline.

Indication Apoplectic stuttering speech.

Method Prick Jinjin and Yuye with a three-edged needle to bleed. Lianquan and Fengfu are needled to the depth of about 3 cm, the reducing method is applied. Retain the needles for 30 minutes.

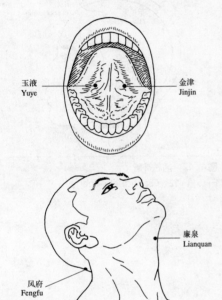

玉液
Yuye

金津
Jinjin

廉泉
Lianquan

风府
Fengfu

图1-14 难言
Fig. 1-14 Nanyan

耳门前脉
Ermenqianmai

组成 本穴组由耳门前的二个点组合而成。

位置　面部，耳轮棘前缘上0.2寸一穴，耳垂下缘相平下0.2寸一穴。

主治　音哑，舌謇。

操作　麦粒灸，灸7壮。

按注　此穴一般多用灸法，时见刺法时可针0.2—0.5寸。局部痛胀感。

Composition　This group of acupoints is composed of the two points anterior to Ermen.

Location　On the face, one is 0.2 cun above the anterior border of the helix, the other is 0.2 cun below the lower border of the earlap.

Indications　Hoarse voice, stiffness of the tongue.

Method　7 wheat-sized moxa cones of moxibustion is applied.

Note　Usually, moxibustion is used more at this acupoint. When needling, the depth may be 0.2—0.5 cun, and the acu-esthesia of pain or distension should be obtained.

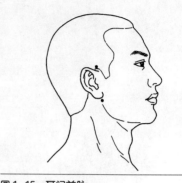

图1-15　耳门前脉
Fig. 1-15　Ermenqianmai

 廉泉三穴
Lianquansanxue

组成　本穴组由廉泉、上廉泉、新廉泉三穴组合而成。

位置　廉泉：喉结上方，当舌骨的下缘凹陷处。

上廉泉：颌下部甲状软骨上凹陷直上1寸点。

新廉泉：颈部正中、甲状软骨与环状软骨之间。

主治　舌强语謇，吞咽困难。

操作　刺法：廉泉、上廉泉针尖向舌根斜刺1~2寸，达舌根部，再提针至皮下，向舌根两侧斜刺，针感舌尖、舌根有发麻感。

新廉泉：针0.2~0.3寸，有针感时可见到针柄搏动。

灸法　麦粒灸3~5壮。

Composition　This group of acupoints is composed of Lianquan(CV23), Shanglianquan and Xinlianquan.

Location　Lianquan：on the neck and anterior midline, above the laryngeal protuberance, in the depression above the lower border of the hyoid bone.

Shanglianquan：1 cun above the depression between the jaw and the thyroid cartilage.

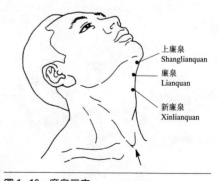

上廉泉
Shanglianquan

廉泉
Lianquan

新廉泉
Xinlianquan

图1-16　廉泉三穴
Fig. 1-16　Lianquansanxue

Xinlianquan: on the midline of the neck, between the thyroid cartilage and the ringed cartilage.

Indications Stiffness of the tongue, stuttering speech, difficulty in swallowing.

Method Acupuncture method: Lianquan and Shanglianquan: the needles are inserted obliquely 1–2 cun towards the tongue root, till the needles reach it. Then lift the needles beneath the skin, insert the needles obliquely towards the two sides of the tongue root. The acu-esthesia of numbness can be felt in the tip and root of the tongue.

Xinlianquan: The needle is inserted 0.2–0.3 cun. When the acu-esthesia is obtained, the trembling of the needle handle can be seen.

Moxibustion method 3–5 wheat-sized moxa cones of moxibustion is applied.

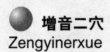

增音二穴
Zengyinerxue

组成 本穴组由增音、增音上二穴组合而成。

位置 增音：颈部甲状软骨切迹上凹与下颌角之中点，当人迎穴上前方。

增音上：颈部甲状软骨上切迹与下颌角连线中点上1厘米处。

主治 音哑音嘶，张口不利。

操作 向咽喉方向刺入0.5～1.2寸，针感咽喉部有发痒或麻、胀感。

Composition This group of acupoints is composed of Zengyin and Zengyinshang.

Location Zengyin: on the neck, at the midpoint of the line connecting the depression above the superior notch of the thyroid cartilage and the mandibular angle, which is anterior and superior to Renying(ST9).

Zengyinshang: on the neck, 1 cm above the midpoint of the line connecting the superior notch of the thyroid cartilage and mandibular angle.

Indications Hoarse voice, inability to open the mouth.

Method The needle is inserted 0.5–1.2 cun towards the throat. The acu-esthesia of itch in the throat or

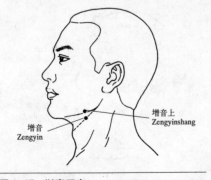

图1-17 增音二穴
Fig. 1-17 Zengyinerxue

numbness or distension can be obtained.

Yiquan

组成　本穴组由下关、颊车、地仓、四白四穴组合而成。

位置　下关：颧弓下缘，下颌骨髁状突之前方，切迹之间凹陷中。合口有孔，张口即闭。

颊车：下颌角前上方一横指凹陷中，咀嚼时咬肌隆起最高点处。

地仓：口角旁0.4寸，巨髎穴直下取之。

四白：目正视，瞳孔直下，当眶下孔凹陷中。

主治　面瘫，面痉。

操作　针法：斜刺，下关透颊车，下关透四白，地仓透颊车，地仓透四白。

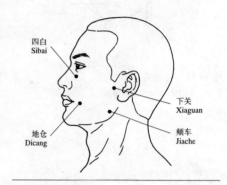

图1-18　一圈
Fig. 1-18　Yiquan

Composition　This group of acupoints is composed of Xiaguan(ST7), Jiache(ST6), Dicang(ST4) and Sibai(ST2).

Location　Xiaguan：in the depression between the lower border of the zygomatic arch and the condyloid process of the mandible. The depression can be felt when the mouth is shut, and will disappear when the mouth is open.

Jiache：in the depression one finger breadth above the mandibular angle, where the masseter muscle is prominent when chewing.

Dicang：0.4 cun lateral to the corner of the mouth, which is directly below Juliao(ST3).

Sibai：directly below the pupil, in the depression of the infraorbital foramen.

Indications　Facial paralysis, facial spasm.

Method　The needles are inserted obliquely, penetrated from Xiaguan to Jiache, Xiaguan to Sibai, Dicang to Jiache and Dicang to Sibai.

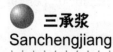
Sanchengjiang

组成　本穴组由承浆穴、挟承浆穴二穴组合而成。

位置　承浆：颏唇沟的中点。

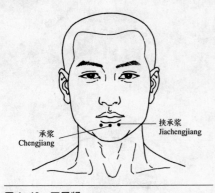

图 1-19 三承浆
Fig. 1-19 Sanchengjiang

挟承浆：承浆穴旁开1寸。

主治 口喎，面颊浮肿，牙痛，面神经麻痹，齿龈溃疡，口唇疔疮，三叉神经痛。

操作 刺法：斜刺0.3～0.5寸。

灸法：温灸5～10分钟。

Composition This group of acupoints is composed of Chengjiang (CV24) and Jiachengjiang.

Location Chengjiang：at the midpoint of the mentolabial sulcus.

Jiachengjiang：1 cun lateral to Chengjiang.

Indications Deviation of the mouth, facial edema, toothache, facial paralysis, gingival ulceration, boil on the lip, trigeminal neuralgia.

Methods Acupuncture：the needle is inserted 0.3–0.5 cun obliquely.

Moxibustion：warm moxibustion for 5–10 minutes.

 三联

Sanlian

组成 本穴组由太阳、下关、地仓三穴组合而成。

位置 太阳：眉梢与目外眦之间向后约1寸凹陷中。

下关：颧弓下缘，下颌骨髁状突之前方，切迹之间凹陷中。合口有孔，张口即闭。

地仓：口角旁0.4寸，巨髎穴直下取之。

主治 面神经麻痹。

操作 平刺或合谷刺，用捻提法，留30分钟，10分钟1次，每日1次。

Composition This group of acupoints is composed of Taiyang(EX-HN5), Xiaguan(ST7) and Dicang(ST4).

Location Taiyang：in the depression 1 cun posterior to the juncture between the lateral end of the eyebrow and the outer canthus.

Xiaguan：in the depression between the lower border of the zygomatic arch and the notch of condyloid process of the mandible. The depression can be felt when the mouth is shut, and will disappear when the mouth is open.

Dicang：0.4 cun lateral to the corner of the mouth,

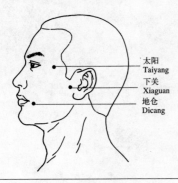

图 1-20 三联
Fig. 1-20 Sanlian

which is directly below Juliao(ST3).

Indication　Facial paralysis.

Method　The needle is inserted horizontally. The techniques of Hegu acupuncture and rotating lifting method are applied. Retain the needles for 30 minutes, manipulate the needles every ten minutes. Treat once every day.

● 齐阳白
Qiyangbai

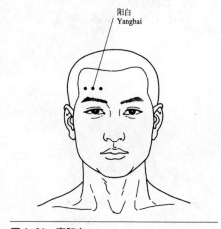

图 1-21　齐阳白
Fig. 1-21　Qiyangbai

组成　本穴组由阳白及其旁二点组合而成。

位置　阳白：目正视，瞳孔直上，眉上1寸。

阳白内外旁开各1寸处二个点。

主治　面神经麻痹，额肌麻痹。

操作　向下平刺0.5~1寸，可接电针仪断续波3分钟，息2分钟，共20分钟。

按注　本穴组有称"上三穴"。

Composition　This group of acupoints is composed of Yangbai (GB14) and two points lateral to it.

Location　Yangbai：directly above the pupil, 1 cun above the eyebrow.

Two points 1 cun lateral to Yangbai.

Indications　Facial paralysis, paralysis of the forehead muscle.

Method　The needle is needled 0.5−1 cun horizontally downwards. The electro-acupuncture can be used with intermittent wave for 3 minutes and 2-minute interval, 20 minutes in all.

Note　This group of acupoints is also called Shangsanxue.

● 齐颧髎下
Qiquanliaoxia

组成　本穴组由颧髎下及其旁二点组合而成。

位置　颧髎下0.5寸处，以及其内外旁开各1寸处。

主治　面神经麻痹。

操作　平刺0.5~1寸，可电针。

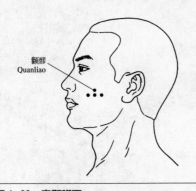

图1-22 齐颧髎下
Fig. 1-22 Qiquanliaoxia

按注 本穴组又称下三穴。

Composition This group of acupoints is composed of Quanliaoxia and two points lateral to it.

Location 0.5 cun below Quanliao (SI18) and 1 cun lateral to Quanliaoxia.

Indication Facial paralysis.

Method The needle is inserted 0.5—1 cun horizontally. The electro-acupuncture can be used.

Note This group of acupoints is also called Xiasanxue.

牵正二穴
Qianzhengerxue

组成 本穴组由牵正穴和中牵正二穴组合而成。

位置 牵正：位于耳垂前方0.5寸，与耳垂中点相平。

中牵正：位于面颊下颌结节前方凹陷与口角外0.4寸连线之中点，也即地仓和颊车穴连线之中点。

主治 面瘫，口角歪斜。

操作 向前斜刺0.3～0.5寸，针感酸麻至颏和颊。

Composition This group of acupoints is composed of Qianzheng and Zhongqianzheng.

Location Qianzheng：0.5 cun anterior to the earlobe, at the level of the midpoint of the earlobe.

Zhongqianzheng：on the face, at the midpoint of the line connecting the depression anterior to the mandibular tubercle and the point 0.4 cun lateral to the corner of the mouth, i.e. at the midpoint of the line connecting Dicang (ST6) and Jiache(ST6).

Indication Facial paralysis, deviation of the mouth.

Method The needle is inserted 0.3—0.5 cun forwards obliquely. The acu-esthesia of soreness and numbness will radiate to the chin and cheek.

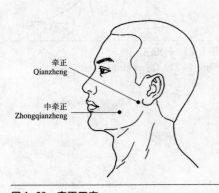

图1-23 牵正二穴
Fig. 1-23 Qianzhengerxue

针风
Zhenfeng

组成 本穴组由风府、百会二穴组合而成。

位置 风府：后发际正中直上1寸。

百会：后发际正中直上7寸。

主治 风疾。

操作 百会沿皮刺0.5~1寸。风府直刺0.5~1寸，得气为度。

Composition This group of acupoints is composed of Fengfu(GV16) and Baihui(GV20).

Location Fengfu：1 cun directly above the midpoint of the posterior hairline.

Baihui：7 cun directly above the midpoint of the posterior hairline.

Indication Diseases due to wind.

Method Baihui：the needle is inserted 0.5—1 cun subcutaneously.

Fengfu：the needle is inserted 0.5—1 cun perpendicularly and manipulated till the acu-esthesia is obtained.

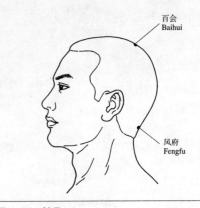

图1-24 针风
Fig. 1-24 Zhenfeng

面八邪
Mianbaxie

组成 本穴组由承光、攒竹、禾髎、人迎左右八穴组合而成。

位置 承光：五处穴后1.5寸。

攒竹：眉头凹陷中。

禾髎：水沟穴旁0.5寸，当鼻孔外缘直下，与水沟穴相平处取穴。

人迎：喉结旁1.5寸，当颈总动脉之后，胸锁乳突肌前缘。

主治 风疾。

操作 点刺出血，或可用三棱针点刺出血。

Composition This group of acupoints is composed of Chengguang(BL6), Zanzhu(BL2), Heliao(LI19) and Renyin (ST9).

Location Chengguang：1.5 cun posterior to Wuchu (BL5).

Cuanzhu：in the depression of the medial end of the eyebrow.

Heliao：0.5 cun lateral to Renzhong (GV26), directly below the lateral border of the nostril, at the level of Shuigou.

Renying：1.5 cun lateral to the laryngeal protuberance,

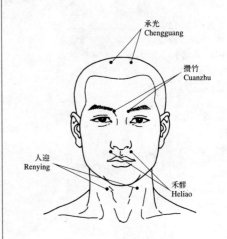

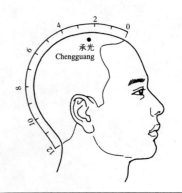

图1-25 面八邪
Fig. 1-25 Mianbaxie

which is posterior to the common carotid artery and anterior to the border of the sternocleidomastoid muscle.

Indication Diseases due to wind.

Method This group of acupoints can be bled by Bian stone or pricked with a three-edged needle.

● 惊痫
Jingxian

组成 本穴组由本神、前顶、囟会、天柱四穴组合而成。

位置 本神：神庭穴（督脉）旁3寸，当神庭穴与头维穴连线的内2/3与外1/3连接点处。

前顶：百会前1.5寸。

囟会：前发际正中直上2寸。

天柱：后发际正中直上0.5寸，旁开1.3寸，当斜方肌外缘凹陷中。

主治 惊恐，惊风。

操作 本神平刺0.5～0.8寸。前顶平刺0.3～0.5寸。天柱直刺0.5～0.8寸。囟会平刺0.2～0.3寸。如小儿囟门未闭者，禁针，改用艾条悬灸5～10分钟。以上诸穴均用单刺法及提插捻转之泻法。

Composition This group of acupoints is composed of Benshen(GB13), Qianding(GV21), Xinhui(GV22) and Tianzhu(BL10).

Location Benshen：3 cun lateral to Shenting (Governor Vessel), at the junction of the medial two thirds and lateral third of the line connecting Shenting and Touwei.

Qianding：1.5 cun anterior to Baihui.

Xinhui：2 cun directly above the midpoint of the anterior hairline.

Tianzhu：1.3 cun lateral to the point and 0.5 directly cun above the midpoint of the posterior hairline, in the depression lateral to the border of trapezius muscle.

Indications Nervousness, convulsion.

Method Benshen is needled 0.5−0.8 cun horizontally, Qianding 0.3−0.5 cun horizontally, Tianzhu 0.5−0.8 cun perpendicularly, Xinhui 0.2−0.3 cun horizontally. Xinhui in infants with open fontanel should not be punctured, suspended moxibustion with moxa roll is appli-

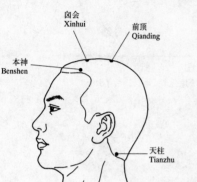

图1-26 惊痫
Fig. 1-26 Jingxian

cable for 5—10 minutes. Single acupuncture and the reducing method of lifting, inserting and rotating can be applied to all the above points.

耳上二穴
Ershangerxue

组成　本穴组由耳上发际和耳上二穴组合而成。

位置　耳上发际：头颞部、耳郭缘之最高点直上方发际处。

耳上：头颞部，卷耳后耳尖直上三横指处。

主治　暴癫。

操作　刺法：针0.1～0.3寸。

灸法：灸3～7壮。

Composition　This group of acupoints is composed of Ershangfaji and Ershang.

Location　Ershangfaji：on the temporal part of the head, at the hairline directly above the ear apex.

Ershang：on the temporal part of the head, three fingers breadth directly above the folded ear apex.

Indication　Sudden insanity.

Method　Acupuncture：the needle is inserted 0.1—0.3 cun.

Moxibustion：3—7 cones of moxibustion can be applied.

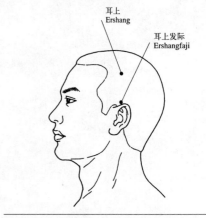

图1-27　耳上二穴
Fig. 1-27　Ershangerxue

颈窦刺组穴
Jingdoucizuxue

组成　本穴组由人迎、水突、气舍三穴组合而成。

位置　人迎：喉结旁1.5寸，当颈总动脉之后，胸锁乳突肌前缘。

水突：人迎穴至气舍穴连线的中点，当胸锁乳突肌前缘。

气舍：人迎直下，锁骨上缘，在胸锁乳突肌的胸骨头与锁骨头之间。

主治　高血压病，瘿气，心血管及内分泌疾病等。

操作　三穴均用齐刺浅刺法，深度为0.1～0.5寸，以针下有感觉为度。

Composition　This group of acupoints is composed of Renying(ST9), Shuitu(ST10) and Qishe(ST11).

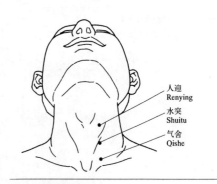

图1-28　颈窦刺组穴
Fig. 1-28　Jingdoucizuxue

Location Renying：1.5 cun lateral to the laryngeal protuberance, which is posterior to the common carotid artery and anterior to the border of the sternocleidomastoid muscle.

Shuitu：at the midpoint of the line connecting Renying and Qishe, which is anterior to the border the sternocleidomastoid muscle.

Qishe：directly below Renying, in the depression between the sternal and clavicular heads of the sternocleidomastoid muscle.

Indications Hypertension, goiter, cardiovascular and endocrine diseases.

Method The needling method of triple needling and shallow needling can be applied to the three acupoints, the depth is 0.1-0.5 cun which is dependent on the arrival of acu-esthesia.

项丛刺穴组
Xiangcongcixuezu

组成 本穴组由项部十二个穴点组合而成。

位置 沿项发际在左右乳突处分成十一等份，计十二点即是。

主治 高血压病，失眠，低智，痴呆，脏躁，癔病、脑病及其后遗症，头痛，目疾等。

操作 直刺0.8~1.2寸，得气为度。

Composition This group of acupoints is composed of the 12 points on the nape.

Location Divide the line along the hairline of the nape between the two mastoid process into equal segments 12 points totally.

Indications Hypertension, insomnia, feeble-mindedness, dementia, Zangzao, hysteria, brain diseases and sequelae, headache, eye diseases, etc..

Method The needle is perpendicularly inserted 0.8-1.2 cun till the acu-esthesia is obtained.

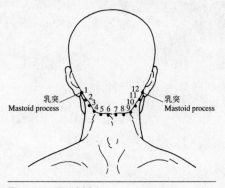

乳突
Mastoid process

乳突
Mastoid process

图1-29 项丛刺穴组
Fig. 1-29 Xiangcongcixuezu

额三针
Esanzhen

组成　本穴组由神庭、上旁神庭二穴点共三穴组合而成。

位置　神庭：前发际正中直上0.5寸。

上旁神庭：神庭上1寸及其旁开各1寸处。

主治　失眠。

操作　直刺至骨膜，不催针，不捻转，留针30分钟，每日1次，6次1疗程。

按注　本穴有书称头三针。

Composition　This group of acupoints is composed of Shenting(GV24) and the two points of shangpangshenting.

Location　Shenting：0.5 cun directly above the midpoint of the anterior hairline.

Shangpangshenting：1 cun superior, and 1 cun lateral to Shenting.

Indication　Insomnia.

Method　The needle is inserted to the periosteum without activating or rotating the needles. Retain the needles for 30 minutes, treat once every day, 6 times as one course of treatment.

Note　This group of acupoints is also called Tousanzhen in some books.

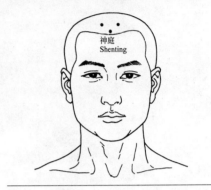

图1-30　额三针
Fig. 1-30　Esanzhen

安眠
Anmian

组成　本穴组由安眠1和安眠2(又名脑清)二穴组合而成。

位置　安眠1：位于头颞部、胸锁乳突肌停止处，乳突下凹陷点前0.5寸处，相当于翳风穴与翳明穴之间。

安眠2：(脑清)位于颞部、项肌隆起外缘凹陷，与胸锁乳突肌停止部乳突下凹陷连线之中点，相当于风池穴与翳明穴之间。

主治　失眠，癫狂痫。

操作　刺法：针0.5~1.5寸，针感酸、麻、热胀。

灸法：麦粒灸3~7壮。

Composition　This group of acupoints is composed of Anmian1 and Anmian2 (also called Naoqing).

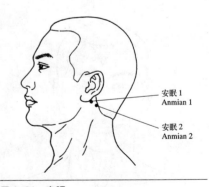

图1-31　安眠
Fig. 1-31　Anmian

Location Anmian1：on the temporal part of the head, at the point where the sternocleidomastoid muscle ends which is 0.5 cun anterior to the depression below the mastoid process, between Yifeng(TE17) and Yiming (EX-HN14).

Anmian2(Naoqing)：on the temporal part of the head, at the midpoint of the line connecting the lateral border of the prominent part of the neck muscle and the depression below the mastoid process where the sternocleidomastoid muscle ends. The point is between Fengchi(GB20) and Yiming.

Indications Insomnia, mania, epilepsy.

Method Acupuncture：the needle is inserted 0.5–1.5 cun. The acu-esthesia may be soreness, numbness, heat or distension.

Moxibustion：3–7 wheat-sized moxa cones of moxibustion is applied.

头三角
Tousanjiao

组成 本穴组由头发际处的三个点组合而成。

位置 由双目内眦直上与发际相交处之点，再由鼻梁正中直上头部取一点，使其与前二点成一等边三角形，该三点是穴。

主治 神经衰弱，失眠。

操作 平刺1厘米，稍捻动，留针1小时，中间捻2～3次，每日1次，10次为1疗程。

Composition This group of acupoints is composed of the three points on the hairline.

Location The first two points are directly above the inner canthus on the anterior hairline. Then select one point on the anterior median line on the head, which can form a equilateral triangle along with the two points before-mentioned. The three points constitute the group.

Indications Neurasthenia, insomnia.

Method The needle is inserted 1 cm horizontally and rotated lightly. Retain the needles for 1 hour and maniputate 2–3 times. Treat once every day, 10 times as one course of treatment.

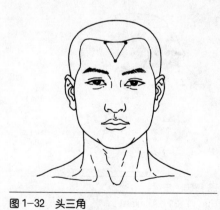

图1-32 头三角
Fig. 1-32 Tousanjiao

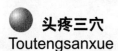 **阳堂**
Yangtang

组成　本穴组由太阳、印堂二穴组合而成。

位置　太阳：眉梢与目外眦之间向后约1寸处凹陷中。

印堂：二眉头连线的中点。

主治　头痛，头晕。

操作　太阳穴：针0.3~0.8寸，针感局部酸、胀。

印堂穴：针向下斜刺0.1~0.3寸，针感酸、胀，向四周放散。

Composition　This group of acupoints is composed of Taiyang(EX-HN5) and Yintang(EX-HN3).

Location　Taiyang：in the depression 1 cun posterior to the juncture between the lateral end of the eyebrow and the outer canthus.

Yintang：at the midpoint of the line connecting the two medial ends of the eyebrows.

Indications　Headache, dizziness.

Method　Taiyang：the needle is inserted 0.3−0.8 cun. The acu-esthesia of soreness and distension can be obtained in this part.

Yintang：the needle is inserted 0.1−0.3 cun obliquely downwards. The acu-esthesia of soreness and distension should be induced and radiate outwards.

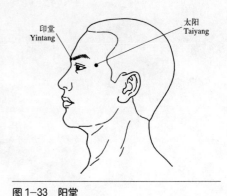

图1-33　阳堂
Fig. 1-33　Yangtang

头疼三穴
Toutengsanxue

组成　本穴组由头疼1、头疼2、头疼3三穴组合而成。

位置　头疼1：位于耳壳后面，折耳向前时耳舟隆起上段尖端至耳根部之中点。

头疼2：耳壳后面，对耳轮窝上端，近耳壳根部。

头疼3：耳壳后面，对耳轮窝上端，折耳向前时，耳舟隆起上段的尖端直下方。

主治　偏头痛，上呼吸道感染。

操作　针0.1~0.2寸，针感局部疼痛，留针20~30分钟。

Composition　This group of acupoints is composed of Touteng 1, Touteng 2 and Touteng 3.

Location　Touteng 1：posterior to the auricle, at the

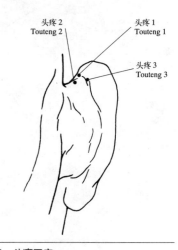

图1-34　头疼三穴
Fig. 1-34　Toutengsanxue

midpoint of the line connecting the tip of the upper part of the scapha prominence and the ear root when the ear is folded forwards.

Touteng 2：posterior to the auricle, in the upper part of the antihelix fossa, close to the auricle root.

Touteng 3：posterior to the auricle, in the upper part of the antihelix fossa, directly below the tip of the upper part of the scapha prominence when the ear is folded forwards.

Indication Migraine, upper respiratory tract infections.

Method The needle is inserted 0.1−0.2 cun. The acu−esthesia is local pain. Retain the needles for 20−30 minutes.

颈三
Jingsan

组成 本穴组由脑清、大椎二穴组合而成。

位置 脑清：胸锁乳突肌上点的后部发际处。

大椎：第七颈椎棘突下。

主治 头晕，失眠，癫痫，癔病。

操作 脑清针0.2～0.5寸，有麻、酸针感时至半侧头部。

大椎针1～1.5寸，针感胀、麻至头，或向腰或向两肩传导。

Composition This group of acupoints is composed of Naoqing and Dazhui(GV14).

Location Naoqing：at the point on the posterior hairline above the upper end of the sternocleidomastoid muscle.

Dazhui：at the point below the spinous process of the 7th cervical vertebra.

Indication Vertigo, insomnia, epilepsy, hysteria.

Method Naoqing：the needle is inserted 0.2−0.5 cun. The acu-esthesia of numbness and soreness will transmit to the half-side head.

Dazhui：the needle is inserted 1−1.5 cun. The acu-esthesia of distension and numbness will transmit to the head, waist or two shoulders.

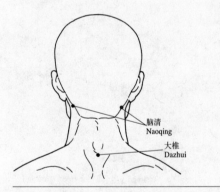

脑清
Naoqing

大椎
Dazhui

图 1−35 颈三
Fig. 1−35 Jingsan

回发五处
Huifawuchu

组成　本穴组由头顶回发中点及周围的四个点共五穴组合而成。

位置　头顶回发中点及前后左右各一穴。

主治　风眩。

操作　刺法：平刺0.5～1寸，局部酸胀，手法用平补平泻法或捻转补泻法。

灸法：间接灸3～5壮，艾条灸5～10分钟。

Composition　This group of acupoints is composed of the midpoint of the gyroidal hair on the vertex and the four points around it.

Location　At the midpoint of the gyroidal hair on the vertex, and the points lateral, anterior and posterior to it.

Indication　Vertigo due to wind.

Method　Acupuncture：the needle is inserted 0.5－1 cun horizontally. The acu-esthesia of soreness and distension should be obtained in this part, the technique of even reinforcing and reducing or the reinforcing and reducing method by rotation is applied.

Moxibustion：3－5 cones of indirect moxibustion or 5－10 minutes' moxibustion with moxa roll can be applied.

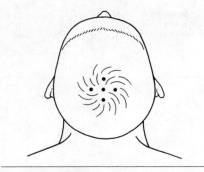

图1-36　回发五处
Fig. 1-36　Huifawuchu

颈三针
Jingsanzhen

组成　本穴组由百劳、大杼、天柱三穴组合而成。

位置　百劳：大椎穴旁开1寸，再直上2寸处。

大杼：第一胸椎棘突下，旁开1.5寸。

天柱：后发际正中直上0.5寸，旁开1.3寸，当斜方肌外缘凹陷中。

主治　颈椎病，眩晕。

操作　取1.5寸30号不锈钢毫针。采用正指直刺，无针左右的直刺法，或采用向颈椎方向斜刺。进针深度依患者的胖瘦程度，一般在0.8～1.2寸之间。留针30分钟，留针时间隔5分钟行针1次。

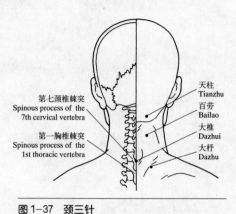

第七颈椎棘突
Spinous process of the
7th cervical vertebra

第一胸椎棘突
Spinous process of the
1st thoracic vertebra

天柱
Tianzhu
百劳
Bailao
大椎
Dazhui
大杼
Dazhu

图1-37　颈三针
Fig. 1-37　Jingsanzhen

Composition　This group of acupoints is composed of Bailao, Dazhu(BL11) and Tianzhu(BL10).

Location　Bailao：2 cun directly above the point 1 cun lateral to Dazhui.

Dazhu：1.5 cun lateral to the spinous process of the 1st thoracic vertebra.

Tianzhu：1.3 cun lateral to the point 0.5 cun directly above the midpoint of the posterior hairline, in the depression lateral to the border of the trapezius muscle.

Indications　Cervical spondylopathy, vertigo.

Method　The filiform needle of 1.5 cun in length and 30 in size is selected. The needle can be inserted perpendicularly without pointing left and right. The needle can also be inserted obliquely towards the direction of the cervical vertebra. The depth is decided according to the patient's build, usually the depth is 0.8-1.2 cun. Retain the needle for 30 minutes, manipulate once every 5 minutes during the retention of the needles.

新识设
Xinshishe

组成　本穴组由新识、新设二穴组合而成。

位置　新识：项部第三、第四颈椎间旁开1.5寸。

新设：项部第四颈椎横突尖端、斜方肌外缘。

主治　项强，角弓反张。

操作　直刺或斜刺0.5～1.2寸，得气为度。

Composition　This group of acupoints is composed of Xinshi and Xinshe.

Location　Xinshi：1.5 cun lateral to the point between the spinous processes of the 3rd and 4th cervical vertebrae.

Xinshe：at the tip of the transverse process of the 4th cervical vertebra, lateral to the border of the trapezius muscle.

Indication　Neck rigidity, opisthotonus.

Method　The needle is inserted 0.5-1.2 cun perpendicularly or obliquely till the acu-esthesia is obtained.

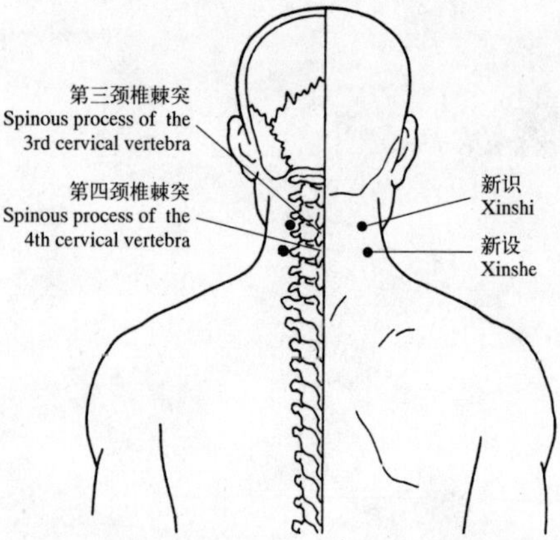

第三颈椎棘突
Spinous process of the
3rd cervical vertebra

第四颈椎棘突
Spinous process of the
4th cervical vertebra

新识
Xinshi

新设
Xinshe

图1-38　新识设
Fig. 1-38　Xinshishe

项三风
Xiangsanfeng

组成　本穴组由风府、风池二穴组合而成。

位置　风府：后发际正中直上1寸。

风池：胸锁乳突肌与斜方肌之间凹陷中，平风府穴处。

主治　颈项强痛，眩晕，目痛，鼻衄，中风，头痛，感冒，癫狂，痫证。

操作　斜刺0.5～1寸(风府向下颌方向，风池向鼻尖方向)得气为度。

Composition　This group of acupoints is composed of Fengfu(GV16) and Fengchi(GB20).

Location　Fengfu: 1 cun directly above the midpoint of the posterior hairline.

Fengchi: in the depression between the sternocleidomastoid and trapezius muscles, at the level of Fengfu.

Indications　Pain and rigidity of the neck, vertigo, ophthalmalgia, epistaxis, apoplexy, headache, common cold, mania, epilepsy.

Method　The needle is inserted 0.5-1 cun obliquely (needling Fengfu toward the jaw, puncturing Fengchi toward the tip of the nose) till the acu-esthesia is obtained.

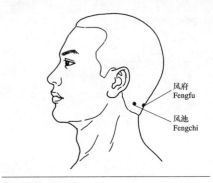

图1-39　项三风
Fig. 1-39　Xiangsanfeng

眼三针
Yansanzhen

组成　本穴组由眼1、眼2、眼3三穴组合而成。

位置　眼1：眶内缘、目内眦上0.2寸处。

眼2：目下0.7寸，直目瞳子，当眼球与眶下缘之间。

眼3：目外眦旁0.1寸，上0.1寸处，当眶内缘与眼球之间。

主治　视神经萎缩，视网膜炎，色盲，近视，远视，斜视弱视，视网膜黄斑变性，早期青光眼，白内障等。

操作　眼1采用轻捻缓进针法进针，将针尖先置于眼皮肤上，再用腕力和指力捻进皮、眼，直刺1.5寸。眼2在进针后直刺5分，然后使针尖朝眶内刺入1寸，共刺入1.5寸深。眼3在进针后针尖向内，使针身与二眼连线夹角为60°，进针0.5寸后，使针身与双眼连线的夹角为45°～50°，再刺入1寸许，共入针1.5寸。

上穴在针刺中务使患者眼球内有得气感，得气大多以胀、

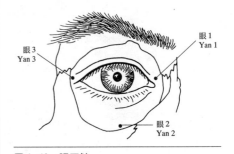

图1-40　眼三针
Fig. 1-40　Yansanzhen

酸、麻为主，偶有轻微疼痛。寻得针感后应留针30分钟，其间每隔10分钟轻捻或插针1次，忌大幅度提插捻转，以防出血或伤及眼球，出针时以棉球轻压针孔。

Composition　This group of acupoints is composed of Yan1, Yan2 and Yan3.

Location　Yan1：in the inner orbital ridge 0.2 cun above the inner canthus.

Yan2：0.7 cun directly below the pupil, between the eyeball and the infraorbital ridge.

Yan3：0.1 cun above the point 0.1 cun lateral to the outer canthus, between the eyeball and the inner orbital ridge.

Indication　Optic atrophy, retinitis, achromatopsia, myopia, hypermetropia, strabismus, amblyopia, macular degeneration, early glaucoma, cataract, etc..

Method　Yan 1: The needle is inserted with the lightly rotating and slowly inserting method. The tip of the needle is put above the skin, then the needle is inserted 1.5 cun perpendicularly into the skin and orbit with the force of fingers and wrist. After the inserting of the needle tip, Yan 2 can be punctured 0.5 cun perpendicularly, then 1 cun more towards the inner orbit, 1.5 cun totally. For Yan 3, the tip of the needle points inwards so that the angle formed by the body of the needle and the line connecting both eyes is 60°. After inserting the needle 0.5 cun, adjust the needling angle to 45°−50°, then insert 1 cun more or so, the depth is 1.5 cun totally.

The acu-esthesia should be obtained during the needling of the above acupoints. The feeling will mostly be distension, soreness and numbness, and will be slightly pain occasionally. Retain the needles for 30 minutes after the acu-esthesia is obtained, rotate or thrust the needles lightly every 10 minutes. It is forbidden to lift, insert or rotate with large amplitude in order to avoid bleeding or hurting the eyeball. Press the acupoints slightly with cotton balls after the withdrawal of the needle.

睛阳鱼
Jingyangyu

组成　本穴组由睛明、太阳、鱼尾三穴组合而成。

位置　睛明：目内眦旁0.1寸。

太阳：眉梢与目外眦之间向后约1寸处凹陷中。

鱼尾：眉外端与眼外眦连线之中点外方0.3寸处。

主治　目疾。

操作　睛明针刺时嘱闭目，并轻推眼球于外固定，慢慢进针，紧靠眶缘直刺0.5~1寸，不捻转，不提插，以眼眶、眼球发酸胀为度，出针后按压针孔片刻，以防出血。太阳、鱼尾可用沿皮刺0.5~0.8寸，得气为度。

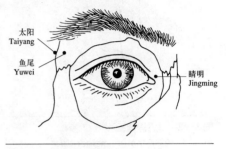

图1-41　睛阳鱼(右眼)
Fig. 1-41　Jingyangyu(right eye)

Composition　This group of acupoints is composed of Jingming(BL1), Taiyang(EX-HN5) and Yuwei.

Location　Jingming：0.1 cun lateral to the inner canthus.

Taiyang：in the depression 1 cun posterior to the juncture between the lateral end of the eyebrow and the outer canthus.

Yuwei：0.3 cun lateral to the midpoint of the line connecting the lateral end of the eyebrow and the outer canthus.

Indication　Eye diseases.

Method　Jingming：ask the patient to close eyes, gently push the eyeball to the lateral side with the left hand, puncture slowly and perpendicularly 0.5−1 cun along the orbital wall without rotating, lifting or inserting the needle till the acu-esthesia of soreness and distension in the eyeball is obtained. Press the needled point slightly with cotton balls after the withdrawal of the needle to avoid bleeding.

Taiyang and Yuwei is inserted 0.5−0.8 cun under the skin till the acu-esthesia is obtained.

耳后静脉三条
Erhoujingmaisantiao

组成　本穴组由耳壳背部之三个点组合而成。

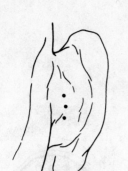

图 1-42　耳后静脉三条
Fig. 1-42　Erhoujingmaisantiao

位置　耳壳背侧三条静脉是穴。

主治　目疗，目赤痛。

操作　三棱针挑刺出血。

Composition　This group of acupoints is composed of the three points on the back of the auricle.

Location　The three veins on the back of auricle constitute the group of acupoints.

Indications　Eye boil, redness and pain of the eyes.

Method　Bleed the points with the pricking method by a three-edged needle.

 听灵
Tingling

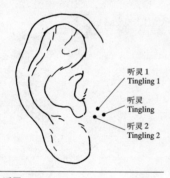

图 1-43　听灵
Fig. 1-43　Tingling

组成　本穴组由听灵、听灵 1、听灵 2 三穴组合而成。

位置　听灵：耳前方、耳屏和耳屏间切迹联线下 3/4 点处，与下颌小头后缘间凹陷处。

听灵 1：耳前方、耳屏和耳屏间切迹之间点与下颌小头后缘之间凹陷近、耳侧 0.2 厘米处。

听灵 2：耳前方、耳屏和耳屏间切迹联线之下 3/4 点近耳侧 0.2 厘米处。

主治　耳鸣，耳聋。

操作　略张口，针直刺 1~1.5 寸，针感为耳中酸、麻。

Composition　This group of acupoints is composed of Tingling, Tingling1 and Tingling2.

Location　Tingling：anterior to the ear, in the depression of the junction of the upper one-fourth and lower three-fourths of the line connecting the tragus and supratragic notch and the posterior border of the manibular capitulum.

Tingling1：anterior to the ear, 0.2 cm lateral to the midpoint of the line connecting the tragus and supratragic notch and the posterior border of the manibular capitulum.

Tingling2：anterior to the ear, 0.2 cm lateral to the junction of the upper one-fourth and lower three-fourths of the line connecting the tragus and supratragic notch.

Indications　Tinnitus and deafness.

Method　Ask the patient to open the mouth slightly. The needle is inserted 1-1.5 cun perpendicularly. The acu-esthesia of soreness and numbness in the ear can be obtained.

耳三针
Ersanzhen

组成　本穴组由完骨、听宫、听会三穴组合而成。

位置　完骨：乳突后下方凹陷中。

听宫：耳屏前，下颌骨髁状突的后缘，张口呈凹陷处。

听会：耳屏间切迹前，下颌骨髁状突的后缘，张口有孔。

主治　耳鸣，耳聋。

操作　先刺完骨，直刺或向下斜刺1~1.2寸，针感向颈后放射；次针听宫、听会，二穴张口取穴，深1~1.5寸，以酸、胀得气为度。

Composition　This group of acupoints is composed of Wangu(GB12), Tinggong(SI19) and Tinghui(GB2).

Location　Wangu：in the depression posterior and inferior to the mastoid process.

Tinggong：anterior to the tragus, in the depression posterior to the border of the condyloid process of the mandible when the mouth is open.

Tinghui：anterior to the intertragic notch, in the depression posterior to the condyloid process of the mandible when the mouth is open.

Indications　Tinnitus and deafness.

Method　Wangu is needled first by inserting the needle 1−1.2 cun perpendicularly or obliquely downwards, the acu-esthesia will radiate to the back of the neck. Then Tinggong and Tinghui are needled when the mouth is open, the depth is 1−1.5 cun till the acu-esthesia of soreness and distension is obtained.

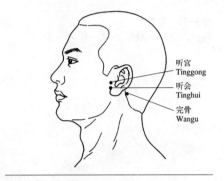

图1-44　耳三针
Fig. 1-44　Ersanzhen

翳听
Yiting

组成　本穴组由听宫、听会、翳风三穴组合而成。

位置　听宫：耳屏前，下颌骨髁状突的后缘，张口呈凹陷处。

听会：耳屏间切迹前，下颌骨髁状突的后缘，张口有孔。

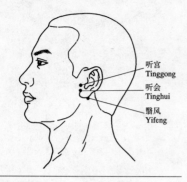

图 1—45 翳听
Fig. 1—45 Yiting

翳风：乳突前下方，平耳垂后下缘的凹陷中。

主治 耳聋，耳鸣，耳气闭塞。

操作 针直刺用泻法，深 0.5～1 寸，留针 15 分钟。

Composition This group of acupoints is composed of Tinggong(SI18), Tinghui(GB2) and Yifeng(TE17).

Location Tinggong：anterior to the tragus, in the depression posterior to the border of the condyloid process of the mandible when the mouth is open.

Tinghui：anterior to the intertragic notch, in the depression posterior to the condyloid process of the mandible when the mouth is open.

Yifeng：anterior and inferior to the mastoid process, in the depression at the level of the posterior and lower border of the earlobe.

Indication Deafness, tinnitus.

Method The needle is inserted 0.5—1 cun perpendicularly with the reducing techniques. Retain the needles for 15 minutes.

 耳后听
Erhouting

组成 本穴组由后听、后听会二穴组合而成。

位置 后听：耳颞部和耳郭内侧面之根部，同耳壳外侧面耳屏和耳屏间切迹之间点，与下颌小头后缘之间凹陷处相平。

后听会：位于耳郭后方，近耳郭缘曲线、颞骨乳突与下颌支后缘间之凹陷上 0.5 寸，相当于"翳风"穴上 0.5 寸凹陷处。

主治 耳鸣，耳聋。

操作 针略向前下方刺入 0.5～1.5 寸，针感耳中酸、胀、热。

Composition This group of acupoints is composed of Houting and Houtinghui.

Location Houting：at the root of the temporal part and inner side of the auricle, i.e. the midpoint between the tragus and intertragic notch of the outer side of the auricle, at the same level of the depression posterior to the border of the mandibular head.

Houtinghui：posterior to the auricle, close to the curve line of the border of the auricle, 0.5 cun superior to the depression between the mastoid process of the

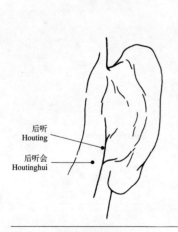

图 1—46 耳后听
Fig. 1—46 Erhouting

temporal bone and the lateral border of the mandible, i.e. in the depression 0.5 cun superior to Yifeng.

Indications   Tinnitus and deafness.

Method   The needle is inserted 0.5–1.5 cun forwards and downwards slightly. The acu-esthesia may be soreness, distension and pyrexia.

翳明下三穴
Yimingxiasanxue

组成   本穴组由翳明下、后翳明、聋通三穴组合而成。

位置   翳明下：位于颞部、胸锁乳突肌停止部、颞骨乳突下凹陷直下0.5寸处。

后翳明：于颞骨乳突凹陷处直后方0.5寸处。

聋通：于颞骨乳突下一横指之点，再向后移一横指处。

主治   耳聋，耳鸣。

操作   针0.5～1.5寸，向耳垂部凹陷处针之，针感耳中酸胀热。

Composition   This group of acupoints is composed of Yingmingxia, Houyiming and Longtong.

Location   Yingmingxia：on the temporal part of the head, at the end of the sternocleidomastoid muscle, 0.5 cun directly below the depression inferior to the mastoid process of the temporal bone.

Houyiming：0.5 cun posterior to the depression of the mastoid process of the temporal bone.

Longtong：one finger breadth inferior and posterior to the mastoid process of the temporal bone.

Indications   Tinnitus and deafness.

Method   The needle is inserted 0.5–1.5 cun towards the depression in the back of the earlobe. The acu-esthesia may be soreness, distension and pyrexia in the ear.

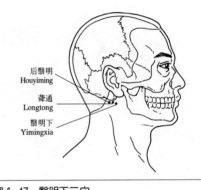

图1-47   翳明下三穴
Fig. 1-47   Yimingxiasanxue

哑穴
Yaxue

组成   本穴组由颈前二点、枕二点共四穴组合而成。

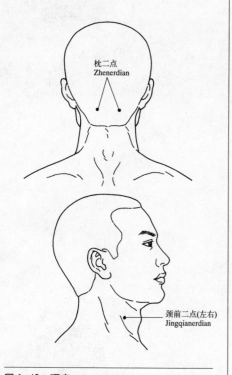

图 1-48 哑穴
Fig. 1-48 Yaxue

位置 颈前二点：位于人迎和水突二穴之间，稍向外斜0.2寸许，于胸锁乳突肌前缘取之左右计二穴。

枕二点：位于风池穴上0.4寸，枕骨下缘、胸锁乳突肌止部，脑空穴直下是穴。

主治 聋哑。

操作 刺法：颈前二点直刺0.5~1寸，枕后二点直刺1~1.5寸。

按注 刺颈前二点时，注意避开颈总动脉，以免意外。

Composition This group of acupoints is composed of Jingqianerdian and Zhenerdian.

Location Jingqianerdian：0.2 cun lateral to the midpoint between Renying(ST9) and Shuitu(ST40), anterior to the border of sternocleidomastoid muscle.

Zhenerdian：0.4 cun above Fengchi(GB20), inferior to the border of the occipa, at the end of the sternocleidomastoid muscle, directly below Naokong(GB19).

Indications Deaf-mutism.

Method Jingqianerdian is needled perpendicularly 0.5−1 cun, Zhenerdian is needled perpendicularly 1−1.5 cun.

Note Avoid puncturing the common carotid artery when Jingqianerdian is needled.

● 迎香二穴
Yingxiangerxue

组成 本穴组由迎香穴、上迎香二穴组合而成。

位置 迎香：鼻翼外缘中点，旁开0.5寸，当鼻唇沟中。

上迎香：鼻根两侧，目内眦下0.5寸。

主治 鼻塞，鼻衄，鼻息肉，鼻炎，鼻窦炎等。

操作 刺法：平刺或斜刺0.3~0.5寸。

灸法：温灸3~5分钟。

Composition This group of acupoints is composed of Yingxiang(LI20) and Shangyingxiang.

Location Yingxiang：at the midpoint of the lateral border of the ala nasi, in the nasolabial groove.

Shangyingxiang：on both side of the root of the nose, 0.5 cun below the inner canthus.

Indications Nasal obstruction, epistaxis, rhinopolypus,

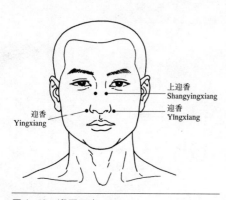

图 1-49 迎香二穴
Fig. 1-49 Yingxiangerxue

rhinitis and nasosinusitis, etc..

Methods Acupuncture：the needle is inserted 0.3—0.5 cun horizontally or obliquely.

Moxibustion：3—5 minutes' warm moxibustion is applied.

三星穴
Sanxingxue

组成　本穴组由督脉的上星、奇穴伴星二穴组合而成。

位置　上星：前发际正中直上1寸。

伴星：前发际上1寸，旁开3寸处。

主治　鼻渊，鼻痔，头痛，眩晕，目赤肿痛，热病。

操作　刺法：平刺0.5～1寸。

灸法：艾炷灸1～3壮，或温灸5～10分钟。

Composition　This group of acupoints is composed of Shangxing(GV23) and the extraordinary points Banxing.

Location　Shangxing：1 cun directly above the midpoint of the anterior hairline.

Banxing：3 cun lateral to the point, 1 cun directly above the midpoint of the anterior hairline.

Indications Rhinitis, rhinopolypus, headache, vertigo, redness, pain and swelling of the eye, febrile diseases.

Method　Acupuncture：the needle is inserted 0.5—1 cun horizontally.

Moxibustion：moxibustion with 1—3 moxa cones or warm moxibustion of 5—10 minutes is applied.

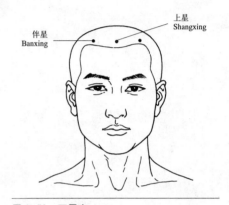

图1-50　三星穴
Fig. 1-50　Sanxingxue

香星
Xiangxing

组成　本穴组由迎香、上星二穴组合而成。

位置　迎香：鼻翼外缘中点，旁开0.5寸，当鼻唇沟中。

上星：前发际正中直上1寸。

主治　鼻塞，不闻香臭。

操作　迎香沿鼻唇沟向睛明方向透刺0.5～1.2寸。上星向额部或囟会方向透刺0.5～1.2寸。各以得气为度。留针30分钟，留针期间可行捻转等手法。

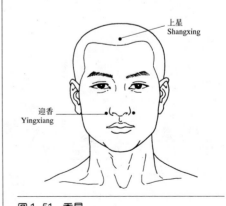

图1-51　香星
Fig. 1-51　Xiangxing

Composition　This group of acupoints is composed of Yingxiang(LI20) and Shangxing(GV23).

Location　Yingxiang：at the midpoint of the lateral border of the ala nasi, in the nasolabial groove.

Shangxing：1 cun directly above the midpoint of the anterior hairline.

Indications　Nasal obstrution and hyposmia.

Method　Yingxiang：the needle is inserted 0.5－1.2 cun towards Jingming along the nasolabial groove.

Shangxing：the needle is inserted 0.5－1.2 cun towards forehead or Xinhui. The acu-esthesia should be obtained in all acupoints, retain the needle for 30 minutes. The rotating techniques may be applied during the retention of the needles.

香风
Xiangfeng

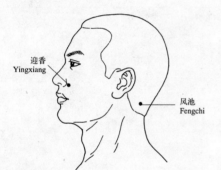

迎香
Yingxiang

风池
Fengchi

图 1-52　香风
Fig. 1-52　Xiangfeng

组成　本穴组由迎香、风池二穴组合而成。

位置　迎香：鼻翼外缘中点，旁开0.5寸，当鼻唇沟中。

风池：胸锁乳突肌与斜方肌之间凹陷中，平风府穴处。

主治　鼻塞，不闻香臭。

操作　迎香沿鼻唇沟刺0.5～0.8寸。风池向中央鼻尖方向刺0.8～1.2寸，得气为度，留针30分钟，留针期间可行捻转手法。

Composition　This group of acupoints is composed of Yingxiang(LI20) and Fengchi(GB20).

Location　Yingxiang：at the midpoint of the lateral border of the ala nasi, in the nasolabial groove.

Fengchi：in the depression between the sternocleidomastoid and trapezius muscles, at the horizontal level of Fengfu.

Indications　Nasal obstruction and hyposmia.

Method　Yingxiang：the needle is inserted 0.5－0.8 cun along the nasolabial groove.

Fengchi：the needle is inserted 0.8－1.2 cun towards the nose tip, till the acu-esthesia is obtained. Retain the needles for 30 minutes. The rotating techniques may be applied during the retention of the needles.

鼻三针
Bisanzhen

组成 本穴组由迎香、鼻通、印堂三穴组合而成。

位置 迎香：鼻翼外缘中点，旁开0.5寸，当鼻唇沟中。

鼻通：鼻唇沟上端尽处。

印堂：二眉头连线的中点。

主治 鼻衄，鼻渊，过敏性鼻炎，急、慢性鼻窦炎。

操作 先取鼻通穴，针尖向鼻根部方向斜刺；再取迎香穴，得气酸胀感；后取印堂穴，针感向鼻尖方向及鼻翼两侧放射。

Composition This group of acupoints is composed of Yingxiang(LI20), Bitong and Yintang(EX-HN3).

Location Yingxiang：at the midpoint of the lateral border of the ala nasi, in the nasolabial groove.

Bitong：at the end of the upper part of the nasolabial groove.

Yintang：at the midpoint of the two inner ends of the eyebrows.

Indications Nasal obstruction, rhinorrhea, allergic rhinitis, acute and chronic nasosinusitis.

Method Bitong is needled first, the tip of the needle is inserted obliquely towards the nose root. Then puncture Yingxiang till the acu-esthesia of soreness and distension is obtained. Yintang is inserted last, and the acu-esthesia will be induced to the tip of nose and both sides of the ala nasi.

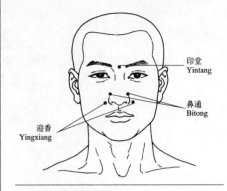

图1-53 鼻三针
Fig. 1-53 Bisanzhen

三龙指鼻
Sanlongzhibi

组成 本穴组由印堂、迎香二穴组合而成。

位置 印堂：两眉头连线的中点。

迎香：鼻翼外缘中点，旁开0.5寸，当鼻唇沟中。

主治 鼻病，胆道蛔虫痛，便秘等。

操作 印堂沿皮向鼻刺。迎香沿鼻唇沟向内眦睛明方向沿皮透刺，深度为0.5~1寸。

Composition This group of acupoints is composed of Yintang(EX-HN3) and Yingxiang(LI20).

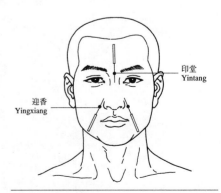

图1-54 三龙指鼻
Fig. 1-54 Sanlongzhibi

Location Yintang: at the midpoint of the two inner ends of the eyebrows.

Yingxiang: at the midpoint of the lateral border of the ala nasi, in the nasolabial groove.

Indications Diseases of nose, biliary ascariasis and constipation.

Method The needle is inserted towards the nose from Yintang under the skin. For Yingxiang, the needle is inserted towards the inner canthus of Jingming under the skin of nasolabial groove, the depth is 0.5−1 cun.

● 开鼻窍
Kaibiqiao

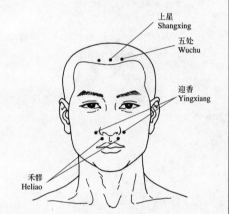

图1-55 开鼻窍
Fig. 1-55 Kaibiqiao

组成 本穴组由迎香、上星、五处、禾髎四穴组合而成。
位置 迎香：鼻翼外缘中点，旁开0.5寸，当鼻唇沟中。
禾髎：水沟穴旁0.5寸，当鼻孔外缘直下，与水沟穴相平处取穴。
上星：前发际正中直上1寸。
五处：曲差穴上0.5寸，距头部正中线1.5寸。
主治 鼻塞，不闻香臭，兼见头痛、口干。
操作 针刺用泻法，留针30分钟。

Composition This group of acupoints is composed of Yingxiang(LI20), Shangxing(GV23), Wuchu(BL5) and Heliao(LI19).

Location Yingxiang: at the midpoint of the lateral border of the ala nasi, in the nasolabial groove.

Heliao: 0.5 cun lateral to Shuigou, directly below the lateral border of the nostril, at the horizontal level of Shuigou.

Shangxing: 1 cun directly above the midpoint of the anterior hairline.

Wuchu: 0.5 cun superior to Quchai, 1.5 cun lateral to the midline of the head.

Indications Nasal obstruction, hyposmia with headache and thirst.

Method Acupuncture: The reducing method is applied, retain the needles for 30 minutes.

气通

Qitong

组成　本穴组由迎香、印堂、上星、通天、风池五穴组合而成。

位置　迎香：鼻翼外缘中点，旁开0.5寸，当鼻唇沟中。

印堂：两眉头连线的中点。

上星：前发际正中直上1寸。

通天：承光穴后1.5寸。

风池：胸锁乳突肌与斜方肌之间凹陷中，平风府穴处。

主治　鼻塞，流涕。

操作　风池斜刺0.8～1.2寸，得气为度。其他各穴可用沿皮刺0.5～1寸不等，各以得气为度。

Composition　This group of acupoints is composed of Yingxiang(LI20), Yintang(EX-HN3), Shangxing(GV23), Tongtian(BL7) and Fengchi(GB20).

Location　Yingxiang：at the midpoint of the lateral border of the ala nasi, in the nasolabial groove.

Yintang：at the midpoint of the two inner ends of the eyebrows.

Shangxing：1 cun directly above the midpoint of the anterior hairline.

Tongtian：1.5 cun posterior to Chengguang.

Fengchi：in the depression between the sternocleido-mastoid and trapezius muscles, at the horizontal level of Fengfu.

Indications　Nasal obstruction and rhinorrhea.

Method　The needle is inserted 0.8−1.2 cun obliquely into Fengchi till the acu-esthesia is obtained. For other acupoints, the needles can be inserted along the skin, the depth is 0.5−1 cun, till the acu-esthesia is obtained.

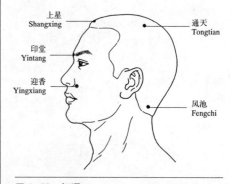

图1-56　气通
Fig. 1-56　Qitong

星会

Xinghui

组成　本穴组由上星、囟会二穴组合而成。

位置　上星：前发际正中直上1寸。

囟会：前发际正中直上2寸。

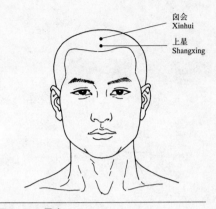

图1-57 星会
Fig. 1-57 Xinghui

主治 鼻衄。

操作 从上星向囟会透刺进针1.5寸，用泻法，血止后停用手法，留针20分钟。

Composition This group of acupoints is composed of Shangxin(GV23) and Xinhui(GV22).

Location Shangxing：1 cun directly above the midpoint of the anterior hairline.

Xinhui：2 cun directly above the midpoint of the anterior hairline.

Indication Epistaxis.

Method The needle is penetrated 1.5 cun from Shangxing to Xinhui, the reducing method is applied till the blood is stanched. Retain the needle for 20 minutes.

星椎
Xingzhui

组成 本穴组由上星、大椎二穴组合而成。

位置 上星：前发际正中直上1寸。

大椎：第七颈椎棘突下。

主治 鼻衄。

操作 上星向额部或向囟会方向沿皮刺0.5~1.2寸。大椎直刺0.5~0.8寸，得气后可行泻法。

Composition This group of acupoints is composed of Shangxing(GV23) and Dazhui(GV14).

Location Shangxing：1 cun directly above the midpoint of the anterior hairline.

Dazhui：at the point below the spinous process of the 7th cervical vertebra.

Indication Epistaxis.

Method Shangxing：the needle is inserted 0.5-1.2 cun towards forehead or Xinhui beneath the skin.

Dazhui：the needle is inserted 0.5-0.8 cun perpendicularly. The reducing method can be applied after the acu-esthesia is obtained.

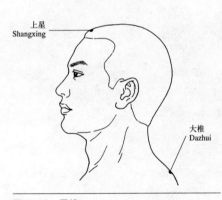

图1-58 星椎
Fig. 1-58 Xingzhui

唇二针
Chunerzhen

组成　本穴组由人中、承浆二穴组合而成。

位置　人中：在人中沟的上1/3与中1/3交界处。

承浆：颏唇沟的中点。

主治　牙痛，喎僻，面肿，癫痫，消渴，以及针刺麻醉镇痛和改善腹膜松弛等。

操作　刺法：斜刺0.3～0.5寸。

灸法：人中穴不灸。承浆穴可温灸5～10分钟。

Composition　This group of acupoints is composed of Renzhong(GV26) and Chengjiang(GV24).

Location　Renzhong：at the junction of the upper one-third and middle one-third of the philtrum.

Chengjiang：at the midpoint of the mentolabial sulcus.

Indications　Toothache, deviation of the mouth, facial edema, epilepsy and diabetes. This group can also be used in acupuncture anesthesia and improving the loose peritoneum.

Method　Acupuncture：the needle is inserted 0.3—0.5 cun obliquely.

Moxibustion：Moxibustion isn't applied to Renzhong；but as to Chengjiang, 5—10 minutes' warm moxibustion can be applied.

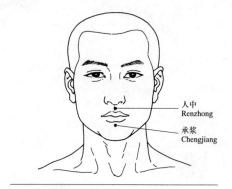

图1-59　唇二针
Fig. 1-59　Chunerzhen

人中
Renzhong
承浆
Chengjiang

唇上下
Chunshangxia

组成　本穴组由唇上、唇下二穴组合而成。

位置　唇上：位于人中沟下端正中，距上唇缘约0.2厘米。

唇下：位于下唇缘中点，距下唇缘约0.5厘米处。

主治　胸腰部及胸腹痛。

操作　以15°角分别斜向上向下进针约0.5和1寸，局部有酸麻重胀感，得气后加用电针。

Composition　This group of acupoints is composed of Chunshang and Chunxia.

Location　Chunshang：in the middle of the lower end of the philtrum, 0.2 cm away from the lip.

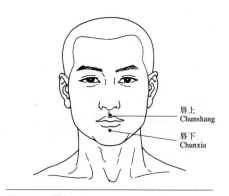

图1-60　唇上下
Fig. 1-60　Chunshangxia

唇上
Chunshang
唇下
Chunxia

Chunxia：at the midpoint of the border of the underlip, 0.5 cm away from the underlip.

Indication Pain in the chest, abdomen and waist.

Method At the angle of 15° the needles are inserted 0.5 cun upwards or 1 cun downwards respectively. The acu-esthesia of soreness, numbness, heaviness and distension will be felt in this part. The electroacupuncture can be applied after the acu-esthesia is obtained.

项背三针
Xiangbeisanzhen

组成 本穴组由定喘、大椎二穴组合而成。

位置 定喘：大椎旁开0.5寸。

大椎：第七颈椎棘突下。

主治 感冒，咳嗽，哮喘，高热。

操作 刺法：针定喘穴斜向椎体刺入1~1.5寸，针感麻、胀并向下传导至背或腰；大椎穴针1~1.5寸，针感为麻、胀传至头，或向腰或向两肩传导。

灸法：5~9壮，艾条灸10~20分钟。

Composition This group of acupoints is composed of Dingchuan(EX-B1) and Dazhui(GV14).

Location Dingchuang：0.5 cun lateral to Dazhui.

Dazhui：at the point below the spinous process of the 7th cervical vertebra.

Indication Common cold, cough, asthma and high fever.

Method Acupuncture：for Dingchuan, the needle is inserted 1−1.5 cun obliquely towards the centrum, the acu-esthesia of numbness and distension will radiate downwards to the back or waist；for Dazhui, the needle is inserted 1−1.5 cun, the acu-esthesia of numbness and distension can radiate to the head, waist or both shoulders.

Moxibustion：5−9 moxa cones or 10−20 minutes' moxibustion with moxa roll can be applied.

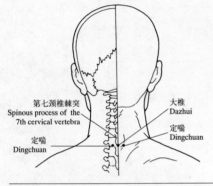

第七颈椎棘突
Spinous process of the
7th cervical vertebra

大椎
Dazhui

定喘
Dingchuan

定喘
Dingchuan

图1-61 项背三针
Fig. 1-61 Xiangbeisanzhen

会椎
Huizhui

组成　本穴组由百会、大椎二穴组合而成。

位置　百会：后发际正中直上7寸。

大椎：第七颈椎棘突下。

主治　低热，骨蒸劳热，午后或夜间热甚。

操作　先灸百会，再灸大椎，各5～7壮。

Composition This group of acupoints is composed of Baihui(GV20) and Dazhui(GV14).

Location Baihui：7 cun directly above the midpoint of the posterior hairline.

Dazhui：at the point below the spinous process of the 7th cervical vertebra.

Indication Low fever, fever due to phthisis, afternoon or night fever.

Method 5-7 cones of moxibustion is applied first to Baihui, then to Dazhui.

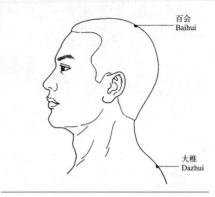

图1-62　会椎
Fig. 1-62　Huizhui

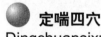

定喘四穴
Dingchuansixue

组成　本穴组由定喘、外定喘、喘息、外喘息四穴组合而成。

位置　定喘：位于颈后部，第七颈椎棘突下旁开0.5寸处。

外定喘：位于颈后部，第七颈椎棘突下旁开1.5寸处。

喘息：位于颈后部，第七颈椎棘突左右旁开各2寸处。

外喘息：位于颈后部，第七颈椎棘突下左右旁开2.5寸处。

主治　咳嗽，哮喘。

操作　刺法：针0.5～1寸，针感为酸麻于颈肩部。

灸法：灸3～5壮。

Composition This group of acupoints is composed of Dingchuan(EX-B1)，Waidingchuan，Chuanxi and Waichuanxi.

Location Dingchuan：on the back of the neck, 0.5 cun lateral to the point below the spinous process of the 7th cervical vertebra.

Waidingchuan：on the back of the neck, 1.5 cun lateral to the point below the spinous process of the 7th

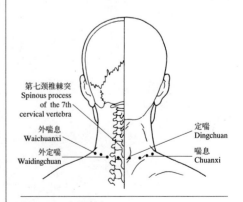

图1-63　定喘四穴
Fig. 1-63　Dingchuansixue

cervical vertebra.

Chuanxi：on the back of the neck, 2 cun lateral to the point below the spinous process of the 7th cervical vertebra.

Waichuanxi：on the back of the neck, 2.5 cun lateral to the point below the spinous process of the 7th cervical vertebra.

Indications Cough and asthma.

Method Acupuncture：the needle is inserted 0.5−1 cun, the acu-esthesia of soreness and numbness will radiate to the neck and shoulders.

Moxibustion：3−5 cones of moxibustion is applied.

郁中
Yuzhong

组成 本穴组由耳轮棘前及耳垂下缘处的二个点组合而成。

位置 耳轮棘前缘一穴，耳垂下缘相平一穴。

主治 哮吼。

操作 麦粒灸，灸3～9壮。

按注 此穴一般多用灸法,有时用刺法时可针0.2～0.5寸,局部感觉痛胀。

Composition This group of acupoints is composed of the two points on the anterior border of the helix and the lower border of the earlobe.

Location One point is on the anterior border of the helix, the other is at the level of the lower border of the earlobe.

Indication Asthma.

Method 3−9 wheat-sized moxa cones of moxibustion is applied.

Note Usually moxibustion is applied to this group of acupoints. Sometimes acupuncture can also be applied by inserting the needle 0.2−0.5 cun till the acu-esthesia of pain and distension is obtained.

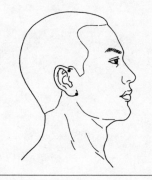

图 1−64 郁中
Fig. 1−64 Yuzhong

大椎四花
Dazhuisihua

组成　本穴组由大椎周围的四个点组合而成。

位置　背部，从第二胸椎棘突下，左右旁开0.6寸的二个点和上下等距0.6寸的二点。

主治　百日咳。

操作　刺法：刺0.5寸，局部有酸胀感，可用平补平泻或捻转补泻法。

灸法：艾炷灸3～5壮，艾条温灸5～15分钟。

Composition　This group of acupoints is composed of the four points around Dazhui.

Location　On the back, the points 0.6 cun lateral, superior and inferior to the point below the 2nd spinous process of the thoracic vertebra.

Indication　Whooping cough.

Method　Acupuncture：the needle is inserted 0.5 cun, the acu-esthesia is soreness and distension in this part. Even reinforcing-reducing techniques or reinforcing and reducing techniques by rotating the needles can be used.

Moxibustion：moxibustion with 3－5 moxa cones, or warm moxibustion with moxa roll for 5－15 minutes.

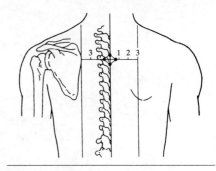

图1-65　大椎四花
Fig. 1-65　Dazhuisihua

百劳四穴
Bailaosixue

组成　本穴组由百劳处的四个穴点组合而成。

位置　一穴在项部，后发际下1寸，从正中线左右旁开各1寸处。

一穴在第七颈椎棘突与第一胸椎棘突之间点，左右旁开各1.3寸处二穴。

主治　瘰病，瘰疬，咳嗽，百日咳，落枕，颈椎病。

操作　刺法：直刺0.5～0.8寸，局部酸胀，平补平泻法。

灸法：艾炷灸或温针灸5～9壮，艾条温灸10～20分钟，或药物灸，也可用累计灸百余壮。

Composition　This group of acupoints is composed of the four points around Bailao.

Location　One point is on the nape, 1 cun below the

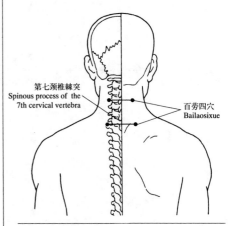

第七颈椎棘突
Spinous process of the 7th cervical vertebra

百劳四穴
Bailaosixue

图1-66　百劳四穴
Fig. 1-66　Bailaosixue

posterior hairline and 1 cun lateral to the midline.

One point at the point between the spinous processes of the 7th cervical vertebra and the 1st thoracic vertebra, two points 1.3 cun lateral to previous point.

Indications Phthisis, scrofula, cough, pertusis, neck rigidity and cervical spondylopathy.

Methods Acupuncture：the needle is inserted 0.5–0.8 cun, the acu-esthesia of soreness and distension in this part should be obtained. The even reinforcing reducing techniques can be applied.

Moxibustion：moxibustion with moxa cone, warm needle moxibustion of 5−9 cones, warm moxibustion with moxa roll for 10−20 minutes or medicated moxibustion can be used. A total of 100 cones of separated moxibustion can also be applied.

八曜
Bayao

组成　本穴组由大椎穴周围之八个点组合而成。

位置　在大椎穴上下左右各外开1寸，斜四方也各外开1寸。

主治　胃病呕吐，妊娠恶阻。

操作　刺法：各针0.5寸，于脊椎旁者则针刺微斜向脊柱刺之。

灸法：灸5～15壮。

Composition This group of acupoints is composed of the eight points around Dazhui.

Location points 1 cun lateral, superior and inferior left-superior, left-inferior right-superior and right-inferior to Dazhui.

Indication Gastric diseases, vomiting and morning sickness.

Method Acupuncture：the needle is inserted 0.5 cun respectively. If the point is close to the vertebra, the needle is inserted obliquely slightly towards the spine.

Moxibustion：5−15 cones.

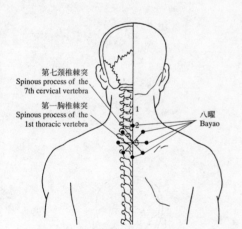

第七颈椎棘突
Spinous process of the 7th cervical vertebra

第一胸椎棘突
Spinous process of the 1st thoracic vertebra

八曜
Bayao

图1−67　八曜
Fig. 1−67　Bayao

聪脑
Congnao

组成　本穴组由后神聪、健脑二穴组合而成。

位置　后神聪：头额正中线，前后发际之中点，当百会后1寸处。

健脑：项后、当胸锁乳突肌与斜方肌间凹陷下缘，约在风池下0.5寸处。

主治　脱发，智力减退，弱智症。

操作　健脑进针0.5~1寸行补法，每日1次，留针15~30分钟，10次为1疗程。

后神聪沿皮刺0.5~1寸，得气为度。

Composition　This group of acupoints is composed of Houshencong and Jiannao.

Location　Houshencong：on the midline of the head, at the midpoint of the anterior and posterior hairline, 1 cun posterior to Baihui.

Jiannao：on the nape, on the lower border of the depression between the sternocleidomastoid and trapezius muscles, about 0.5 cun below Fengchi(GB20).

Indications　Trichomadesis, decreased intelligence and feeble-mindedness.

Method　Jiannao：the needle is inserted 0.5-1 cun, the reinforcing techniques are applied. Treat once every day, retain the needles for 15-30 minutes, 10 times as a course of treatment.

Houshencong：the needle is inserted 0.5-1 cun under the skin till the acu-esthesia is obtained.

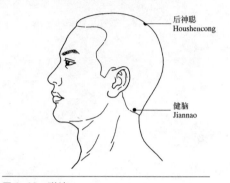

图1-68　聪脑
Fig. 1-68　Congnao

耳屏外三穴
Erpingwaisanxue

组成　本穴组由耳屏外的三个点组合而成。

位置　头部耳郭之耳舟中，计三穴：对耳屏外上方凹陷处一穴，对耳屏外方凹陷处一穴，对耳屏外下方凹陷处，近耳垂下方一穴。

主治　疟腮，耳聋，耳鸣，聤耳，咽痛，咽肿。

操作　针0.2~0.5寸，以不穿过对侧皮肤为度，针后痛

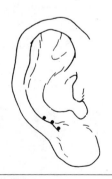

图1-69　耳屏外三穴
Fig. 1-69　Erpingwaisanxue

感较烈。

Composition This group of acupoints is composed of three points lateral to the tragus.

Location In the scapha of the auricle on the head, three points on each side: one point in the depression lateral and superior to the antitragus, one point in the depression lateral and inferior to the antitragus, one point close to the lower part of the earlobe.

Indications Parotitis, deafness, tinnitus, otorrhea and sore throat.

Method The needle is inserted 0.2—0.5 cun without penetrating to the opposite skin. The acu-esthesia of pain is severe.

 耳阑尾点
Erlanweidian

组成 本穴组由耳阑尾1、耳阑尾2、耳阑尾3三穴组合而成。

位置 耳阑尾1：耳舟上端，耳轮与耳轮上脚交界处的耳舟部。

耳阑尾2：耳舟中端，当耳脚上端延伸至耳舟延长线上。

耳阑尾3：耳舟下端，当耳甲腔最凹陷处相平的耳舟下部。

主治 急慢性阑尾炎。

操作 针0.1～0.2寸，针感局部疼痛，留针20～30分钟。

Composition This group of acupoints is composed of Erlanwei1, Erlanwei2 and Erlanwei3.

Location Erlanwei 1: in the upper part of the scapha which is in the juncture of the helix and the superior antihelix crus.

Erlanwei 2: in the middle part of the scapha, on the extended line from the ear crus to the scapha.

Erlanwei 3: in the lower part of the scapha, at the level the of lowest point of the depression in the cavum concha.

Indication Acute and chronic appendicitis.

Method The needle is inserted 0.1—0.2 cun. The acu-esthesia is pain in this part. Retain the needles for 20—30 minutes.

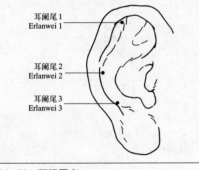

耳阑尾 1
Erlanwei 1

耳阑尾 2
Erlanwei 2

耳阑尾 3
Erlanwei 3

图1-70 耳阑尾点
Fig. 1—70 Erlanweidian

耳会阴
Erhuiyin

组成　本穴组由耳会阴1、耳会阴2二穴组合而成。

位置　耳会阴1：耳垂背面外上方，耳舟隆起下缘与对耳轮窝下缘之间点。

耳会阴2：耳垂背面外上方，近耳舟隆起下缘。

主治　痔，前列腺疾和月经不调。

操作　针0.1～0.2寸，局部疼痛感，针20～30分钟。

Composition　This group of acupoints is composed of Erhuiyin 1 and Erhuiyin 2.

Location　Erhuiyin 1：lateral and superior to the back of the earlobe, at the point between the lower border of the prominence of the scapha and the lower border of the antihelix fossa.

Erhuiyin 2：lateral and superior to the back of the earlobe, close to the lower border of the prominence of the scapha.

Indication　Hemorrhoids, prostate diseases and irregular menstruation.

Method　The needle is inserted 0.1−0.2 cun. The acu-esthesia is pain in this part. Retain the needles for 20−30 minutes.

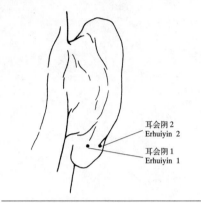

图1-71　耳会阴
Fig. 1-71 Erhuiyin

第二章　躯干部组合穴

CHAPTER 2 COMPOSED ACUPOINTS ON THE TRUNK

 肺道
Feidao

组成　本穴组由肺俞、陶道二穴组合而成。

位置　肺俞：第三胸椎棘突下，旁开1.5寸。

陶道：第一胸椎棘突下。

主治　发热时行温热病。

操作　肺俞向脊柱方向斜刺0.5～0.8寸。陶道针0.5～1寸。各以得气为度。

Composition　This group of acupoints is composed of Feishu(BL13) and Taodao(GV13).

Location　Feishu：1.5 cun lateral to the point below the 3rd spinous process of the thoracic vertebra.

Taodao：at the point below the 1st spinous process of the thoracic vertebra.

Indication　Febrile diseases.

Method　Feishu：the needle is inserted 0.5－0.8 cun obliquely towards the spine till the acu-esthesia is obtained. Taodao：the needle is inserted 0.5－1 cun till the acu-esthesia is obtained.

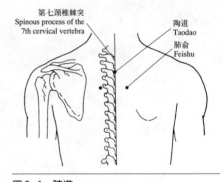

图2-1　肺道
Fig. 2-1　Feidao

 感冒灸
Ganmaojiu

组成　本穴组由大椎、风门、肺俞三穴组合而成。

位置　大椎：第七颈椎棘突下。

肺俞：第三胸椎棘突下，旁开1.5寸。

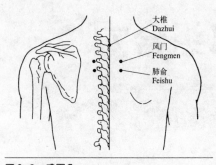

大椎
Dazhui

风门
Fengmen

肺俞
Feishu

图2-2 感冒灸
Fig. 2-2 Ganmaojiu

风门 第二胸椎棘突下，旁开1.5寸。

主治 感冒(灸)，哮喘。

操作 刺法：治哮喘可用针法。肺俞、风门可向脊椎方向斜刺0.5~0.8寸。大椎直刺0.8~1.2寸，得气后留针20分钟，行针2~3分钟，也可针后拔罐。

灸法：治感冒以艾条灸雀啄法10~20分钟，皮肤焮红微为度。治哮喘可用麦粒灸5~9壮。

Composition This group of acupoints is composed of Dazhui(GV14), Fengmen(BL12) and Feishu(BL13).

Location Dazhui：at the point below the 7th spinous process of the cervical vertebra.

Feishu：1.5 cun lateral to the point below the 3rd spinous process of the thoracic vertebra.

Fengmen：1.5 cun lateral to the point below the 2nd spinous process of the thoracic vertebra.

Indications Common cold (moxibustion) and asthma.

Method Acupuncture：When treating asthma, the acupuncture method is applied. For Feishu and Fengmen, the needles can be inserted 0.5−0.8 cun obliquely towards the spine. For Dazhui, the needle can be inserted 0.8−1.2 cun perpendicularly. Retain the needles for 20 minutes after the acu-esthesia is obtained. Manipulate the needles for 2−3 minutes. Cupping may be applied after acupuncture.

Moxibustion：Sparrow-pecking moxibustion with moxa roll for 10−20 minutes is applied till the skin appears reddish when treating common cold. Moxibustion of 5−9 wheat-sized moxa cones can be applied when treating asthma.

 针嗽

Zhensou

组成 本穴组由肺俞、风门二穴组合而成。

位置 肺俞：第三胸椎棘突下，旁开1.5寸。

风门：第二胸椎棘突下，旁开1.5寸。

主治 咳嗽。

操作 刺法：向脊柱方向斜刺0.5~0.8寸，得气为度。

灸法：艾炷灸5~9壮，艾条温灸10~20分钟。

Composition　This group of acupoints is composed of Feishu(BL13) and Fengmen(BL12).

Location　Feishu：1.5 cun lateral to the point below the 3rd spinous process of the thoracic vertebra.

Fengmen：1.5 cun lateral to the point below the 2nd spinous process of the thoracic vertebra.

Indication　Cough.

Method　Acupuncture：the needle is inserted 0.5−0.8 cun obliquely towards the spine till the acu-esthesia is obtained.

Moxibustion：moxibustion with 5−9 moxa cones, warm moxibustion with moxa roll for 10−20 minutes can be applied.

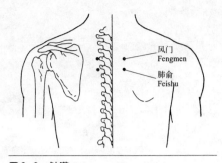

图2-3　针嗽
Fig. 2-3　Zhensou

背五柱
Beiwuzhu

组成　本穴组由督脉之身柱、陶道、大椎和膀胱经之风门，再加两侧风门之中央点共六穴组合而成。

位置　身柱：第三胸椎棘突下。

陶道：第一胸椎棘突下。

大椎：第七颈椎棘突下。

风门：第二胸椎棘突下，旁开1.5寸。

风门之中央点：二风门之中央点即第二胸椎棘突下。

主治　咳嗽。

操作　刺法：针0.5寸，脊旁二穴向脊柱方向斜刺0.5～0.8寸，局部酸胀，平补平泻手法。

灸法：艾炷灸3～5壮，艾条温灸5～10分钟。

Composition　This group of acupoints is composed of Shenzhu(GV12), Taodao(GV13), Dazhui(GV14) of Govenor Vessel, Fengmen(BL13) of the Bladder Meridian and the midpoint of the line connecting both Fengmen, 6 points in all.

Location　Shenzhu：below the spinous process of the 3rd thoracic vertebra.

Taodao：below the spinous process of the 1st thoracic vertebra.

Dazhui：below the spinous process of the 7th cervical vertebra.

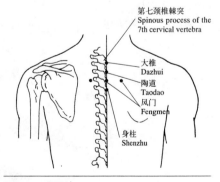

第七颈椎棘突
Spinous process of the 7th cervical vertebra

大椎
Dazhui

陶道
Taodao

风门
Fengmen

身柱
Shenzhu

图2-4　背五柱
Fig. 2-4　Beiwuzhu

Fengmen：1.5 cun lateral to the point below the spinous process of the 2nd thoracic vertebra.

Fengmenzhizhongyangdian：at the midpoint of the line connecting both Fengmen, i.e. below the spinous process of the 2nd thoracic vertebra.

Indication   Cough.

Method   Acupuncture：the needle is inserted 0.5 cun. For the two points lateral to the spine, the needles are inserted obliquely 0.5−0.8 cun towards the spine. The acu-esthesia of soreness and distension should be obtained. The even reinforcing reducing techniques are applied.

Moxibustion：moxibustion with 3−5 moxa cones, or warm moxibustion with moxa roll for 5−10 minutes can be applied.

● 背三针
Beisanzhen

组成   本穴组由大杼、风门、肺俞三穴组合而成。

位置   大杼：第一胸椎棘突下，旁开1.5寸。

风门：第二胸椎棘突下，旁开1.5寸。

肺俞：第三胸椎棘突下，旁开1.5寸。

主治   哮喘，咳嗽，背痛等。

操作   刺法：针尖向下与背呈45°角斜向背柱慢慢向下捻入，深0.5～0.8寸，酸胀感觉。

灸法：哮喘缓解后可用艾炷直接灸或化脓灸背三针各穴3～9壮。

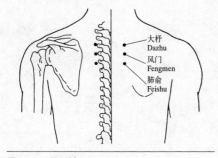

图2−5 背三针
Fig. 2−5 Beisanzhen

Composition   This group of acupoints is composed of Dazhu(BL11), Fengmen(BL12) and Feishu(BL13).

Location   Dazhu：1.5 cun lateral to the point below the spinous process of the 1st thoracic vertebra.

Fengmen：1.5 cun lateral to the point below the spinous process of the 2nd thoracic vertebra.

Feishu：1.5 cun lateral to the point below the spinous process of the 3rd thoracic vertebra.

Indications   Asthma, cough and backache, etc..

Method   Acupuncture：The needle is inserted obliquely at 45° angle formed by the needle and the back towards the spine slowly with rotating method, the depth is 0.5−0.8 cun. The acu-esthesia is soreness or distension.

Moxibustion：3−9 cones of direct moxibustion with moxa cone or scar-forming moxibustion may be applied to Beisanzhen after the symptom is relieved.

解喘
Jiechuan

组成　本穴组由"上次髎"外1寸处四点组合而成。

位置　骶部，平第一、第二骶背侧孔外侧约1寸处，当"上髎"、"次髎"穴外侧约1寸处。

主治　哮喘。

操作　刺法：针1～1.5寸，局部酸胀。

灸法：艾炷灸，温针灸3～5壮，艾条灸5～10分钟。

Composition　This group of acupoints is composed of four points 1 cun lateral to Shangliao(BL31) and Ciliao (BL32).

Location　On the sacrum, about 1 cun lateral to the 1st and 2nd posterior sacral foramen, 1 cun lateral to Shangliao and Ciliao.

Indication　Asthma.

Method　Acupuncture：The needle is inserted 1−1.5 cun. The acu-esthesia in this part is soreness and distension.

Moxibustion：3−5 cones of moxibustion with moxa cone or warm needle moxibustion, or moxibustion with moxa roll for 5−10 minutes is applied.

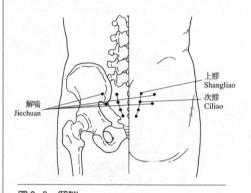

图2-6　解喘

Fig. 2-6　Jiechuan

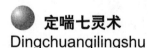
定喘七灵术
Dingchuanqilingshu

组成　本穴组由督脉之腰俞、腰阳关穴和二穴之间的腰、骶椎棘五点共七穴组合而成。

位置　腰俞：当骶管裂孔处。

腰阳关：第四腰椎棘突下。

腰骶棘五点：在上二穴间的腰骶椎棘突间。

主治　咳嗽，哮喘息，腰痛。

操作　刺法：第一针由腰俞穴进针向上沿皮斜刺，第二针

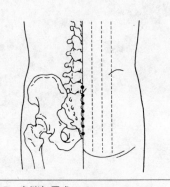

图2-7 定喘七灵术
Fig. 2-7 Dingchuanqilingshu

依法在棘突间向上斜刺，如此法共七针，针0.3～0.5寸，局部酸、麻、胀感。

灸法：灸3～9壮，艾条灸10～20分钟。

Composition This group of acupoints is composed of Yaoshu(GV2), Yaoyangguan(GV3) of the Governor Vessel, and five points on the spinous processes of the lumbar vertebrae and sacrum between above two points, 7 points in all.

Location Yaoshu：at the point of the sacral hiatus.

Yaoyangguan：below the spinous process of the 4th lumbar vertebra.

Yaodijiwudian：at the points of the spinous processes of the lumbar vertebrae and sacrum between above two points.

Indications Cough, asthma and low back pain.

Method Acupuncture：The first needle is inserted upwards obliquely under the skin from Yaoshu, the second is inserted upwards obliquely between the spinous processes with above method. 7 needles in all, the depth is 0.3−0.5 cun, the acu-esthesia of this part is soreness, numbness and distension.

Moxibustion：3−9 cones of moxibustion or 10−20 minutes' moxibustion with moxa roll is applied.

魄膏

Pogao

组成 本穴组由魄户、膏肓二穴组合而成。

位置 膏肓：第四胸椎棘突下，旁开3寸。

魄户：第三胸椎棘突下，旁开3寸。

主治 痨瘵。

操作 艾炷灸5～9壮，艾条温灸10～30分钟。

Composition This group of acupoints is composed of Pohu(BL42) and Gaohuang(BL43).

Location Gaohuang：3 cun lateral to the point below the spinous process of the 4th thoracic vertebra.

Pohu：3 cun lateral to the point below the spinous process of the 3rd thoracic vertebra.

Indication Phthisis.

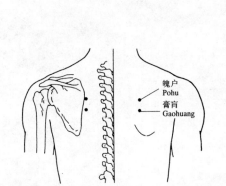

魄户
Pohu
膏肓
Gaohuang

图2-8 魄膏
Fig. 2-8 Pogao

Method　Moxibustion with 5−9 moxa cones or moxibustion with moxa roll for 10−30 minutes is applied.

⬤ 双结核
Shuangjiehe

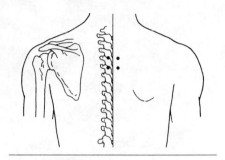

图2-9　双结核
Fig. 2-9　Shuangjiehe

组成　本穴组由第二、第三胸椎棘突左右旁开0.5寸处的四个点组合而成。

位置　背部，第二胸椎棘突旁开0.5寸处各一穴；第三胸椎棘突旁开0.5寸处各一穴。

主治　肺结核。

操作　刺法：针0.5~0.8寸，局部酸、胀感。

灸法：艾炷灸5~9壮，或灸100~300壮(累计灸)。

Composition　This group of acupoints is composed of the four points 0.5 cun lateral to the spinous processes of the 2nd and 3rd thoracic vertebrae.

Location　On the back, 0.5 cun lateral to the spinous process of the 2nd thoracic vertebra on each side, and 0.5 cun lateral to the spinous process of the 3rd thoracic vertebra on each side.

Indication　Pulmonary tuberculosis.

Method　Acupuncture：the needle is inserted 0.5−0.8 cun. The acu-esthesia in this part is soreness and distension.

Moxibustion：Moxibustion with 5−9 moxa cones each time or a total of 100−300 cones of separated moxibustion can be applied.

⬤ 四花
Sihua

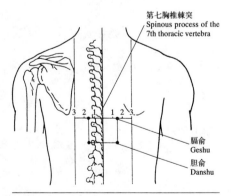

第七胸椎棘突
Spinous process of the 7th thoracic vertebra

膈俞
Geshu
胆俞
Danshu

图2-10　四花
Fig. 2-10　Sihua

组成　本穴组由膈俞、胆俞二穴组合而成。

位置　膈俞：第七胸椎棘突下，旁开1.5寸。

胆俞：第十胸椎棘突下，旁开1.5寸。

主治　劳瘵，咳嗽，哮喘，虚弱羸瘦。

操作　艾炷灸5~9壮。

Composition　This group of acupoints is composed of Geshu(BL17) and Danshu(BL19).

Location Geshu：1.5 cun lateral to the point below the spinous process of the 7th thoracic vertebra.

Danshu：1.5 cun lateral to the point below the spinous process of the 10th thoracic vertebra.

Indications Phthisis, cough, asthma and emaciation due to general deficiency.

Method Moxibustion with 5-9 moxa cones is applied.

四花患门
Sihuahuanmen

组成 本穴组由第五、第七、第十胸椎棘突下旁开1.5寸之六个点组合而成。

位置 背部，第五胸椎棘突下，第七胸椎棘突下，第十胸椎棘突下各旁开1.5寸。

主治 肺痨，咳嗽，喘息，虚弱羸瘦。

操作 艾炷灸9~15壮或随年壮灸。

按注 本穴实为足太阳膀胱经穴心俞、膈俞、胆俞三者的组合。由膈俞、胆俞组合者名为四花穴，也为常用奇穴。

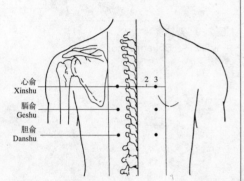

心俞
Xinshu

膈俞
Geshu

胆俞
Danshu

图2-11 四花患门
Fig. 2-11 Sihuahuanmen

Composition This group of acupoints is composed of the six points 1.5 cun lateral to the points below the spinous processes of the 5th, 7th and 10th thoracic vertebrae.

Location On the back, at the points 1.5 cun lateral to the points below the 5th, 7th and 10th spinous processes of the thoracic vertebrae.

Indications Pulmonary tuberculosis, cough, asthma and emaciation due to general deficiency.

Method Moxibustion with 9-15 moxa cones can be applied. The number of cones can also be based on the patient's age.

Note This group of acupoints is the group of Xinshu (BL15), Geshu(BL17) and Danshu(BL19) of the Bladder Meridian of Foot Tai-yang.

The group of Geshu and Danshu is called Sihua, which is also a commonly used extraordinary acupoint.

五花针
Wuhuazhen

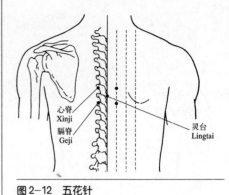

图2-12 五花针
Fig. 2-12 Wuhuazhen

组成 本穴组由灵台、心脊、膈脊三穴组合而成。

位置 灵台：第六胸椎棘突下。

心脊：第五、第六胸椎棘突间旁开1寸处。

膈脊：第七、第八胸椎棘突间旁开1寸处。

主治 肺病，胁肋疼痛。

操作 灵台进针后向上斜刺1~1.5寸。心脊穴及膈脊穴四针均向脊柱斜刺1~1.5寸，局部酸、胀感。

Composition This group of acupoints is composed of Lingtai(GV10), Xinji and Geji.

Location Lingtai：below the spinous process of the 6th thoracic vertebra.

Xinji：1 cun lateral to the point between the spinous processes of the 5th and 6th thoracic vertebrae.

Geji：1 cun lateral to the point between the spinous processes of the 7th and 8th thoracic vertebrae.

Indication Pulmonary diseases, pain in the hypochondric region.

Method After the insertion of Lingtai, the needle is inserted upwards obliquely 1−1.5 cun. For Xinji and Geji, the four needles are all inserted 1−1.5 cun obliquely towards the spine. The acu−esthesia in this part is soreness and distension.

八华
Bahua

组成 本穴组由背部的八个点组合而成。

位置 背部以患者两乳头间之距离折作8寸，以2寸为一边，作成等边三角形的纸片，将此等边三角形纸片之一角置于大椎穴上，将底边放成水平，其余二边所指之处是穴，再将此三角形放在上一三角形底边之中点上，其下二角也是穴，如此再量一次，计八穴。

主治 虚弱羸瘦，骨节疼痛，咳嗽，盗汗。

操作 灸5~9壮。

按注 本穴去最下面两点，称六华穴，临床每多用于灸治。

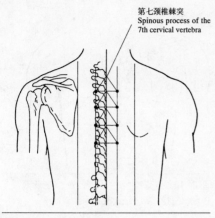

第七颈椎棘突
Spinous process of the
7th cervical vertebra

图2-13 八华
Fig. 2-13 Bahua

Composition This group of acupoints is composed of eight points on the back.

Location On the back. The distance between the two nipples of the patient is 8 cun. Cut a paper equilateral triangle of 2 cun each side. Put one angle of this paper triangle on Dazhui, and adjust the base to horizontal level, the other two sides are two points of this group. Then put one angle of this paper triangle on the midpoint of the base of the above triangle, the lower two angles are another two points of this group. Locate the points again with the above method, 8 points in all.

Indications Emaciation due to general deficiency, pain in the joints, cough and night sweating.

Method 5-9 cones of moxibustion is applied.

Note Liuhua is contained in this group of acupoints. Moxibustion is applied more in clinical use to this group.

经门之六穴(经六)
Jingmenzhiliuxue (Jingliu)

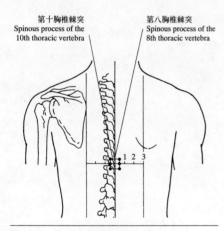

第十胸椎棘突
Spinous process of the
10th thoracic vertebra

第八胸椎棘突
Spinous process of the
8th thoracic vertebra

图2-14 经门之六穴(经六)
Fig. 2-14 Jingmenzhiliuxue (Jingliu)

组成 本穴组由背部第九胸椎周围的六个刺激点组合而成。

位置 当第九胸椎棘突之高点两侧各0.5寸处2点,此二穴上下各0.5寸处又4点。

主治 肺结核,喘息,支气管炎,虚弱。

操作 艾炷灸1～3壮,或温灸5～10分钟。

Composition This group of acupoints is composed of the six points around the 9th thoracic vertebra.

Location Two points are the two points 0.5 cun lateral to the prominence of the 9th thoracic vertebra, another four points are 0.5 cun superior and inferior to the above two points.

Indications Pulmonary tuberculosis, asthma, bronchitis, and emaciation.

Methods Moxibustion with 1-3 moxa cones or warm moxibustion for 5-10 minutes can be applied.

阶段灸
Jieduanjiu

组成　本穴组由第七至第十一胸椎棘突旁2寸之五个点组合而成。

位置　第七至第十一胸椎棘突旁开各2寸之两侧线上，左右计十穴。

主治　肺痨，咳嗽，失眠，体弱及呼吸系消化系疾患，脊髓疾患。

操作　各灸5～9壮，可轮番使用。

Composition　This group of acupoints is composed of the five points 2 cun lateral to the spinous processes from the 7th to 11th of the thoracic vertebrae.

Location　On the lines 2 cun lateral to the spinous processes of the thoracic vertebrae from 7th to 11th, 10 points on both sides in all.

Indications　Pulmonary tuberculosis, cough, insomnia, emaciation, diseases of pulmonary and digestive systems, spinal cord disease.

Method　5−9 cones of Moxibustion for each point. The points may be used alternatively.

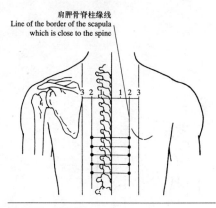

肩胛骨脊柱缘线
Line of the border of the scapula which is close to the spine

图2-15　阶段灸
Fig. 2−15　Jieduanjiu

传尸痨
Chuanshilao

组成　本穴组由肺俞、厥阴俞、心俞、肝俞、三焦俞、肾穴，各穴上下各1寸处的十二个点组合而成。

位置　背部正中线，左右旁开各1.5寸，即当肺俞(第三胸椎棘突下，旁开1.5寸)、厥阴俞(第四胸椎棘突下，旁开1.5寸)、心俞(第五胸椎棘突下，旁开1.5寸)、肝俞(第九胸椎棘突下，旁开1.5寸)、三焦俞(第一腰椎棘突下，旁开1.5寸；间点平高)、肾俞(第二腰椎棘突下，旁开1.5寸间点平高)，各穴之上下各1寸处是穴，左右计二十四穴。

主治　痨瘵，寄生虫病。

操作　各灸5～9壮，每日灸四穴，按次序分六日灸之。即第一日灸心俞上下各1寸处，第二日灸肺俞上下各1寸处，余以此类推。

Composition　This group of acupoints is composed of

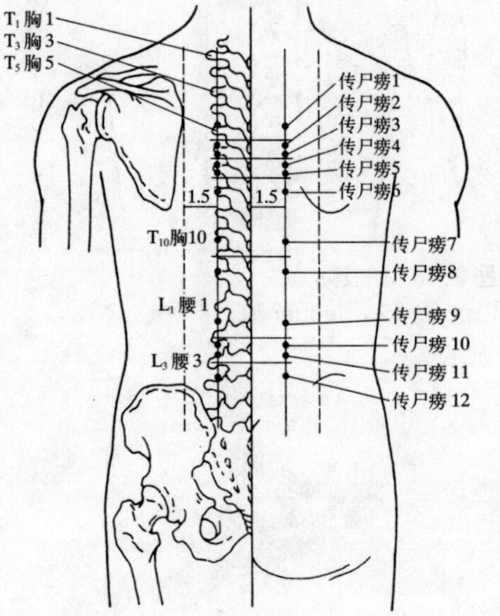

12 points respectively 1 cun superior and inferior to Feishu(BL13), Jueyinshu(BL14), Xinshu(BL15), Ganshu (BL18), Sanjiaoshu(BL22) and Shenshu(BL23).

Location   On the line 1.5 cun lateral the posterior midline of the back, 1 cun superior and inferior to Feishu (1.5 cun lateral to the point below the spinous process of the 3rd thoracic vertebra), Jueyinshu (1.5 cun lateral to the point below the spinous process of the 4th thoracic vertebra), Xinshu (1.5 cun lateral to the point below the spinous process of the 5th thoracic vertebra), Ganshu (1.5 cun lateral to the point below the spinous process of the 9th thoracic vertebra), Sanjiaoshu (1.5 cun lateral to the point below the spinous process of the 1st lumbar vertebra) and Shenshu (1.5 cun lateral to the point below the spinous process of the 2nd lumbar vertebra), 24 points on both sides.

Indications   Phthisis, verminosis.

Method   5—9 cones of moxibustion for each point, 4 points in turn every day, thus moxibustion can be applied to all points within six days, i.e. moxibustion is applied to the points 1 cun superior and inferior to Xinshu on the first day, to the points superior and inferior to Feishu on the second day, and the like.

图 2-16　传尸痨
Fig. 2-16　Chuanshilao

腰部八穴
Yaobubaxue

组成　本穴组由腰骶部的八个点组合而成。

位置　腰骶部。令患者示、中和环指并拢，以指中央关节横长为一边，作成等边三角形纸片五块，然后于命门穴下1寸处划一横线，将三块纸片平排于此横线下，三角形的二角在上，顶角向下，中间一块三角形的顶点对准脊柱中线，其上缘共得四点，即为四穴位；再于上排三个三角形的顶点上平排两块纸片，也得四穴。

主治　虚痨羸瘦，身体衰弱。

操作　灸9~15壮，或以强壮保健穴累计灸百壮。

按注　此穴为强壮穴，灸之其强壮保健之功更佳。

Composition   This group of acupoints is composed of eight points on the lower back and the sacrum.

Location   On the lower back and sacrum. Ask the patient to level the index, middle and ring fingers, the transverse breadth of the middle joints of the fingers is one side of a equilateral triangle. Cut five such paper triangles. Draw a transverse line below Mingmen, arrange three paper triangles horizontally below this line with each triangle's two angles up and one angle down, align the central triangle's vertex to the midline of the spine, thus four points can be located on its upper border; arrange two paper triangles horizontally again on the vertex of the above three vertex to locate another 4 points.

Indication：Emaciation due to general deficiency.

Method   9—15 cones of moxibustion can be applied. A total of 100 cones of separated moxibustion may be applied to nourish health.

Note   This group of acupoints can improve health. The function is better when moxibustion is applied.

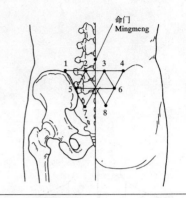

图2-17　腰部八穴
Fig. 2-17　Yaobubaxue

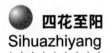

四花至阳
Sihuazhiyang

组成　本穴组由四花、至阳共五穴组合而成。

位置　四花：即由左右膈俞和胆俞组合而成。

至阳：第七胸椎棘突下。

主治　呃逆。

操作　先直刺，膈俞0.3～0.4寸，得气后，将针沿皮向胆俞透刺，并使针感向四周扩散；再以至阳分透膈俞，留针20分钟。

Composition   This group of acupoints is composed of Sihua and Zhiyang(GV9).

Location   Sihua：composed of Geshu(BL17) and Danshu (BL19).

Zhiyang：below the spinous process of the 7th thoracic vertebra.

Indication   Hiccup.

Method   Geshu is punctured 0.3—0.4 cun first. After the acu-esthesia is obtained, penetrate the needle towards Danshu, and the acu-esthesia should spread

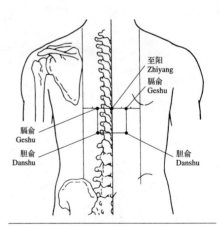

图2-18　四花至阳
Fig. 2-18　Sihuazhiyang

outwards. Then the needle is penetrated from Zhiyang to Geshu. Retain the needle for 20 minutes.

六之灸
Liuzhijiu

组成　本穴组由膈俞、肝俞、脾俞三穴组合而成。

位置　膈俞：第七胸椎棘突下，旁开1.5寸。

肝俞：第九胸椎棘突下，旁开1.5寸。

脾俞：第十一胸椎棘突下，旁开1.5寸。

左右计六穴。

主治　胃病，胃痛，胃癌，呃逆，食欲不振，消化不良等。

操作　各灸7～15壮。

Composition　This group of acupoints is composed of Geshu(BL17), Ganshu(BL18) and Pishu(BL20).

Location　Geshu：1.5 cun lateral to the point below the spinous process of the 7th thoracic vertebra.

Ganshu：1.5 cun lateral to the point below the spinous process of the 9th thoracic vertebra.

Pishu：1.5 cun lateral to the point below the spinous process of the 11th thoracic vertebra.

Sixpoints on both sides.

Indications　Gastric diseases, stomachache, stomach cancer, hiccup, anorexia and indigestion.

Method　7—15 cones of moxibustion is applied to each point.

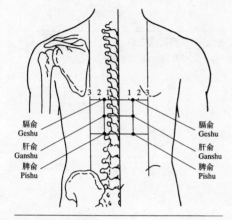

膈俞 Geshu
肝俞 Ganshu
脾俞 Pishu

图2-19　六之灸
Fig. 2-19　Liuzhijiu

斜差
Xiecha

组成　本穴组由左肝俞、右脾俞二穴组合而成。

位置　肝俞：第九胸椎棘突下旁开1.5寸。

脾俞：第十一胸椎棘突下，旁开1.5寸。

主治　肝胃疾病，小儿胃肠病。

操作　刺法：向脊柱方向斜刺0.5～0.8寸，局部酸胀感。

灸法：灸5～15壮，艾条温灸10～20分钟。

Composition　This group of acupoints is composed of left-side Ganshu(BL18) and right-side Pishu(BL20).

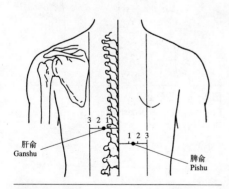

肝俞 Ganshu
脾俞 Pishu

图2-20　斜差
Fig. 2-20　Xiecha

Location Ganshu：1.5 cun lateral to the point below the spinous process of the 9th thoracic vertebra.

Pishu：1.5 cun lateral to the point below the spinous process of the 11th thoracic vertebra.

Indications Hepatic and gastric diseases, pediatric gastroin testinal diseases.

Methods Acupuncture：the needle is inserted 0.5−0.8 cun obliquely towards the spine, the acu-esthesia is soreness and distension in this part.

Moxibustion：5−15 cones of moxibustion, or warm moxibustion with moxa roll for 10−20 minutes can be applied.

胆纲
Dangang

组成 本穴组由胆俞、阳纲二穴组合而成。

位置 胆俞：第十胸椎棘突下，旁开1.5寸。

阳纲：第十胸椎棘突下，旁开3寸。

主治 目黄。

操作 胆俞向脊柱方向斜刺0.5~0.8寸。阳纲向上沿皮刺0.5~0.8寸。各以得气为度。

Composition This group of acupoints is composed of Danshu(BL10) and Yanggang(BL48).

Location Danshu：1.5 cun lateral to the point below the spinous process of the 10th thoracic vertebra.

Yanggang：3 cun lateral to the point below the spinous process of the 10th thoracic vertebra.

Indication Yellowish sclera.

Method Danshu is needled 0.5−0.8 cun obliquely towards the spine. Yanggang is needled 0.5−0.8 cun upwards beneath the skin till the acu−esthesia is obtained.

脾横
Piheng

组成 本穴组由第十一胸椎棘突上及旁之二个点共三穴组合而成。

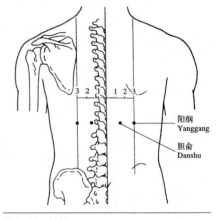

图 2−21 胆纲
Fig. 2−21 Dangang

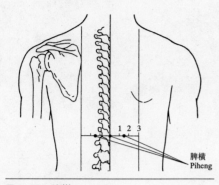

图2-22 脾横
Fig. 2-22 Piheng

位置　背部，第十一胸椎棘突上一穴，及左右旁开1.5寸二穴。

主治　身黄，寒热，腰疼痛，腹满，食呕，舌强。

操作　三处各灸5～9壮。

Composition　This group of acupoints is composed of three points respectively superior and lateral to the spinous process of the 11th thoracic vertebra.

Location　On the back, one point is above the spinous process of the 11th thoracic vertebra, the other two points are 0.5 cun lateral to previous point.

Indications　Jaundice, chills and fever, pain in the lower back, fullness of the abdomen, vomiting after meals, stiffness of the tongue.

Method　5-9 cones of moxibustion can be applied to each point.

肝三针
Gansanzhen

组成　本穴组由肝区背后的三个刺激点组合而成。

位置　约当第九胸椎棘突下旁开3寸处的魂门穴点，及其左右旁开1寸处各一点。

主治　肝区痛及肝肿大。

操作　刺法：斜刺0.5～0.8寸。

灸法：艾炷灸5～9壮，温灸10～20分钟。

Composition　This group of acupoints is composed of the three points on the back opposite to the hepatic region.

Location　Hunmen, which is about 3 cun lateral to the point below the spinous process of the 9th thoracic vertebra and two points 1 cun lateral to Hunmen.

Indications　Hepatalgia and hepatomegaly.

Methods　Acupuncture：the needle is inserted 0.5-1 cun obliquely.

Moxibustion：moxibustion with 5-9 moxa cones, or warm moxibustion for 10 to 20 minutes can be applied.

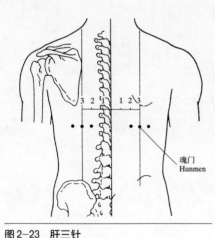

图2-23 肝三针
Fig. 2-23 Gansanzhen

下字灸
Xiazijiu

组成 本穴组由腰部的五个穴点组合而成。

位置 第二腰椎棘突下一穴,第三腰椎棘突之高点一穴,第四腰椎棘突下一穴,平二腰椎棘突下点两侧各0.5寸处各一穴。

主治 腹部疾病。

操作 灸5~15壮。

Composition This group of acupoints is composed of the five points on the lower back.

Location One point below the spinous process of the 2nd lumbar vertebra, one point on the prominence of the spinous process of the 3rd lumbar vertebra, one point below the spinous process of the 4th lumbar vertebra, and the two points 0.5 cun lateral to the point below the spinous process of the 2nd lumbar vertebra.

Indication Abdominal diseases.

Method 5—15 cones of moxibustion is applied.

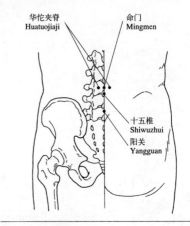

图2-24 下字灸
Fig. 2-24 Xiazijiu

胃管下俞三穴
Weiguanxiashusanxue

组成 本穴组由奇穴八椎下及胃管下俞二穴共三穴组合而成。

位置 八椎下:位于第八胸椎棘突下凹陷中。

胃管下俞:位于第八胸椎棘突下旁开1.5寸处。

主治 消渴,咽喉干。

操作 刺法:直刺或斜刺0.5~0.8寸。

灸法:艾炷灸3~5壮,或温灸5~10分钟。

Composition This group of acupoints is composed of extraordinary acupoints Bazhuixia and Weiguanxiashu.

Location Bazhuixia:in the depression below the spinous process of the 8th thoracic vertebra.

Weiguanxiashu:1.5 cun lateral to the point below the spinous process of the 8th thoracic vertebra.

Indication Diabetes and dryness of the throat.

Methods Acupuncture:the needle is inserted 0.5—

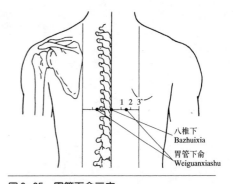

图2-25 胃管下俞三穴
Fig. 2-25 Weiguanxiashusanxue

0.8 cun perpendicularly or obliquely.

Moxibustion: moxibustion with 3—5 moxa cones, or warm moxibustion for 5—10 minutes is applied.

八髎
Baliao

组成　本穴组由上髎、次髎、中髎、下髎左右八穴组合而成。

位置　上髎：第一骶后孔中，约当髂后上棘与督脉的中点。

次髎：第二骶后孔中，约当髂后上棘下与督脉的中点。

中髎：第三骶后孔中，约当中膂俞与督脉之间。

下髎：第四骶后孔中，约当白环俞与督脉之间。

主治　泌尿生殖系统疾患、痢疾等。

操作　刺法：针0.5～1寸，局部酸胀感，如针1～2寸，针感可扩散至腰骶部，如以60°～70°角向下部耻骨联合方向进针，能通向骶前孔到达盆腔，应也可向前少腹及阴部放散。

灸法：灸5～9壮，艾条温灸5～15分钟。

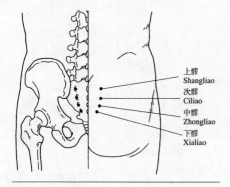

图2-26　八髎
Fig. 2-26　Baliao

Composition　This group of acupoints is composed of Shangliao(BL31), Ciliao(BL32), Zhongliao(BL33) and Xialiao (BL34), 8 points on both sides.

Location　Shangliao: in the 1st posterior sacral foramen, at the midpoint between the posteriosuperior iliac spine and the posterior midline.

Ciliao: in the 2nd posterior sacral foramen, at the midpoint between the posterioinferior iliac spine and the posterior midline.

Zhongliao: in the 3rd posterior sacral foramen, between Zhonglushu and the posterior midline.

Xialiao: in the 4th posterior sacral foramen, about between Baihuanshu and the posterior midline.

Indication　Diseases of urogenital system and dysentery.

Method　Acupuncture: the needle is inserted 0.5—1 cun, the acu-esthesia is soreness and distension in this part. If the depth is 1—2 cun, the acu-esthesia will spread to the lower back and the sacrum region. If the needle is inserted at the angle of 60°—70° towards the symphysis pubis beneath, the acu-esthesia will spread to the pelvis through the anterior sacral foramen. The feeling may also radiate to the lower abdomen and perineum region.

Moxibustion：5－9 cones of moxibustion, or warm moxibustion with moxa roll for 5－15 minutes can be applied.

 骶屏组穴
Dipingzuxue

组成　本穴组由八髎及八髎外 1 寸处之八穴共十六穴组合而成。

位置　八髎：见八髎穴。

八髎外穴：八髎外 1 寸。

主治　泌尿生殖系病证，内分泌失调，前列腺病证等。

操作　先取八髎刺之(其刺法见八髎)，再取八髎外侧 1 寸处之八穴，与八髎穴平行刺之，得气为度。

Composition　This group of acupoints is composed of Baliao and 8 points 1 cun lateral to Baliao.

Location　Baliao：See "Baliao".

Baliaowai：1 cun lateral to Baliao.

Indications　Diseases of urogenital system, endocrine dyscrasia, prostate diseases.

Method　Baliao is inserted first (See Acupuncture method of Baliao). Then locate the 8 points 1 cun lateral to Baliao, the points are needled parallel to Baliao till the acu-esthesia is obtained.

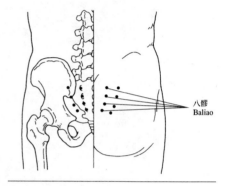

图 2－27　骶屏组穴
Fig. 2－27　Dipingzuxue

 膂阳
Lüyang

组成　本穴组由中膂俞、会阳二穴组合而成。

位置　中膂俞：第三骶椎棘突下，旁开 1.5 寸。

会阳：尾骨尖旁开 0.5 寸。

主治　阳痿。

操作　从中膂俞呈 70°角缓缓向下方刺入，经臀大肌，通过坐骨大孔时，针下有沉紧感，当出现针感向下腹及会阴部扩散时，即为得气。会阴穴针尖向耻骨联合方向针刺，以针感向下腹及会阴部扩散为度，二穴各留针 20 分钟。

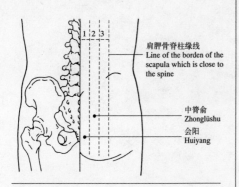

图 2-28 臀阳
Fig. 2-28 Lüyang

Composition This group of acupoints is composed of Zhonglushu(BL29) and Huiyang(BL35).

Location Zhonglushu：at the horizontal level of the 3rd posterior sacral foramen, 1.5 cun lateral to the medial sacral crest.

Huiyang：0.5 cun lateral to the tip of the coccyx.

Indication Impotence.

Method The needle is inserted downwards at the angle of 70° slowly. When the needle passes the greatest gluteal muscle and great sciatic foramen, heavy and tense feeling can be sensed under the needle. The acu-esthesia is obtained when the feeling radiates towards to the lower abdomen and the perineum region.

For Huiyang, the tip of the needle is inserted towards the symphysis pubis till the acu-esthesia spreads towards the lower abdomen and the perineum region. Retain the needles for 20 minutes.

淋泉
Linquan

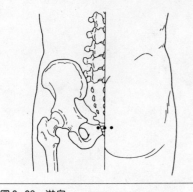

图 2-29 淋泉
Fig. 2-29 Linquan

组成 本穴组由尾骨尖上的三个点组合而成。

位置 臀裂下际尾骨部，尾骨尖上0.5寸处一穴，其左右各0.5寸处各一穴。

主治 淋证。

操作 灸5~9壮。

Composition This group of acupoints is composed of three points on the tip of the coccyx.

Location On the coccyx region below the gluteal cleft, one point is 0.5 cun superior to the tip of the coccyx, 2 points are 0.5 cun lateral to previous point.

Indication Stranguria.

Method 5-9 cones of moxibustion can be applied.

营卫四穴
Yingweisixue

组成 本穴组由骶外左右八点组合而成。

位置　骶部，第一、第二、第三、第四后孔相平处旁开中线2寸。

主治　二便不利，腹痛。

操作　灸9～15壮，或用累计灸百壮。

Composition　This group of acupoints is composed of the eight points lateral to the sacrum.

Location　On the sacrum, respectively at the level with the 1, 2, 3, 4 posterior sacral foramen, 2 cun lateral to the midline.

Indications　Dysuria and constipation.

Method　9–15 cones of moxibustion, or separated moxibustion up to one hundred cones can be applied.

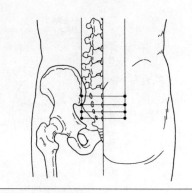

图2-30　营卫四穴
Fig. 2-30　Yingweisixue

闾上
Lüshang

组成　本穴组由骶部第二骶椎棘突上及旁二点共三穴组合而成。

位置　骶部，第二骶椎棘突上一穴，左右旁开1.5寸各一穴。

主治　痔疮，便血。

操作　灸5～9壮。

按注　本穴临床独用灸法。

Composition　This group of acupoints is composed of the three points respectively superior and lateral to the spinous process of the 2nd sacral vertebra.

Location　On the sacrum. One point is on the spinous process of the 2nd sacral vertebra, and two points lateral to previous point, 3 points in all.

Indications　Hemorrhoids and intestinal hemorrhage.

Method　5–9 cones of moxibustion is applied.

Note　Only moxibustion can be applied to this group in clinic.

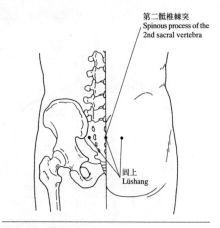

第二骶椎棘突
Spinous process of the 2nd sacral vertebra

闾上
Lüshang

图2-31　闾上
Fig. 2-31　Lüshang

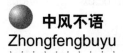

中风不语
Zhongfengbuyu

组成　本穴组由第一、第四胸椎棘突下之二穴组合而成。

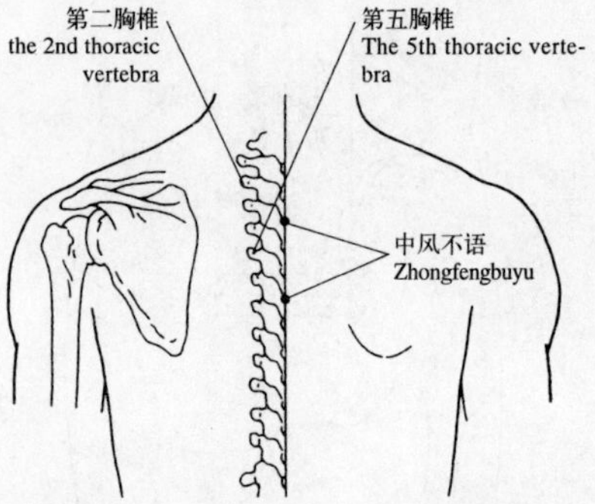

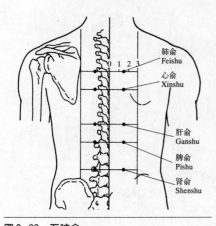

第二胸椎 the 2nd thoracic vertebra
第五胸椎 The 5th thoracic vertebra
中风不语 Zhongfengbuyu

图2-32 中风不语
Fig. 2-32 Zhongfengbuyu

位置　背部正中线，第一胸椎棘突下一穴，第四胸椎棘突下一穴。

主治　中风不语。

操作　灸5~9壮(同时施灸)。

Composition　This group of acupoints is composed of the points respectively below the spinous processes of the 1st and 4th thoracic vertebrae.

Location　On the midline of the back, one point is below the spinous process of the 1st thoracic vertebra, the other is below the spinous process of the 4th thoracic vertebra.

Indication　Post-apoplectic aphasia.

Method　5-9 cones of moxibustion is applied to both acupoints at the same time.

五脏俞
Wuzangshu

组成　本穴组由肺俞、心俞、肝俞、脾俞、肾俞五穴组合而成。

位置　肺俞：第三胸椎棘突下，旁开1.5寸。

心俞：第五胸椎棘突下，旁开1.5寸。

肝俞：第九胸椎棘突下，旁开1.5寸。

脾俞：第十一胸椎棘突下，旁开1.5寸。

肾俞：第二腰椎棘突下，旁开1.5寸。

主治　风疾，中毒，面庞胀如黑云，或遍身锥利痛或二手顽麻。

操作　按肺、心、肝、脾、肾之次序，各灸50壮，周而复始，病愈为度。

Composition　This group of acupoints is composed of Feishu(BL13), Xinshu(BL15), Ganshu(BL18), Pishu(BL20) and Shenshu(BL23).

Location　Feishu：1.5 cun lateral to the point below the spinous process of the 3rd thoracic vertebra.

Xinshu：1.5 cun lateral to the point below the spinous process of the 5th thoracic vertebra.

Ganshu：1.5 cun lateral to the point below the spinous process of the 9th thoracic vertebra.

Pishu：1.5 cun lateral to the point below the spinous

肺俞 Feishu
心俞 Xinshu
肝俞 Ganshu
脾俞 Pishu
肾俞 Shenshu

图2-33 五脏俞
Fig. 2-33 Wuzangshu

汉 英 对 照

process of the 11th thoracic vertebra.

Shenshu：1.5 cun lateral to the point below the spinous process of the 2nd lumbar vertebra.

Indications Diseases due to wind, poisoning, blackish facial edema, severe pain all over the body or numbness of the upper limbs.

Method 50 cones of moxibustion is applied to the acupoints in the order of lung, heart, live, spleen and kidney respectively and repeatedly, till the disease is cured.

 脊背五穴
Jibeiwuxue

组成 本穴组由脊背腰骶部的五个点组合而成。

位置 五个穴位分别位于背腰骶部，第二胸椎棘突之高点一穴；骶骨尖端一穴；第十二胸椎棘突下一穴；第三腰椎棘突平，左右旁开各4寸处各一穴。

主治 癫痫，小儿惊风，痉挛。

操作 灸5~9壮。

Composition This group of acupoints is composed of five points on the back, waist and sacrum.

Location The five points are all on the back, waist and sacrum. They are the point on the prominence of the spinous process of the 2nd thoracic vertebra, the point on the tip of the sacrum, the point below the spinous process of the 12th thoracic vertebra, and two points 4 cun lateral to the prominence of the spinous process of the 3rd lumbar vertebra.

Indication Epilepsy and infantile convulsion.

Method 5-9 cones of moxibustion is applied.

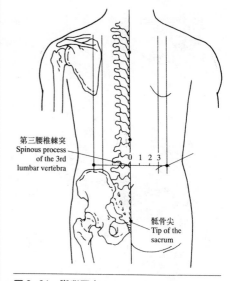

第三腰椎棘突
Spinous process
of the 3rd
lumbar vertebra

0 1 2 3

骶骨尖
Tip of the
sacrum

图2-34 脊背五穴
Fig. 2-34 Jibeiwuxue

心神
Xinshen

组成 本穴组由心俞、神道二穴组合而成。

位置 心俞：第五胸椎棘突下，旁开1.5寸。

神道：第五胸椎棘突下。

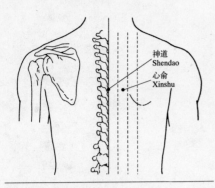

图2-35 心神
Fig. 2-35 Xinshen

主治 风痫。

操作 刺法：心俞向脊柱方向斜刺0.5~0.8寸。神道由下向上刺0.5~0.8寸。

灸法：艾炷灸3~5壮。

Composition This group of acupoints is composed of Xinshu(BL15) and Shendao(GV11).

Location Xinshu：1.5 cun lateral to the point below the spinous process of the 5th thoracic vertebra.

Shendao below the spinous process of the 5th thoracic vertebra.

Indication Epilepsy due to wind.

Method Acupuncture：Xinshu is needled 0.5-0.8 cun obliquely towards the spine. Shendao is needled 0.5-0.8 cun upwards.

Moxibustion：Moxibustion with 3-5 moxa cones is applied.

● 齐天宗
Qitianzong

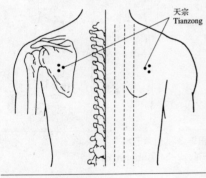

图2-36 齐天宗
Fig. 2-36 Qitianzong

组成 本穴组由天宗及其旁二点共三穴组合而成。

位置 天宗：肩胛骨冈下窝的中央。

天宗及其外0.5寸处上下各一穴（使三针呈一锐角形）。

主治 头痛，肩胛疼痛。

操作 直刺0.5~1寸，留10~15分钟，拔罐。

按注 本穴也称天宗三穴。

Composition This group of acupoints is composed of Tianzong(SI11) and two points beside Tianzong.

Location Tianzong：in the centre of the subscapular fossa of the scapula.

The two points superior and inferior to the point 0.5 cun lateral to Tianzong (Three points will form an acute triangle).

Indication Headache and pain in the scapula.

Method The needle is inserted 0.5-1 cun. Retain the needles for 10-15 minutes, then perform cupping.

Note This group of acupoints is also called Tianzongsanxue.

飞翅
Feichi

组成　本穴组由上飞翅、翅根、下飞翅三穴组合而成。

位置　上飞翅：肩胛冈内端上缘，平第二胸椎距脊柱2寸处。

翅根：肩胛冈内侧边缘，平第五胸椎距脊柱3寸处。

下飞翅：肩胛冈下角，平第七胸椎距脊柱4寸处。

主治　颈项强痛，肩胛痛，肩臂痛，肩背拘急，胃痛，呃逆，食管炎，乳腺炎，胆囊炎。

操作　沿皮透刺0.5寸，留针20分钟。

Composition　This group of acupoints is composed of Shangfeichi, Chigen and Xiafeichi.

Location　Shangfeichi：on the upper border of the inner end of the scapular spine, 2 cun lateral to the spine, at the level of the 2nd thoracic vertebra.

Chigen：on the inner border of the scapular spine, 3 cun lateral to the spine, at the level of the 5th thoracic vertebra.

Xiafeichi：on the lower angle of the scapula, 4 cun lateral to the spine, at the level of the 7th thoracic vertebra.

Indication　Pain and rigidity of the neck, pain in the scapula, pain in the shoulder and arm, rigidity of the shoulder and arm, stomachache, hiccup, esophagitis, mastitis and cholecystitis.

Method　The needle is inserted 0.5 cun beneath the skin. Retain the needles for 20 minutes.

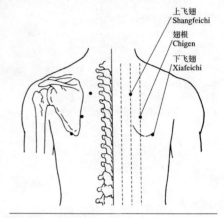

图2-37　飞翅
Fig. 2-37　Feichi

肩痛点
Jiantongdian

组成　本穴组由肩痛1、肩痛2、肩痛3、肩痛4、肩痛5点组合而成。

位置　肩痛1：肩胛角内上角上方的斜方肌处，当肩井穴下约1.5寸处。

肩痛2：肩胛角冈上窝，近内侧端，内上角的下方与肩胛冈之端，当曲垣穴稍外侧。

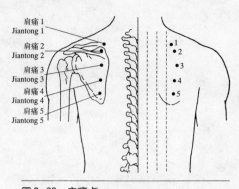

图 2-38 肩痛点
Fig. 2-38 Jiantongdian

肩痛3：肩胛骨近脊柱缘处，肩胛骨下角直上方，下角与肩胛冈联线的上1/4点，当天宗处斜上内方。

肩痛4：肩胛骨近脊柱缘处，肩胛骨下角直上方，下角与肩胛冈联线之中心点当天宗穴斜下内方。

肩痛5：肩胛骨下角稍上方约1寸处。

主治　肩背痛。

操作　肩痛1针0.3～0.5寸，肩痛2～肩痛5针0.5～1寸。

针感局部酸麻胀感传至肩。

Composition This group of acupoints is composed of Jiantong 1-Jiantong 5.

Location Jiantong1：on the trapezius muscle superior to the medial side of the superior angle of the scapula, roughly 1.5 cun inferior to Jianjing.

Jiantong2：in the inner end of the suprascapular fossa of the scapula, superior to the medial upper angle, at the end of the scapular spine, i.e. a bit lateral to Quyuan.

Jiantong3：at the border of the scapula near the spine, directly above the lower angle of the scapula, at the upper fourth point of the line connecting the lower angle and the scapular spine, superior to the medial side of Tianzong.

Jiantong4：at the border of the scapula near the spine, directly above the lower angle of the scapular, at the midpoint of the line connecting the lower angle and the scapular spine, inferior to the medial side of Tianzong.

Jiantong5：1 cun superior to the lower angle of the scapula.

Indication Pain in the shoulder and back.

Method Jiantong1 is needled 0.3-0.5 cun. Jiantong 2-Jiantong 5 are needled 0.5-1cun. The acu-esthesia of soreness, numbness and distension in this part will spread to the shoulder.

 脊三
Jisan

组成　本穴组由脊部三穴组合而成。
位置　脊1：哑门穴下1寸。

脊 2：第一胸椎棘突下陷中。

脊 3：十七椎(第五腰椎棘突下陷中)下陷中。

主治 腰酸背楚。

操作 刺法：斜刺针 0.3～0.5 寸，从背侧面，针尖略向上刺入。

灸法：各灸 3 壮，艾条温灸 5～10 分钟。

Composition This group of acupoints is composed of three points on the spine.

Location Ji1：1 cun below Yamen(GV15).

Ji2：in the depression below the spinous process of the 1st thoracic vertebra.

Ji3：in the depression below the spinous process the 17th vertebra (the 5th lumbar vertebra).

Indication Pain in the back and waist.

Method Acupuncture：The needle is inserted 0.3–0.5 cun obliquely. The tip of the needle is inserted upwards slightly.

Moxibustion：3 cones of moxibustion is applied to each point, or warm moxibustion with moxa roll for 5–10 minutes is applied.

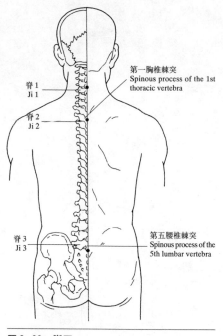

脊 1 Ji 1
脊 2 Ji 2
脊 3 Ji 3
第一胸椎棘突 Spinous process of the 1st thoracic vertebra
第五腰椎棘突 Spinous process of the 5th lumbar vertebra

图 2-39 脊三
Fig. 2-39 Jisan

腰三针
Yaosanzhen

组成 本穴组由肾俞、命门二穴组合而成。

位置 肾俞：第二腰椎棘突下，旁开 1.5 寸。

命门：第二腰椎棘突下。

主治 腰痛，腰扭伤。

操作 刺法：肾俞穴针 1～2 寸，针感为腰部胀、麻感，或触电样感觉向下放散至足；命门穴针 0.5～1 寸，针感为腰部胀、麻感。

灸法：艾炷灸或温针灸 5～9 壮，艾条灸 10～20 分钟。

Composition This group of acupoints is composed of Shenshu(BL23) and Mingmen(GV4).

Location Shenshu：1.5 cun lateral to the point below the spinous process of the 2nd lumbar vertebra.

Mingmen：below the spinous process of the 2nd lumbar vertebra.

Indications Pain in the lower back and lumbar sprain.

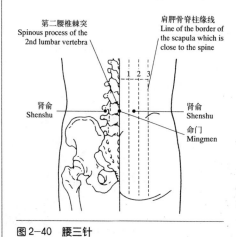

第二腰椎棘突 Spinous process of the 2nd lumbar vertebra
肩胛骨脊柱缘线 Line of the border of the scapula which is close to the spine
1 2 3
肾俞 Shenshu
肾俞 Shenshu
命门 Mingmen

图 2-40 腰三针
Fig. 2-40 Yaosanzhen

Methods Acupuncture: Shenshu is needled 1–2 cun. The acu–esthesia of distension, numbness or electric shock will spread downwards to the foot.

Mingmen is needled 0.5–1 cun. The acu-esthesia of distension and numbness can be obtained in the lower back.

Moxibustion: 5–9 cones of moxibustion or warm needle moxibustion, or moxibustion with moxa roll 10–20 minutes is applied.

 腰骶五处
Yaodiwuchu

组成　本穴组由腰骶部的五个点组合而成。

位置　腰骶关节部，第五腰椎棘突高点一穴，旁开左右2寸和4寸处各二穴。

主治　一切腰间疾病。

操作　刺法：针0.8～1.2寸，局部酸胀感，或向下放射麻电感。

灸法：艾炷灸5～9壮，艾条温灸5～15分钟。

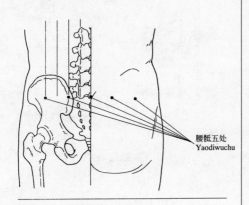

图2-41　腰骶五处
Fig. 2-41　Yaodiwuchu

Composition This group of acupoints is composed of five points on the waist and sacrum.

Location On the joint of the waist and sacrum, one point on the prominence of the spinous process of the 5th lumbar vertebra, and two points 2 cun, two points 4 cun lateral to the above point.

Indication Diseases in the lower back.

Method Acupuncture: the needle is inserted 0.8–1.2 cun. The acu-esthesia may be soreness and distension in this part, or electric shock radiates downwards.

Moxibustion Moxibustion with 5–9 moxa cones, or warm moxibustion with moxa roll for 5–15 minutes is applied.

 尾穷骨
Weiqlonggu

组成　本穴组由尾骨上的三个点组合而成。

位置　臀裂下端、尾骨上1寸处及左右旁开各1寸处。

主治　闪腰痛，腰尻疼痛，肛门痛，淋证，便秘，尿闭，痔疮。

操作　艾炷灸5～9壮，艾条灸5～15分钟。

Composition　This group of acupoints is composed of three points on the coccyx.

Location　On the lower part of the gluteal cleft, the point 1 cun above the coccyx and the two points 1 cun lateral to the coccyx.

Indication　Pain due to lumbar sprain, pain in the waist and buttocks, pain in the anus, stranguria, constipation, dysuria and hemorrhoids.

Method　Moxibustion with 5−9 moxa cones, or moxibustion with moxa roll for 5−15 minutes is applied.

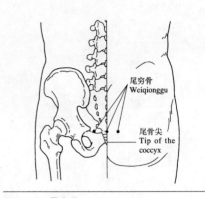

图2−42　尾穷骨
Fig. 2−42　Weiqionggu

上字灸
Shangzijiu

组成　本穴组由腰部的五个穴点组合而成。

位置　命门：第二腰椎棘突下凹陷处。

十五椎：第三腰椎棘突下凹陷处。

华佗夹脊：平第四腰椎棘突下点两侧0.5寸。

腰阳关：第四腰椎棘突下凹陷处。

主治　腰尻痛，脊背痛，酸寒痛，下肢麻痹，下肢疼痛，关节炎，妇科疾患。

操作　灸5～15壮。

Composition　This group of acupoints is composed of five points on the waist.

Location　One point below the spinous process of the 2nd lumbar vertebra, one point on the prominence of the spinous process of the 3rd lumbar vertebra, one point below the spinous process of the 4th lumbar vertebra, and two points 0.5 cun lateral to the point below the spinous process of the 4th lumbar vertebra, 5 points in all. i.e. this group is composed of Mingmen, Shiwuzhui, Yaoyangguan and Huatuojiaji beside Yaoyangguan.

Indications　Pain in the waist and buttocks, pain in the back, pain due to cold, paralysis, pain of the lower extremities, arthritis and gynecological diseases.

Method　5−15 cones of moxibustion is applied.

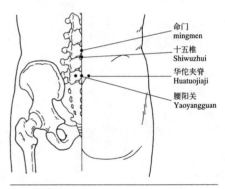

图2−43　上字灸
Fig. 2−43　Shangzijiu

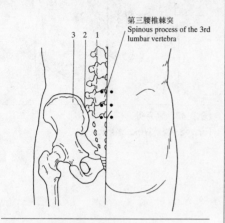

第三腰椎棘突
Spinous process of the 3rd
lumbar vertebra

3 2 1

图2-44 奇腰三针
Fig. 2-44 Qiyaosanzhen

奇腰三针
Qiyaosanzhen

组成　本穴组由第三至第五腰椎的三个夹脊穴组合而成。

位置　第三腰椎至第五腰椎棘突下旁开0.5寸。

主治　坐骨神经痛(根性)，腰痛。

操作　针2～3寸深，令针感向下放射为度。

Composition　This group of acupoints is composed of three Jiaji points beside 3rd—5th Lumbar vertebrae.

Location　0.5 cun lateral to the point below the spinous process of the 3rd—5th lumbar vertebrae.

Indication　Sciatica of nerve root type, pain in the lower back.

Method　The needle is inserted 2—3 cun till the acuesthesia spreads downwards.

臀髂三针
Tunqiasanzhen

组成　本穴组由秩边、环跳、髂尾点三穴组合而成。

位置　秩边：第四骶椎棘突下，旁开3寸。

环跳：股骨大转子高点与骶管裂孔连线的外1/3与内2/3交界处。

髂尾点：髂后上棘与尾骨尖连线的中点。

主治　坐骨神经痛，腰骶痛。

操作　取5寸长针或芒针直刺3～4寸，以麻电感或下肢有抽动感为度。

Composition　This group of acupoints is composed of Zhibian(BL54), Huantiao(GB30) and Qiaweidian.

Location　Zhibian：3 cun lateral to the point below the spinous process of the 4th lumbar vertebra.

Huantiao：at the junction of the lateral one-third and medial two-thirds of the line connecting the prominence of the great trochanter and the sacral hiatus.

Qiaweidian：at the midpoint of the line between the posterior superior illiac spine and the tip of the coccyx.

Indication　Sciatica and pain in the lower back.

Method　The needle of 5 cun is selected and inserted

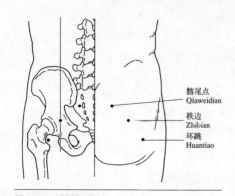

髂尾点
Qiaweidian

秩边
Zhibian

环跳
Huantiao

图2-45 臀髂三针
Fig. 2-45 Tunqiasanzhen

3—4 cun till the acu-esthesia of electric shock or twicthing on the lower limb is obtained.

一条
Yitiao

组成　本穴组由背部正中线上共十七个穴点组合而成。

位置　背部正中线，自第七颈椎至第五腰椎每两棘突之间是穴。计十七穴。当督脉的大椎、陶道、身柱、神道、灵台、至阳、筋缩、中枢、命门、阳关等十二穴同位。

主治　瘫痪，四肢疼痛。

操作　针1～1.5寸，针感有向上下传电感觉。

Composition　This group of acupoints is composed of 17 points on the midline of the back.

Location　On the midline of the back, points between every two spinous process from the 7th cervical vertebra to the 5th lumbar vertebra, 17 points in all. This group includes the following 12 acupoints of Governor Vessel: Dazhui, Taodao, Shendao, Lingtai, Zhiyang, Jingsuo, Zhongshu, Mingmen and Yangguan.

Indication　Paralysis, pain in the four limbs.

Method　The needle is inserted 1—1.5 cun. The acu-esthesia of electric shock will spread upwards and downwards.

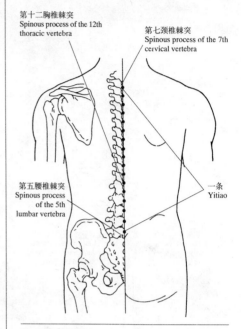

图2—46　一条
Fig. 2—46　Yitiao

两边
Liangbian

组成　由第七颈椎至第五腰椎旁开1寸的十八穴点组合而成。

位置　背部正中线两侧旁开1寸，自第七颈椎至第五腰椎。与每一棘突下缘相平，每侧十八穴。左右计三十六穴。

主治　瘫痪，四肢疼痛。

操作　斜刺，向脊椎方向刺1.5寸，针感酸、胀可放散到胸、腹及四肢。

Composition　This group of acupoints is composed of 18 points 1 cun lateral to the spine from the 7th cervical vertebra to the 5th lumbar vertebra.

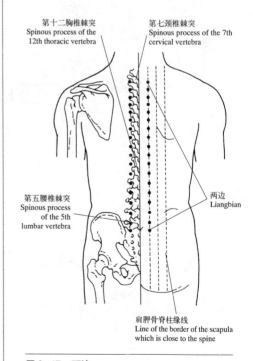

图2—47　两边
Fig. 2—47　Liangbian

Location   Points 1 cun lateral to the midline of the back, from the 7th cervical vertera to the 5th lumbar vertebra, at the same levels of each spinous process, 18 points on each side, 36 points on both sides.

Indications   Paralysis and pain of the four limbs.

Method   The needle is inserted 1.5 cun obliquely towards the spine. The acu-esthesia of soreness and distension will transmit to the chest, abdomen and four limbs.

医瘫
Yitan

组成   本穴组由双数胸腰椎下缘旁开 0.3 寸之八点组合而成。

位置   位于第二、第四、第六、第八、第十、第十二胸椎，第二、第四腰椎下缘两侧旁开 0.3 寸。左右计十六穴。

主治   瘫痪。

操作   针 1~1.5 寸，针感局部胀、麻。

Composition   This group of acupoints is composed of the eight points 0.3 cun lateral to the lower borders of thoracic and lumbar vertebrae of even numbers.

Location   0.3 cun lateral to the lower border of the 2nd, 4th, 6th, 8th, 10th, 12th thoracic vertebrae and 2nd, 4th lumbar vertebrae, 16 points on both sides.

Indication   Paralysis.

Method   The needle is inserted 1−1.5 cun. The acu-esthesia of distension and numbness should be obtained in this part.

脑脊三
Naojisan

组成   本穴组由后发际下 0.5 寸、第二胸椎、第五腰椎棘突各旁开 0.5 寸之六个点组合而成。

位置   上穴在项部正中线旁开 0.5 寸，后发际下 0.5 寸处，左右二穴；

中穴在第二胸椎棘突高点旁开 0.5 寸处，左右二穴；

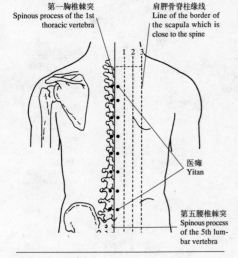

第一胸椎棘突
Spinous process of the 1st thoracic vertebra

肩胛骨脊柱缘线
Line of the border of the scapula which is close to the spine

1 2 3

医瘫
Yitan

第五腰椎棘突
Spinous process of the 5th lumbar vertebra

图 2-48 医瘫
Fig. 2-48 Yitan

下穴在第五腰椎棘突高点旁开0.5寸处，左右二穴。

主治　脑炎后遗症，大脑发育不良，腰背痛。

操作　针法：针尖向椎体方向斜刺1～1.5寸，针感局部胀。

灸法：灸3～5壮。

Composition　This group of acupoints is composed of the six points which are 0.5 cun lateral to the point 0.5 cun below the posterior hairline, to the spinous process of the 2nd thoracic vertebra and the 5th lumbar vertebra.

Location　The upper points：0.5 cun lateral to the midline of the nape and 0.5 cun below the midpoint of posterior hairline, two points on both sides.

The middle points　0.5 cun lateral to the spinous process of the 2nd thoracic vertebra, two points on both sides.

The lower points　0.5 cun lateral to the spinous process of the 5th lumbar vertebra, two points on both sides.

Indications　Cephalitis sequela, cerebral hypogenesis, pain in the back and waist.

Methods　Acupuncture：The tip of the needle is inserted 1－1.5 cun obliquely towards the vertebral body, the acu-esthesia of distension in this part can be obtained.

Moxibustion：3－5 cones of moxibustion is applied.

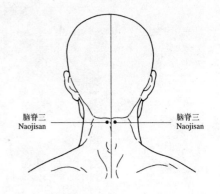

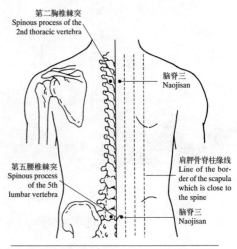

脑脊三　Naojisan
脑脊三　Naojisan
第二胸椎棘突　Spinous process of the 2nd thoracic vertebra
脑脊三　Naojisan
第五腰椎棘突　Spinous process of the 5th lumbar vertebra
肩胛骨脊柱缘线　Line of the border of the scapula which is close to the spine
脑脊三　Naojisan

图2-49　脑脊三
Fig. 2-49　Naojisan

 ## 背四穴
Beisixue

组成　本穴组由长强、命门、至阳、大椎四穴组合而成。

位置　长强：尾骨尖下0.5寸，约当尾骨尖端与肛门的中点。

命门：第二腰椎棘突下。

至阳：第七胸椎棘突下。

大椎：第七颈椎棘突下。

主治　小儿麻痹，脑炎后遗症，脑发育不全，多发性神经根炎。

操作　透刺、长强透命门，命门透至阳，至阳透大椎，抽插3～5次，再向左右透刺，得气为度，每日1次。

Composition　This group of acupoints is composed of

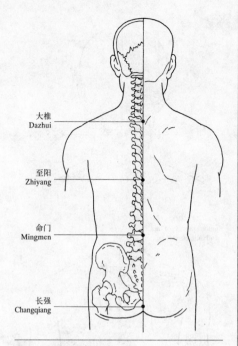

图 2-50　背四穴

Fig. 2-50　Beisixue

Changqiang(GV1), Mingmen(GV4), Zhiyang(GV9) and Dazhui(GV14).

Location　Changqiang：0.5 cun below the tip of the coccyx, at the midpoint of the line connecting the tip of the coccyx and anus.

Mingmen：below the spinous process of the 2nd lumbar vertebra.

Zhiyang：below the spinous process of the 7th thoracic vertebra.

Dazhui：below the spinous process of the 7th cervical vertebra.

Indications　Infantile paralysis, syphilitics sequela, encephalon hypoplasia, polyradiculoneuritis.

Method：The needles are penetrated from Changqiang to Mingmen, Mingmen to Zhiyang, Zhiyang to Dazhui. Lift and insert the needles for 3-5 times, then penetrate the needles towards left and right till the acu-esthesia is obtained. One treatment every day may be applied.

脊缝
Jifeng

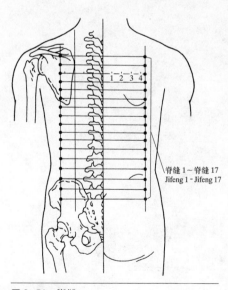

脊缝1～脊缝17
Jifeng 1 - Jifeng 17

图 2-51　脊缝

Fig. 2-51　Jifeng

组成　本穴组由躯干背腰部三十四点组合而成。

位置　背部正中线，左右旁开各4.5寸之两侧线上，从第一胸椎棘突下方起至第五腰椎棘突下方止，与每一棘突下方相平，左右相对二穴。

主治　龟背，脊痹。

操作　针0.3～0.5寸，局部有沉胀感。

按注　此穴与华佗扶脊穴相似，唯佗脊穴系在第一至第十七椎下左右旁开各0.5寸处。

Composition　This group of acupoints is composed of thirty-four points on the back and waist.

Location　On the line 4.5 cun lateral to the posterior midline, from the 1st thoracic vertebra to 5th lumbar vertebra, at the same level of each spinous process 2 points on both sides and 34 points in all.

Indication　Kyphosis, pain and numbness of the spine.

Method　The needle is inserted 0.3-0.5 cun. The acu-esthesia of distension will be obtained.

Note This group of acupoints is similar to Huatuojiaji. The only difference is that Huatuojiaji is 0.5 cun lateral to the points below the spinous processes from the 1st vertebra to the 17th vertebra.

九连环
Jiulianhuan

组成 本穴组由背腰部九个点组合而成。

位置 背部正中线，第一、第三、第五、第七、第九、第十一胸椎棘突与第一、第三、第五腰椎棘突之下方凹陷中，计九穴，自上至下，分别命名为九连环1、2、3、4、5、6、7、8、9。

主治 脊髓疾患，慢性疾病。

操作 刺法：直刺0.5～0.8寸，局部酸胀感，可用捻转等补法。

灸法：艾炷灸5～9壮，艾条温灸10～20分钟。

Composition This group of acupoints is composed of nine points on the back and waist.

Location On the posterior midline, in the depressions below the spinous processes of the 1st, 3rd, 5th, 7th, 11th thoracic vertebrae and the 1st, 3rd and 5th lumbar vertebrae, 9 points in all. The points are respectively named Jiulianhuan1, 2, 3, 4, 5, 6, 7, 8, 9 from the top.

Indication Spinal cord diseases, chronic diseases.

Methods Acupuncture：the needle is inserted 0.5−0.8 cun. The acu-esthesia of distension in this part will be obtained. The reinforcing techniques by rotation may be applied.

Moxibustion：moxibustion with 5−9 cones or warm moxibustion with moxa roll for 10−20 minutes is applied.

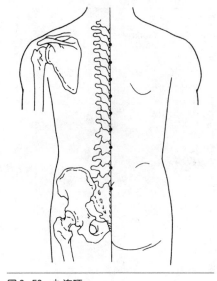

图2-52 九连环
Fig. 2-52 Jiulianhuan

背穴
Beixue

组成 由第六、第五胸椎棘突高点处的主、次二穴组合而成。

位置 背部正中线，第六胸椎棘突高点为主穴，第五胸椎

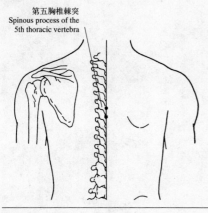

第五胸椎棘突
Spinous process of the
5th thoracic vertebra

图2-53 背穴
Fig. 2-53 Beixue

棘突高点为次穴。

主治 外科疮、毒、皮炎、癣，背痛，胃痛，小腹胀痛，气管炎，哮喘，脑震荡后遗症，高血压，低血压，癫狂痫，失眠健忘，偏头痛，痹证，偏瘫。

操作 用2寸长特制粗针(直径1～1.2毫米)。左手示指固定穴位，右手持针，以40°～45°的角度斜向下方，用示指加压，迅速刺入皮肤后，再将针倾斜成5°～10°沿脊柱正中，在皮肤与皮下组织之间向下斜刺。先针次穴，进皮后不推针；接着针主穴，进皮后斜刺1.5寸左右，然后再推进次穴针，进针1寸左右，但两针不要穿透。一般留针20～30分钟。患者脊柱有烧灼感觉。

Composition This group of acupoints is composed of the primary and secondary acupoints on the prominence of the spinous processes of the 6th and 5th thoracic vertebrae.

Location On the midline of the back, the primary acupoint is on the prominence of the spinous process of the 6th thoracic vertebra, the secondary acupoint is on the prominence of the spinous process of the 5th thoracic vertebra.

Indications Skin diseases including furuncle, dermatitis, and tinea, backache, stomachache, distension and pain of the lower abdomen, tracheitis, asthma, cerebral concussion sequela, hypertension, hypotension, mania, epilepsy, insomnia and poor memory, migraine, Bi syndromes and hemiplegia.

Method Select 2 cun long thick needle (diameter: 1–1.2 mm). Fix the location of the acupoint with the indexfinger of the left hand, hold the needle with the right hand and insert it obliquely downwards at the angle of 40°−45°, press the needle with the index finger. After the needle is inserted into the skin, the angle is adjusted to 5°−10° and the needle is inserted between the skin and the subcutaneous tissues along the spine. The secondary acupoint is needled first without pushing the needle after the needle being inserted into the skin, then the primary acupoint is needled 1.5 cun obliquely after the needle being inserted into the skin, and then the needle in the secondary acupoint is inserted about 1 cun. Do not penetrate the two needles. Usually the needles are retained for 20—30 minutes. The acu-esthesia is the feeling of scalding the spine.

三乳
Sanru

组成　本穴组由乳源、乳泉、乳海三穴组合而成。

位置　乳源：乳线上第二、第三肋间。

乳泉：腋前线上平膻中之交点处。

乳海：乳线上第六、第七肋间。

主治　乳少。

操作　刺法：向乳头平刺1寸，留20～30分钟，每日1次。

灸法：艾条温灸10～20分钟，以乳部感温热为度。

Composition　This group of acupoints is composed of Ruyuan, Ruquan and Ruhai.

Location　Ruyuan：between the 2nd and 3rd ribs, on the vertical line of the nipple.

Ruquan：at the level of Danzhong, on the anterior axillary line.

Ruhai：between the 6th and 7th ribs, on the vertical line of the nipple.

Indication　Insufficient lactation.

Method　Acupuncture：the needle is inserted 1 cun horizontally. Retain the needle for 20—30 minutes, treat once every day.

Moxibustion：Warm moxibustion with moxa roll for 10—20 minutes is applied till the warm feeling on the breast is obtained.

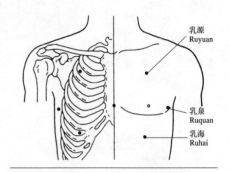

图2-54　三乳

Fig. 2-54　Sanru

通乳术（胸三针）
Tongrushu(Xiongsanzhen)

组成　本穴组由乳根、膻中二穴组合而成。

位置　乳根：第五肋间隙，乳头直下。

膻中：前正中线，平第四肋间隙。

主治　乳少，乳痈，乳汁不通。

操作　从乳根穴呈30°角向乳中方向斜刺0.5～0.8寸，再从膻中向乳中方向呈15°角沿皮透刺，得气为度。

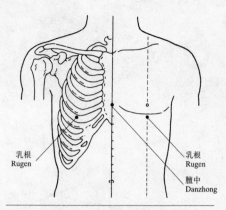

乳根
Rugen

乳根
Rugen

膻中
Danzhong

图2-55 通乳术(胸三针)
Fig. 2-55 Tongrushu(Xiongsanzhen)

按注 膻中穴针刺方向也可向上下或左右斜刺或沿皮刺。

Composition This group of acupoints is composed of Rugen(ST18) and Danzhong(CV17).

Location Rugen: directly below the nipple, in the 5th intercostal space.

Danzhong: on the anterior midline, at the level of the 4th intercostal space.

Indication Insufficient lactation, mastitis, obstruction of lactation.

Method The needle is inserted 0.5－0.8 cun obliquely at the angle of 30° from Rugen to Ruzhong, then another needle is penetrated at the angle of 15° under the skin from Danzhong to Ruzhong till the acu-esthesia is obtained.

Note Usually, Danzhong can also be needled upwards, downwards, outwards or subcutaneously.

催乳术
Cuirushu

组成 本穴组由乳上、乳中、乳下三穴组合而成。
位置 乳中：乳头中央。
乳上、乳下：在乳中穴上1寸和下1寸处。
主治 乳少，乳汁不通，乳痈等。
操作 刺法：取乳上和乳下穴呈30°角向乳中刺0.5～1寸，得气为度。
灸法：艾炷灸3～5壮，或温灸10～20分钟。

Composition This group of acupoints is composed of Rushang, Ruzhong(ST17) and Ruxia.

Location Ruzhong: at the centre of the nipple.

Rushang, Ruxia: one cun respectively above and below Ruzhong.

Indication Insufficient lactation, obstruction of lactation, mastitis, etc..

Methods Acupuncture: Rushang and Ruxia are needled 0.5－1 cun at the angle of 30° towards Ruzhong till the acu-esthesia is obtained.

Moxibustion: moxibustion with 3－5 moxa rolls or warm moxibustion for 10－20 minutes is applied.

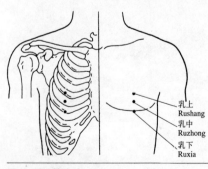

乳上
Rushang
乳中
Ruzhong
乳下
Ruxia

图2-56 催乳术
Fig. 2-56 Cuirushu

天膻

Tiandan

组成　本穴组由天突、膻中二穴组合而成。

位置　天突：胸骨上窝正中。

膻中：前正中线，平第四肋间隙。

主治　喘嗽。

操作　刺法：天突横刺0.5寸。

膻中沿皮刺0.5～1寸，得气为度。

灸法　艾炷灸5～9壮，艾条温灸10～20分钟。

按注　天突一穴，有经验者可深刺至1～3寸，但一般医者不必追求过深，以免发生医疗事故。

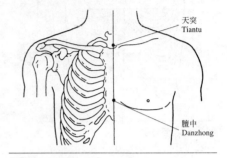

图2-57　天膻

Fig. 2-57　Tiandan

Composition　This group of acupoints is composed of Tiantu(CV22) and Danzhong(CV17).

Location　Tiantu：in the centre of the suprasternal fossa.

Danzhong：on the anterior midline, at the level of the 4th intercostal space.

Indications　Asthma and cough.

Methods　Acupuncture：Tiantu：the needle is inserted 0.5 cun transversely.

Danzhong：the needle is inserted 0.5-1 cun beneath the skin, till the acu-esthesia is obtained.

Moxibustion：moxibustion with 5-9 moxa cones or warm moxibustion with moxa roll for 10-20 minutes is applied.

Note　Tiantu can be inserted to the depth of 1-3 cun by experienced practitioners. For practitioners without much experience, do not needle the acupoint too deep in case of medical accidents.

 五柱灸

Wuzhujiu

组成　本穴组由巨阙、中脘、下脘和左右梁门五穴组合而成。

位置　巨阙：脐上6寸。

中脘：脐上4寸。

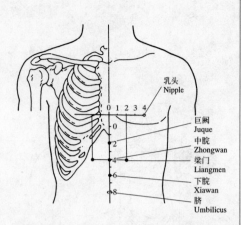

图 2-58　五柱灸
Fig. 2-58　Wuzhujiu

下脘：脐上 2 寸。

梁门：脐上 4 寸，前正中线旁开 2 寸。

主治　哮喘，脘腹部疾病。

操作　灸 3～5 壮。

Composition　This group of acupoints is composed of Juque(CV14), Zhongwan(CV12), Xiawan(CV10) and both Liangmen(ST21).

Location　Juque：6 cun above the centre of the umbilicus.

Zhongwan：4 cun above the centre of the umbilicus.

Xiawan：2 cun above the centre of the umbilicus.

Liangmen：4 cun above the centre of the umbilicus and 2 cun lateral to the anterior midline.

Indications　Asthma and abdominal diseases.

Method　3-5 cones of moxibustion is applied.

舒心术
Shuxinshu

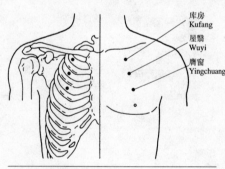

图 2-59　舒心术
Fig. 2-59　Shuxinshu

组成　本穴组由库房、屋翳、膺窗三穴组合而成。

位置　库房：第一肋间隙，前正中线旁开 4 寸。

屋翳：第二肋间隙，前正中线旁开 4 寸。

膺窗：第三肋间隙，前正中线旁开 4 寸。

左右计六穴。

主治　心悸心痛，胸闷，喘咳，呼吸不利等。

操作　取六穴沿肋间隙沿皮透刺至肾经或任脉，得气为度。

Composition　This group of acupoints is composed of Kufang(ST14), Wuyi(ST15) and Yingchuang(ST16).

Location　Kufang：in the 1st intercostal space, 4 cun lateral to the anterior midline.

Wuyi：in the 2nd intercostal space and 4 cun lateral to the anterior midline.

Yingchuang：in the 3rd intercostal space and 4 cun lateral to the anterior midline.

Indications　Palpitation, cardiac pain, stuffy chest, asthma and cough, difficulty in breathing.

Method　The six points are penetrated towards the Kidney Meridian or Conception Vessel beneath the skin in the intercostal spaces till the acu-esthesia is obtained.

宽胸理气术
Kuanxiongliqishu

组成　本穴组由神封、灵墟、神藏、彧中四穴组合而成。

位置　神封：第四肋间隙，前正中线旁开2寸。

灵墟：第三肋间隙，前正中线旁开2寸。

神藏：第二肋间隙，前正中线旁开2寸。

彧中：第一肋间隙，前正中线旁开2寸。

左右计八穴。

主治　胸闷胸痛，心悸喘咳，吞咽，呼吸不利。

操作　各穴沿肋间隙沿皮透刺至中线，得气为度。

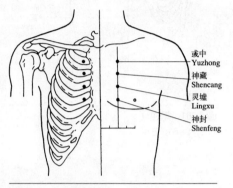

图 2-60　宽胸理气术
Fig. 2-60　Kuanxiongliqishu

Composition　This group of acupoints is composed of 4 points of Shenfeng(KI23), Lingxu(KI24), Shencang(KI25) and Yuzhong(KI26).

Location　Shenfeng：in the 4th intercostal space and 2 cun lateral to the anterior midline.

Lingxu：in the 3rd intercostal space and 2 cun lateral to the anterior midline.

Shencang：in the 2nd intercostal space and 2 cun lateral to the anterior midline.

Yuzhong：in the 1st intercostal space and 2 cun lateral to the anterior midline.

8 points on both sides in all.

Indications　Stuffy chest, pain in the chest, palpitation, asthma and cough, difficulty in swallowing and breathing.

Method　The needle is penetrated to the midline subcutaneously in the intercostal space till the acu-esthesia is obtained.

呃逆
Eni

组成　本穴组由期门、膻中、中脘三穴组合而成。

位置　期门：乳头直下，第六肋间隙。

膻中：前正中线，平第四肋间隙。

中脘：脐上4寸。

主治　气逆上冲，喉间呃逆连声，声短而频，不能自制。

操作　期门、膻中、中脘，三穴均用艾炷灸7～14壮。

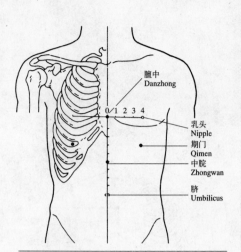

图2-61 呃逆
Fig. 2-61 Eni

Composition   This group of acupoints is composed of Qimen(LR14), Danzhong(CV17) and Zhongwan(CV12).

Location   Qimen：directly below the nipple, in the 6th intercostal space.

Danzhong：on the anterior midline, at the level of the 4th intercostal space.

Zhongwan：4 cun above the centre of the umbilicus.

Indications   Reverse of qi, short, frequent and involuntary hiccup.

Method   Moxibustion with 7-14 moxa cones is applied to Qimen, Danzhong and Zhongwan.

针吐
Zhentu

组成   本穴组由中脘、气海、膻中三穴组合而成。

位置   中脘：脐上4寸。

气海：脐下1.5寸。

膻中：前正中线，平第四肋间隙。

主治   吐疾。

操作   中脘、气海各针0.5~1.2寸。膻中沿皮刺0.5~1寸。各以得气为度。

Composition   This group of acupoints is composed of Zhongwan(CV12), Qihai(CV6) and Danzhong(CV17).

Location   Zhongwan：4 cun above the centre of the umbilicus.

Qihai：1.5 cun below the centre of the umbilicus.

Danzhong：on the anterior midline, at the level of the 4th intercostal space.

Indication   Vomiting.

Method   Zhongwan and Qihai are needled 0.5-1.2 cun.

Danzhong is needled 0.5-1 cun subcutaneously. Stop manipulating the needles till the acu-esthesia is obtained in every point.

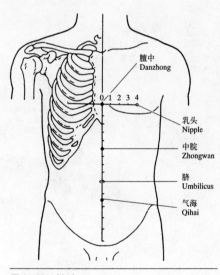

图2-62 针吐
Fig. 2 62 Zhentu

上下气海
Shangxiaqihai

组成　本穴组由膻中、气海二穴组合而成。

位置　膻中：前正中线，平第四肋间隙。

气海：脐下1.5寸。

主治　气疾。

操作　见针吐穴。

Composition　This group of acupoints is composed of Danzhong(CV17) and Qihai(CV6).

Location　Danzhong：on the anterior midline, at the level of the 4th intercostal space.

Qihai：1.5 cun below the centre of the umbilicus.

Indication　Diseases due to qi.

Method　See "Zhentu".

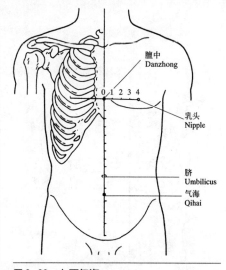

图 2-63　上下气海
Fig. 2-63　Shangxiaqihai

吐泻
Tuxie

组成　本穴组由中脘、天枢、气海三穴组合而成。

位置　中脘：脐上4寸。

气海：脐下1.5寸。

天枢：脐旁2寸。

主治　发病急骤，吐泻不止。

操作　先直刺中脘1~1.5寸，再直刺天枢1.5~2寸，行针1~2次，留针30分钟。气海针刺用补法，留针30分钟；同时，气海穴加温灸30分钟。

Composition　This group of acupoints is composed of Zhongwan(CV12), Tianshu(ST25) and Qihai(CV6).

Location　Zhongwan：4 cun above the centre of the umbilicus.

Qihai：1.5 cun below the centre of the umbilicus.

Tianshu：2 cun lateral to the centre of the umbilicus.

Indication　Sudden vomiting and diarrhea.

Method　Zhongwan is needled 1−1.5 cun perpendicularly first, then Tianshu is needled 1.5−2 cun perpendicularly. Manipulate the needles once or twice and retain them for 30 minutes. Qihai is needled with

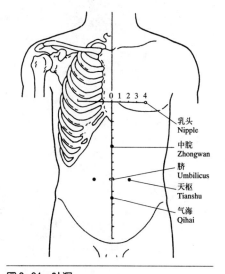

图 2-64　吐泻
Fig. 2-64　Tuxie

reinforcing methods for 30 minutes, and at the same time, warm moxibustion is applied to Qihai for 30 minutes.

三脘(三管)
Sanwan(sanguan)

组成　本穴组由上、中、下脘三穴组合而成。

位置　上脘：脐上5寸。

中脘：脐上4寸。

下脘：脐上2寸。

主治　各种胃病。

操作　刺法：取上脘针稍向下呈70°角，中脘直刺，下脘直刺深1～1.5寸。各以得气为度。

灸法：艾炷灸5～9壮，温灸10～30分钟。

Composition　This group of acupoints is composed of Shangwan(CV13), Zhongwan(CV12) and Xiawan(CV10).

Location　Shangwan：5 cun above the centre of the umbilicus.

Zhongwan：4 cun above the centre of the umbilicus.

Xiawan：2 cun above the centre of the umbilicus.

Indication　All kinds of gastric diseases.

Method　Acupuncture：Shangwan is needled downwards at the angle of 70°, Zhongwan is needled perpendicularly, Xiawan is needled perpendicularly, the depth is 1−1.5 cun till the acu-esthesia is obtained.

Moxibustion：moxibustion with 5−9 moxa cones, or warm moxibustion for 10−30 minutes is applied.

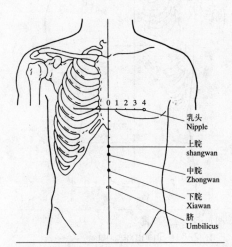

图2-65　三脘
Fig. 2-65　Sanwan(sanguan)

乳头　Nipple
上脘　shangwan
中脘　Zhongwan
下脘　Xiawan
脐　Umbilicus

梅花
Meihua

组成　本穴组由上腹部五个点组合而成。

位置　以中脘为梅花的中点，加上阴都穴上下各0.5寸处四穴。

主治　各种胃病，消化不良，食欲不振。

操作　刺法：直针0.3～0.5寸，局部沉紧酸胀感。或中间一针刺0.5～1寸，旁四针斜刺或沿皮刺0.5～1寸，可稍用盘摇之术。

灸法：艾炷灸3～5壮，艾条温针5～10分钟。

Composition　This group of acupoints is composed of the five points on the upper abdomen.

Location　Zhongwan(CV12) is the centre of Meihua, the other four points are 0.5 cun superior and inferior to Yindu(KI19).

Indication　All kinds of gastric diseases, indigestion and anorexia.

Method　Acupuncture：the needle is inserted 0.3−0.5 cun and the acu-esthesia of heaviness and tense feeling is obtained. Or the central point is needled 0.5−1 cun, the four points around it are needled 0.5−1 cun obliquely or subcutaneously. The circling and shaking methods may be applied.

Moxibustion：moxibustion with 3−5 moxa cones or warm moxibustion for 5−10 minutes is applied.

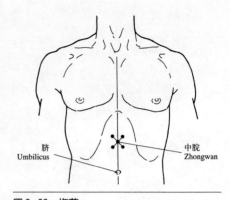

图2-66　梅花
Fig. 2-66　Meihua

中脘梅花
Zhongwanmeihua

组成　本穴组以中脘为中心，加上、下、左、右各一穴共五穴点组合而成。

位置　中脘：脐上4寸。

中脘上下左右各穴：取中脘上下左右各1寸处为穴。

主治　各种胃病。

操作　针法：取中脘和其他四点直刺之，深1～1.2寸，得气为度。

灸法：艾炷灸3～5壮，或温灸10～20分钟。

Composition　This group of acupoints is composed of the five points of Zhongwan(CV12) and the points superior, inferior and lateral to Zhongwan.

Location　Zhongwan：4 cun above umbilicus.

The points around Zhongwan：1 cun superior, inferior and lateral to Zhongwan.

Indication　All kinds of gastric diseases.

Method　Acupuncture：Zhongwan and the other four points are needled perpendicularly, the depth is 1−1.2 cun till the acu-esthesia is obtained.

Moxibustion：moxibustion with 3−5 moxa cones or

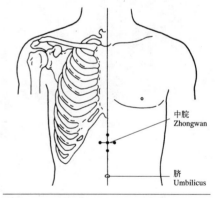

图2-67　中脘梅花
Fig. 2-67　Zhongwanmeihua

warm moxibustion for 10−20 minutes is applied.

升胃
Shengwei

组成　本穴组由升胃主穴和升胃1、升胃2、升胃3、升胃4穴和升胃5穴组合而成。

位置　升胃主穴：位于右幽门穴下0.5寸。

升胃1、升胃2、升胃3、升胃4穴：分别在脐左侧旁开0.5寸、1寸、1.5寸、2寸处。

升胃5穴：位于胃下极下1寸。

主治　胃下垂。

操作　用长针或芒针，在升胃主穴进针，与腹壁呈35°角快速刺入皮下0.3寸，然后沿皮下进针过中脘向升胃1、升胃2、升胃3、升胃4，直至胃下极下1寸之升胃5穴。留针45分钟，以饭后30~50分钟治疗为佳，治疗后卧床休息15分钟。隔日1次。

Composition　This group of acupoints is composed of Shengweizhuxue, Shengwei 1, Shengwei 2, Shengwei 3, Shengwei 4 and Shengwei 5.

Location　Shengweizhuxue：0.5 cun below Youmen on the right side.

Shengwei 1, Shengwei 2, Shengwei 3, Shengwei 4：0.5, 1, 1.5, 2 cun lateral to the left side of the umbilicus respectively.

Shengwei5：1 cun below the lower border of the stomach.

Indication　Gastroptosis.

Method　Select long needle. Insert the needle 0.3 cun swiftly into the skin in Shengweizhuxue, the angle formed by the needle and the abdomen is 35°. Then insert the needle to Shengwei1, 2, 3, 4 through Zhongwan beneath the skin, till the needle reach Shengwei 5 which is 1 cun below the lower border of the stomach. Retain the needles for 45 minutes. The best time for treatment is 30−50 minutes after meal. Lie in bed to rest for 15 minutes after the treatment. Treat once every other day.

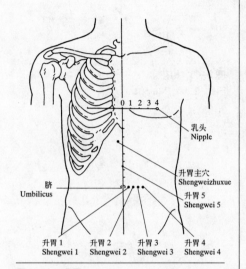

图2-68　升胃
Fig. 2-68　Shengwei

上腹三角
Shangfusanjiao

组成　本穴组由中脘及左右腹哀三穴组合而成。

位置　中脘：脐上4寸。

腹哀：大横穴上3寸，前正中线旁开4寸。

主治　胃病，胃下垂，上腹痛。

操作　中脘稍向下呈70°角刺，腹哀由外向内上方呈45°角斜刺，深度为1～1.5寸，得气为度。

Composition　This group of acupoints is composed of Zhongwan(CV12) and Fuai(SP16) on both sides.

Location　Zhongwan：4 cun above the centre of the umbilicus.

Fuai：3 cun above Daheng, 4 cun lateral to the anterior midline.

Indication　Gastric diseases, gastroptosis, pain in the upper abdomen.

Method　Zhongwan is needled downwards slightly at the angle of 70°. Fuai is needled obliquely at the angle of 45° inwards. The depth is 1−1.5 cun till the acuesthesia is obtained.

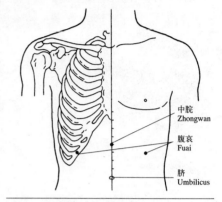

图2-69　上腹三角
Fig. 2-69　Shangfusanjiao

腹上三针
Fushangsanzhen

组成　本穴组由胃上、中脘二穴组合而成。

位置　胃上：脐上2寸，旁开4寸。

中脘：脐上4寸。

主治　胃下垂，上腹痛。

操作　刺法：针胃上穴向脐部表皮横向透刺1～2寸，针感腹部胀；中脘穴直刺1～2寸，针感为上腹部胀、麻，下传至小腹部。

灸法：艾炷灸或温针灸5～9壮，艾条灸10～20分钟。

Composition　This group of acupoints is composed of Weishang and Zhongwan(CV12).

Location　Weishang：4 cun lateral to the point 2 cun above the centre of the umbilicus.

Zhongwan：4 cun above the centre of the umbilicus.

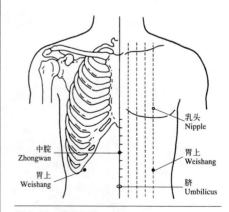

图2-70　腹上三针
Fig. 2-70　Fushangsanzhen

Indication   Gastroptosis, pain in the upper abdomen.

Methods   Acupuncture：Weishang is penetrated traversely 1—2 cun towards the epidermis in the umbilicus region. The acu-esthesia is distension in the abdomen. Zhongwan is needled 1—2 cun perpendicularly. The acuesthesia is distension and numbness in the upper abdomen which will spread to the lower abdomen.

Moxibustion   5—9 cones of moxibustion or warm needle moxibustion, or moxibustion with moxa roll for 10—20 minutes is applied.

胃三关
Weisanguan

组成   本穴组由不容、天枢、鸠尾、神阙四穴组合而成。

位置   不容：脐上6寸，前正中线旁开2寸。

天枢：脐旁2寸。

鸠尾：剑突下，脐上7寸。

神阙：脐的中间。

主治   奔豚气，胃脘痛，腹泻，胸痛，呃逆等。

操作   刺法：透刺。不容透天枢，鸠尾透神阙，留针30分钟。

灸法：艾条温灸10～20分钟，以腹部皮肤呈红晕状一片为度。

Composition   This group of acupoints is composed of Burong(ST19), Tianshu(ST25), Jiuwei(CV15) and Shenque(CV8).

Location   Burong：6 cun above the umbilicus, 2 cun lateral to the anterior midline.

Tianshu：2 cun lateral to the centre of the umbilicus.

Jiuwei：below the xiphoid process, 7 cun above the centre of the umbilicus.

Shenque：in the centre of the umbilicus.

Indications   Bentun syndrome epigastric pain, diarrhea, pain in the chest and hiccup.

Method   Acupuncture：penetration. Burong to Tianshu, Jiuwei to Shenque. Retain the needles for 30 minutes.

Moxibustion：warm moxibustion with moxa roll for 10~20 minutes is applied till the abdomen skin appears

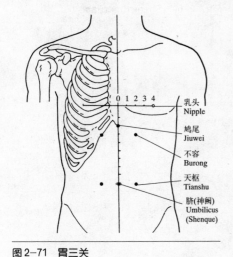

图2-71 胃三关
Fig. 2-71 Weisanguan

汉 英 对 照

reddish.

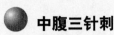

中腹三针刺
Zhongfusanzhenci

组成　本穴组由气海、左右天枢三穴组合而成。

位置　气海：脐下1.5寸。

天枢：脐旁2寸。

主治　脐腹痛，腹泻，痢疾等肠胃病。

操作　天枢稍向脐呈70°角刺之，气海稍向下方呈70°角刺之。各以得气为度。

Composition　This group of acupoints is composed of Qihai(CV6) and Tianshu(ST25).

Location　Qihai：1.5 cun below the centre of the umbilicus.

Tianshu：2 cun lateral to the centre of the umbilicus.

Indications　Pain in the umbilicus and abdomen, diarrhea, dysentery and other intestinal and gastric diseases.

Method　Tianshu is needled towards the umbilicus slightly at the angle of 70°, Qihai is needled downwards slightly at the angle of 70° till the acu-esthesia is obtained.

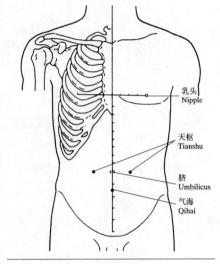

图2-72　中腹三针刺
Fig. 2-72　Zhongfusanzhenci

卒腹痛
Cufutong

组成　本穴组由脐周的四个穴点组合而成。

位置　腹中部、脐上下左右各0.5寸处是穴。

主治　卒腹痛。

操作　艾炷灸3~5壮，艾条温针10~20分钟。

Composition　This group of acupoints is composed of the four points around the umbilicus.

Location　On the central region of the abdomen, 0.5 cun superior, inferior and lateral to the centre of the umbilicus.

Indication　Sudden pain in the abdomen.

Method　Moxibustion with 3-5 moxa cones, or warm

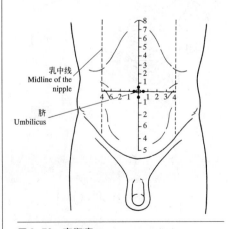

图2-73　卒腹痛
Fig. 2-73　Cufutong

needle moxibustion with moxa roll for 10~20 minutes is applied.

脐三针
Qisanzhen

组成　本穴组由天枢、止泻二穴组合而成。

位置　天枢：脐旁2寸。

止泻：脐下2.5寸处。

主治　腹泻，痢疾。

操作　刺法：天枢穴针1~2寸，针感胀向两侧及小腹放散。止泻穴针1~2寸，针感抽胀至尿道。

灸法：艾炷灸或温针灸5~9壮，艾条灸10~20分钟。

Composition　This group of acupoints is composed of Tianshu(ST25) and Zhixie.

Location　Tianshu：2 cun lateral to the centre of the umbilicus.

Zhixie：2.5 cun below the centre of the umbilicus.

Indications　Diarrhea and dysentery.

Method　Acupuncture：Tianshu is needled 1−2cun. The acu-esthesia will radiate towards both sides and lower abdomen. Zhixie is needled 1−2 cun. The acu-esthesia of twitching and distension will spread to the urethra.

Moxibustion　5−9 cones of moxibustion or warm needle moxibustion, or moxibustion with moxa roll for 10−20 minutes is applied.

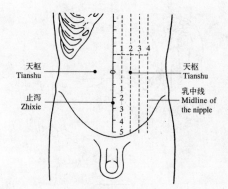

图2-74　脐三针

Fig. 2-74　Qisanzhen

表四灵
Biaosiling

组成　本穴组由滑肉门、大巨二穴组合而成。

位置　滑肉门：脐上1寸，前正中线旁开2寸。

大巨：脐下2寸，前正中线旁开2寸。

主治　肠炎。

操作　灸3~5壮。

Composition　This group of acupoints is composed of Huaroumen(ST24) and Daju(ST27).

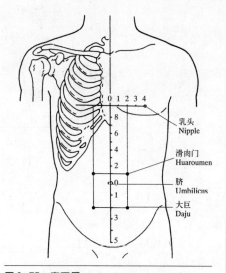

图2-75　表四灵

Fig. 2-75　Biaosiling

Location Huaroumen：1 cun above the centre of the umbilicus, 2 cun lateral to the anterior midline.

Daju：2 cun below the centre of the umbilicus, 2 cun lateral to the anterior midline.

Indication Enteritis.

Method 3-5 cones of moxibustion is applied.

关枢
Guanshu

组成 本穴组由左右天枢及关元共三穴组合而成。

位置 天枢：脐旁2寸。

关元：脐下3寸。

主治 腹泻。

操作 刺法：直刺1～1.5寸，得气为度。

灸法：艾炷灸5～9壮，艾条温灸10～30分钟。

Composition This group of acupoints is composed of Tianshu(ST25) and both Guanyuan(GV4).

Location Tianshu：2 cun lateral to the centre of the umbilicus.

Guanyuan：2 cun below the centre of the umbilicus.

Indication Diarrhea.

Method Acupuncture：the needle is inserted 1-1.5 cun perpendicularly till the acu-esthesia is obtained.

Moxibustion moxibustion with 5-9 moxa cones or warm moxibustion with moxa roll for 10-30 minutes is applied.

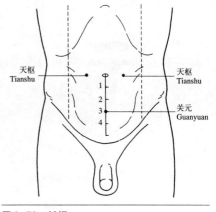

图2-76 关枢
Fig. 2-76 Guanshu

腹四穴(腹四种)
Fusixue (Fusizhong)

组成 本穴组由脐之上、下、左、右各1.5寸处之四个点组合而成。

位置 腹中部，脐上、下、左、右各1.5寸处。

主治 急、慢性痢疾，泄泻，消化不良，食物中毒。

操作 刺法：针2～3寸，针感下腹部酸、麻、胀、热。

灸法：灸5～9壮，艾条灸10～20分钟。

Composition This group of acupoints is composed of

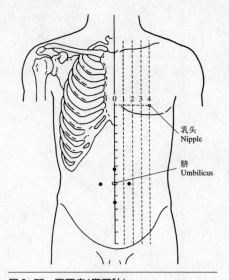

图 2-77 腹四穴(腹四种)
Fig. 2-77 Fusixue(Fusizhong)

four points 1.5 cun respectively superior, inferior and lateral to the umbilicus.

Location On the middle part of the abdomen, 1.5 cun superior, inferior and lateral to the centre of the umbilicus.

Indications Acute and chronic diarrhea, indigestion and food poisoning.

Method Acupuncture: the needle is inserted 2-3 cun. The acu-esthesia of soreness, numbness, distension and pyrexia can be felt in the lower abdomen.

Moxibustion 5-9 cones of moxibustion or moxibustion with moxa roll for 10-20 minutes is applied.

脐上下
Qishangxia

组成 本穴组由脐上下1.5寸的二穴组合而成。

位置 腹中部正中线上,脐上1.5寸一穴,脐下1.5寸一穴。

主治 黄疸,下痢,胃痛,腹痛,体虚。

操作 刺法:直刺1~1.5寸,局部酸胀,可扩散至外阴部。

灸法:艾炷灸或温针灸5~9壮,艾条灸10~20分钟,或药物天灸。强身保健则采用瘢痕灸,每年1次,或间接灸5~9壮,或温灸至局部温热舒适,每日1次,每月20次。本穴也常采用累计灸法百余壮。

按注 本穴脐下一穴实为气海穴,故也有强壮保健之功。本穴单用可名为脐上或脐下。

Composition This group of acupoints is composed of two points respectively superior and inferior to the umbilicus.

Location On the midline of the middle part of the abdomen, one point is 1.5 cun above the centre of the umbilicus, the other point is 1.5 cun below the centre of the umbilicus.

Indication Jaundice, diarrhea, stomachache, pain in the abdomen and weak constitution.

Method Acupuncture: the needle is inserted 1-1.5 cun perpendicularly. The soreness and distension in this

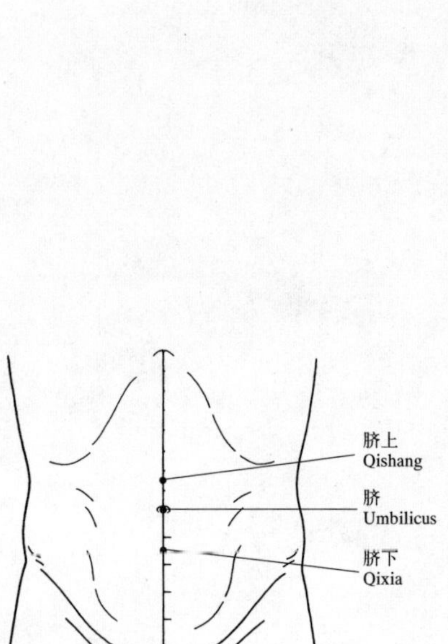

图 2-78 脐上下
Fig. 2-78 Qishangxia

part may spread to the vulva.

Moxibustion: 5−9 cones of moxibustion or warm needle moxibustion, or moxibustion with moxa roll for 10−20 minutes, or medicated moxibustion can be applied. Scarred moxibustion can be applied for the purpose of cultivating health and improving the physique, treat once every year. 5−9 cones of indirect moxibustion, or warm moxibustion till the warm and comfortable feeling obtained in this part can also be applied, treat once every day, 20 times every month. Seperated moxibustion up to about one hundred cones is applied too.

Notes The point below the umbilicus in this group is actually the acupoint of Qihai, and has the function of cultivating health and improving the physique. This group of acupoints can be used singly, and the name is Qishang or Qixia.

● 下腹三角
Xiafusanjiao

组成 本穴组由关元、左右归来共三穴组合而成。

位置 关元：脐下3寸。

归来：脐下4寸，前正中线旁开2寸。

主治 遗精阳痿，月经不调，带多，阴挺，尿频急或遗溺等。

操作 各穴稍向下呈70°角刺之，深度1～2寸，以针感向阴部及二侧少腹部放射为佳。

Composition This group of acupoints is composed of Guanyuan(CV4) and both Guilai(ST29).

Location Guanyuan: 3 cun below the centre of the umbilicus.

Guilai: 4 cun below the centre of the umbilicus, 2 cun lateral to the anterior midline.

Indication Spermatorrhea, impotence, irregular menstruation, excessive leukorrhea, prolapse of the uterus, frequent urination, enuresis, etc.

Method The needle is inserted downwards at the angle of 70°. The depth is 1−2 cun. It is ideal if the acu-esthesia radiates to the vulva and the lower abdomen

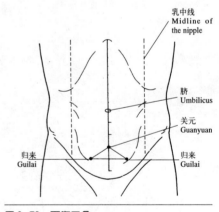

图2-79 下腹三角
Fig. 2−79 Xiafusanjiao

on both sides.

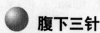

腹下三针
Fuxiasanzhen

组成　本穴组由子宫、中极二穴组合而成。

位置　子宫：中极穴旁开3寸。

中极：脐下4寸。

主治　遗精，阳痿，白带过多，月经不调，阴挺，尿频，尿急，遗尿。

操作　刺法：子宫穴针1～2寸，针感会阴部向上抽动；中极穴针1～2寸，针感麻、胀、抽感至外阴部。

灸法：艾炷灸或温针灸5～9壮，艾条灸10～20分钟。

Composition　This group of acupoints is composed of Zigong(EX-CA1) and Zhongji(CV3).

Location　Zigong：3 cun lateral to Zhongji.

Zhongji：4 cun below the centre of the umbilicus.

Indication　Spermatorrhea, impotence, excessive leukorrhea, irregular menstruation, prolapse of the uterus, frequent urination, urgent urination and enuresis.

Method　Acupuncture：Zhongji is needled 1-2 cun. The acu-esthesia of numbness, distension and twitching feeling will transmit to the vulva.

Moxibustion：5-9 cones of moxibustion with moxa cones or warm needle moxibustion, or moxibustion with moxa roll for 10-20 minutes is applied.

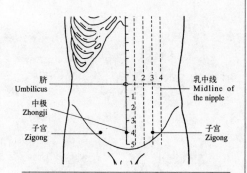

图2-80　腹下三针
Fig. 2-80　Fuxiasanzhen

上中极三角
Shangzhongjisanjiao

组成　本穴组由中极、气穴二穴组合而成。

位置　中极：脐下4寸。

气穴：脐下3寸，前正中线旁开0.5寸。

主治　遗精，阳痿，月经不调，带多，阴挺，尿频急或遗溺等。

操作　二穴各呈70°角刺1～2寸，以针感向前阴及两侧少腹部放散为佳。

Composition　This group of acupoints is composed of

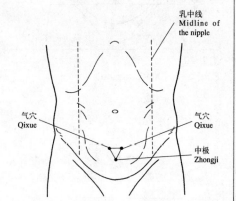

图2-81　上中极三角
Fig. 2-81　Shangzhongjisanjiao

Zhongji(CV3) and Qixue(KI13).

Location　Zhongji：4 cun below the centre of the umbilicus.

Qixue：3 cun below the centre of the umbilicus, 0.5 cun lateral to the anterior midline.

Indications　Spermatorrhea, impotence, irregular menstruation, excessive leukorrhea, prolapse of the uterus, frequent and urgent urination, enuresis, etc..

Method　The three points are needled 1−2 cun at the angle of 70° respectively, it is ideal if the acu-esthesia radiates to the pubes and the lower abdomen on both sides.

● 下中极三角
Xiazhongjisanjiao

组成　本穴组由中极、横骨二穴组合而成。

位置　中极：脐下4寸。

横骨：脐下5寸，耻骨联合上际，前正中线旁开0.5寸。

主治　同上中极三角。

操作　同上中极三角。

Composition　This group of acupoints is composed of Zhongji(CV3) and Henggu(KI11).

Location　Zhongji：4 cun below the centre of the umbilicus.

Henggu：5 cun below the centre of the umbilicus, on the upper border of the symphysis pubis and 0.5 cun lateral to the anterior midline.

Indication　See Shangzhongjisanjiao.

Method　See Shangzhongjisanjiao.

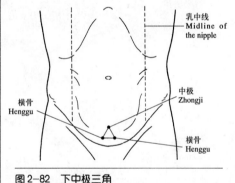

图 2-82　下中极三角
Fig. 2-82　Xiazhongjisanjiao

● 阴毛间
Yinmaojian

组成　本穴组由曲骨、横骨、气冲三穴组合而成。

位置　曲骨：耻骨联合上缘中点处。

横骨：脐下5寸，耻骨联合上际，前正中线旁开0.5寸。

气冲：脐下5寸，前正中线旁开2寸。

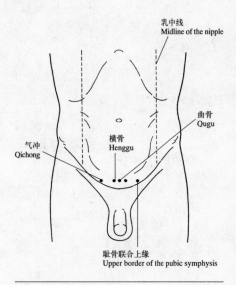

图2-83 阴毛间
Fig. 2-83 Yinmaojian

主治 阳痿早泄，带多阴挺，遗尿等。

操作 直刺深1～1.5寸，以针感向前阴及二侧腹股沟放散为佳。

Composition This group of acupoints is composed of Qugu(CV2), Henggu(KI11) and Qichong(ST30).

Location Qugu：at the midpoint of the upper border of the pubic symphysis.

Henggu：5 cun below the centre of the umbilicus, on the upper border of the symphysis pubis and 0.5 cun lateral to the anterior midline.

Qichong：5 cun below the centre of the umbilicus, 2 cun lateral to the anterior midline.

Indications Impotence, premature ejaculation, excessive leukorrhea, prolapse of the uterus, enuresis, etc..

Method The needle is inserted 1−1.5 cun, it is ideal if the acu-esthesia radiates to the pubes and the two groins on both sides.

 带元

Daiyuan

组成 本穴组由带脉、关元二穴组合而成。

位置 带脉：第十一肋端直下平脐处。

关元：脐下3寸。

主治 肾虚，肾败。

操作 艾炷灸5～9壮，艾条温灸10～30分钟。

Composition This group of acupoints is composed of Daimai(GB26) and Guanyuan(CV4).

Location Daimai：directly below the tip of the 11th rib, at the level of the umbilicus.

Guanyuan：3 cun below the centre of the umbilicus.

Indication Deficiency and failure of the kidney.

Method Moxibustion with 5−9 moxa cones, or moxibustion with moxa roll for 10−30 minutes is applied.

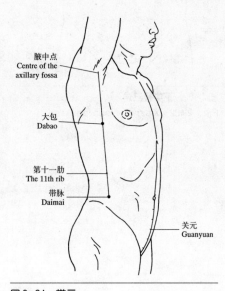

图2-84 带元
Fig. 2-84 Daiyuan

倒八针
Daobazhen

组成　本穴组由少腹部天枢、外陵、大巨、水道左右共八穴组合而成。

位置　天枢：脐旁2寸。

外陵：脐下1寸，前正中线旁开2寸。

大巨：脐下2寸，前正中线旁开2寸。

水道：脐下3寸，前正中线旁开2寸。

主治　癃闭。

操作　以45°方向向肾经针刺，形似"倒形之八字"，得气后通电针。

Composition　This group of acupoints is composed of both Tianshu(ST25), Wailing(ST26), Daju(ST27) and Shuidao(ST28).

Location　Tianshu：2 cun lateral to the centre of the umbilicus.

Wailing：1 cun below the centre of the umbilicus, 2 cun lateral to the anterior midline.

Daju：2 cun below the centre of the umbilicus, 2 cun lateral to the anterior midline.

Shuidao：3 cun below the centre of the umbilicus, 2 cun lateral to the anterior midline.

Indication　Retention of urine.

Method　The needle is inserted at the angle of 45° towards the Kidney Meridian. Two needles form a reversed "八". Electroacupuncture is applied after the acuesthesia is obtained.

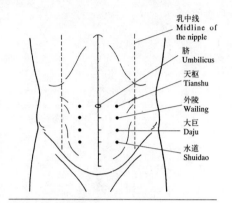

图2-85　倒八针
Fig. 2-85　Daobazhen

肓骨
Huanggu

组成　本穴组由肓俞、横骨二穴组合而成。

位置　肓俞：脐旁0.5寸。

横骨：脐下5寸，耻骨联合上际，前正中线旁开0.5寸。

主治　五淋久积。

操作　直刺0.8~1.5寸，得气感应以向前阴放射者为佳。

Composition　This group of acupoints is composed of

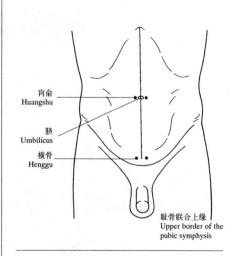

图2-86　肓骨
Fig. 2-86　Huanggu

Huangshu(KI16) and Henggu(KI11).

Location   Huangshu：0.5 cun lateral to the centre of the umbilicus.

Henggu：5 cun below the centre of the umbilicus, on the upper border of the symphysis pubis and 0.5 cun lateral to the anterior midline.

Indication   Chronic stranguria.

Method   The needle is inserted 0.8−1.5 cun. It is ideal if the acu-esthesia spreads to the pubes.

关寸
Guancun

组成　本穴组由脐下少腹部的三个点组合而成。

位置　脐下4.5寸处为一穴。脐下3.5寸左右旁开各1寸二穴。

主治　赤白带下，疝痛，泄泻，腹痛，子痛，遗精，遗尿，月经不调，尿急尿痛。

操作　刺法：直刺1～1.5寸，局部酸胀感，可放散至生殖器及会阴部。

灸法：艾炷灸或温针灸5～9壮，艾条灸10～20分钟或药物天灸。

Composition   This group of acupoints is composed of the three points on the lower abdomen.

Location   One point is 4.5 cun below the centre of the umbilicus, the other two points are 1.2 cun lateral to the point 3.5 cun below the centre of the umbilicus.

Indications   Morbid leukorrhea, pain due to hernia, diarrhea, pain in the abdomen, orchitis and epididymitis, spermatorrhea, enuresis, irregular menstruation, urgent and painful urination.

Methods   Acupuncture：the needle is inserted 1−1.5 cun perpendicularly. The acu-esthesia of soreness and distension in this part will radiate to the genitals and the perincum.

Moxibustion   5−9 cones of moxibustion or warm needle moxibustion is applied. Moxibustion with moxa roll for 10−20 minutes or medicated moxibustion can also be applied.

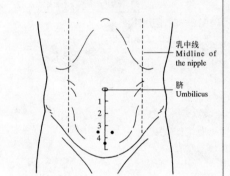

图2-87　关寸
Fig. 2-87　Guancun

疝气穴(三角灸)
Shanqixue(Sanjiaojiu)

组成　本穴组由神阙穴与其下两侧两个刺激点组合而成。

位置　以患者两口角的长度为一边,作一等边三角形。将顶角置于患者脐中为一穴,底边呈水平线,于两底角处为另二穴。

主治　疝气,奔豚,绕脐疼痛,妇人不孕,冷气心痛。

操作　艾炷灸3~7壮,或温灸10~20分钟。

按注　本穴又名三角灸或脐下三角。

Composition　This group of acupoints is composed of Shenque(CV8) and two points below it.

Location　Take the distance between the two corners of the mouth of the patient as one side and make a equilateral triangle. Put one angle on the centre of the umbilicus of the patient to locate one acupoint, adjust the bottom line to the horizontal level, and the two angles at each end of this line are the other two points.

Indications　Hernia, Bentun syndrome, pain around the umbilical region, sterility, cardiac pain due to cold.

Method　Moxibustion with 3−7 moxa cones or warm moxibustion for 10−20 minutes is applied.

Note　This group is also called sanjiaojiu or Qixiasanjiao.

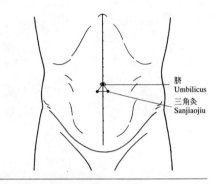

图2-88　疝气穴(三角灸)
Fig. 2-88　Shanqixue(Sanjiaojiu)

肝神
Ganshen

组成　本穴组由剑突下斜沿右肋弓下的三个点组合而成。

位置　右侧上腹部肋弓下缘,由剑突尖下斜沿右肋弓下缘0.5寸处一穴,1.5寸处一穴,2.5寸处一穴。

主治　内耳眩晕症。

操作　针0.5~1寸,局部酸、胀感,当针下有阻力感时,再稍加指力,有穿透薄皮样感觉。

灸法:艾炷灸3~5壮,艾条温灸5~15分钟。

Composition　This group of acupoints is composed of three points along the lower border of the right costal arch below the xiphoid process.

Location　On the lower border of the costal arch of

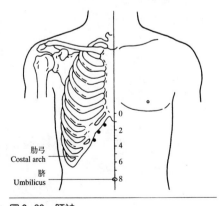

图2-89　肝神
Fig. 2-89　Ganshen

the right upper abdomen, 0.5 cun, 1.5 cun and 2.5 cun lateral to the tip of the xiphoid process along the right costal arch.

Indication   Meniere's disease.

Method   The needle is inserted 0.5–1 cun. The acuesthesia of soreness and distension will be obtained. When the resistance under the needle is felt, the finger strength should be increased, and the feeling of needling through thin skin will be sensed.

Moxibustion：Moxibustion with 3–5 moxa cones or warm moxibustion for 5–15 minutes is applied.

● 理中灸
Lizhongjiu

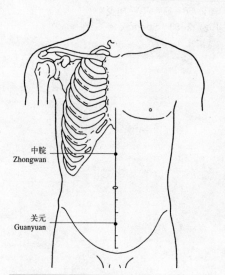

中脘
Zhongwan

关元
Guanyuan

图2-90 理中灸
Fig. 2-90 Lizhongjiu

组成   本穴组由中脘、关元二穴组合而成。

位置   中脘：脐上4寸。

关元：脐下3寸。

主治   头昏脚软，四肢倦怠，心下痞闷，食欲不振。

操作   灸中脘、关元各7～14壮。

Composition   This group of acupoints is composed of Zhongwan(CV12) and Guanyuan(GV4).

Location   Zhongwan：4 cun above the centre of the umbilicus.

Guanyuan：3 cun below the centre of the umbilicus.

Indications   Vertigo, weakness of the four limbs, stuffy chest, anorexia.

Method   7–14 cones of moxibustion is applied to Zhongwan and Guanyuan respectively.

● 璇海
Xuanhai

组成   本穴组由璇玑、气海二穴组合而成。

位置   气海：脐下1.5寸。

璇玑：前正中线，胸骨柄的中央。

主治   虚损瘦弱，久病不愈。

操作   见"上下气海"。

汉 英 对 照

Composition This group of acupoints is composed of Xuanji(CV21) and Qihai(CV6).

Location Qihai：1.5 cun below the centre of the umbilicus.

Xuanji：on the anterior midline, in the centre of the sternal handle.

Indications Emaciation, slow recovery after illness.

Method See "Shangxiaqihai".

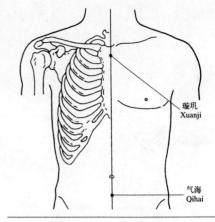

图 2-91 璇海
Fig. 2-91 Xuanhai

延寿
Yanshou

组成 本穴组由关元、气海、命关、中脘四穴组合而成。

位置 关元：脐下3寸。

气海：脐下1.5寸。

中脘：脐上4寸。

命关：上腹部乳头直下与中脘穴相平处。

主治 年老气血虚弱之症。

操作 依次灸关元、气海、中脘、命关，每穴灸10~15分钟或灸5~10壮，亦可用针，均浅刺1.6厘米左右。

Composition This group of acupoints is composed of Guanyuan(CV4), Qihai(CV6), MingGuan and Zhongwan (CV12).

Location Guanyuan：3 cun below the centre of the umbilicus.

Qihai：1.5 cun below the centre of the umbilicus.

Zhongwan：4 cun above the centre of the umbilicus.

Mingguan：the point directly below the nipples and at the same level of Zhongwan.

Indication Qi and blood deficiency due to senility.

Method Moxibustion is applied to Guanyuan, Qihai, Zhongwan and Mingguan in turn, 10—15 minutes' or 5—10 cones of moxibustion each point. Acupuncture is applicable too. The needle is inserted superficially, the depth is about 1.6 cm.

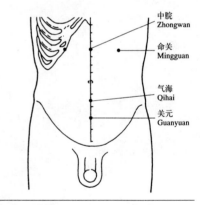

图 2-92 延寿
Fig. 2-92 Yanshou

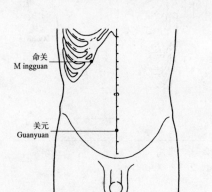

图 2-93 火灸
Fig. 2-93 Huojiu

火灸
Huojiu

组成　本穴组由关元、命关二穴组合而成。

位置　关元：脐下3寸。

命关：见延寿中命关穴。

主治　素体阳虚或病后伤及脾肾之阳，致使元阳衰微，见有神昏，手足厥冷，目合，口张，口吐涎沫，遗尿。

操作　关元、命关均用灸法。先灸关元，不拘壮数，再灸命关5～10壮。

Composition　This group of acupoints is composed of Guanyuan(CV4) and MingGuan.

Location　Guanyuan：3 cun below the centre of the umbilicus.

Mingguan：see Mingguan in Yanshou.

Indications　Yang deficiency constitution, or yang deficiency of Spleen and Kidney loss of consciousness, cold limbs, closing eyes, open mouth, foam on the lips, enuresis.

Method　Moxibustion is applied to Guanyuan and Mingguan. Moxibustion is applied to Guanyuan first without calculating the number of cones. Then 5–10 cones of moxibustion is applied to Mingguan.

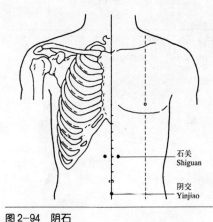

图 2-94 阴石
Fig. 2-94 Yinshi

阴石
Yinshi

组成　本穴组由阴交、石关二穴组合而成。

位置　阴交：脐下1寸。

石关：脐上3寸，前正中线旁开0.5寸。

主治　不育症。

操作　灸柱间接灸5～9壮，艾条温灸10～30分钟，每日或隔日进行1次，需长期坚持，或可有效。

Composition　This group of acupoints is composed of Yinjiao(CV7) and Shiguan(KI18).

Location　Yinjiao：1 cun below the centre of the umbilicus.

Shiguan：3 cun above the centre of the umbilicus, 0.5

cun lateral to the anterior midline.

Indication Sterility.

Method Indirect moxibustion with 5-9 moxa cones, or warm moxibustion with moxa roll for 10-30 minutes is applied. Treat once every day or every other day. It may take effect if the treatment is given for a long time.

梅花三针
Meihuasanzhen

组成 本穴组由护宫、关元二穴组合而成。

位置 护宫：脐下1.5寸，旁开2.6寸处。

关元：脐下3寸。

主治 不孕症，附件炎，卵巢囊肿，睾丸炎。

操作 刺法：针1～2寸，针感局部或向下抽、胀可达前阴。

灸法：艾炷灸或温针灸5～9壮，艾条灸10～20分钟。

Composition This group of acupoints is composed of Hugong and Guanyuan(CV4).

Location Hugong：2.6 cun lateral to the point 1.5 cun below the centre of the umbilicus.

Guanyuan：3 cun below the centre of the umbilicus.

Indications Sterility, annexitis, ovarian cyst, orchitis.

Methods Acupuncture：the needle is inserted 1-2 cun. The acu-esthesia of distension and twitch may be felt only in this part or may radiate to pubes.

Moxibustion：moxibustion with moxa cone or 5-9 cones of warm needle moxibustion, or moxibustion with moxa roll for 10-20 minutes is applied.

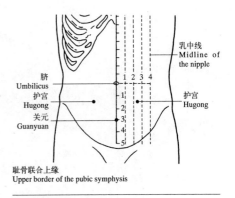

图2-95 梅花三针
Fig. 2-95 Meihuasanzhen

新肋头
Xinleitou

组成 本穴组由第一至第三肋骨部的左右四个点组合而成。

位置 胸部、胸骨两侧，第一、第二肋骨间各一穴，第二、第三肋骨间各一穴。

主治 瘰疬，肋间痛，胸闷，咳嗽，气窒，喘息，呃逆。

操作 灸3～7壮。

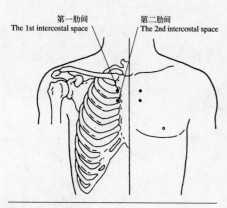

第一肋间
The 1st intercostal space

第二肋间
The 2nd intercostal space

图2-96 新肋头

Fig. 2-96 Xinleitou

按注 本穴主要用于灸治，如欲针时可针刺0.5～0.8寸。

Composition   This group of acupoints is composed of four points in the region of the 1st to 3rd ribs.

Location   On the chest and on both sides of the sternum, one point between the 1st and 2nd ribs on each side, one point between the 2nd and 3rd ribs on each side, 4 points in all.

Indications   Hypochondriac lump, pain in the intercostal region, stuffy chest, cough, obstruction of qi, asthma, hiccup.

Method   3-7 cones of moxibustion is applied.

Note   Moxibustion is applied to this group of acupoints mainly. The depth may be 0.5-0.8 cun if acupuncture is applied.

● 小儿龟胸
Xiaoerguixiong

组成 本穴组由足阳明胃经的乳中、膺窗、屋翳三穴各内侧1.5寸处的六个点组合而成。

位置 胸部正中线，左右旁开各2.5寸之线上，第二、第三、第四肋间隙处，当乳中穴内侧1.5寸处左右二穴；膺窗穴内侧1.5寸处左右二穴；屋翳穴各内侧1.5寸处，左右二穴。

主治 小儿龟胸。

操作 六穴各灸3壮，春夏从下一穴起向上灸。秋冬从上一穴起向下灸。

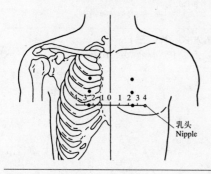

4 3 2 1 0 1 2 3 4

乳头
Nipple

图2-97 小儿龟胸

Fig. 2-97 Xiaoerguixiong

Composition   This group of acupoints is composed of six points respectively 1.5 cun medial to Ruzhong(ST17), Yingchuang(ST16) and Wuyi(ST15).

Location   On the line 2.5 cun lateral to the midline of the chest, in the 1st, 2nd, 3rd and 4th intercostal spaces, 1.5 cun medial to Ruzhong. 1.5 cun medial to Yingchang, 1.5 cun medial to Wuyi, 6 points in all.

Indication   Pigeon breast in children.

Method   3 cones of moxibustion is applied to six acupoints respectively. In spring and summer, moxibustion is applied upwards from the lowest acupoint, and in autumn and winter, the moxibust is applied downwards from the highest acupoint.

脐上下0.5寸
Qishangxia 0.5 cun

组成　本穴组由脐上下各0.5寸的二个点组合而成。

位置　腹中部，脐上0.5寸与脐下0.5寸处。

主治　小儿囟门不合，泄泻，下痢，肠鸣，腹痛腹胀，水肿，疝痛。

操作　刺法：直刺0.5～1寸，局部酸胀沉重感，脐下一穴可有向下抽动感。

灸法：艾炷灸3～5壮，艾条温灸3～9壮，小儿也可日累计灸百壮。

按注　本穴单用可名为脐上0.5寸或脐下0.5寸。

Composition　This group of acupoints is composed of two points 0.5 cun respectively superior and inferior to the centre of the umbilicus.

Location　On the middle part of the abdomen, 0.5 cun superior and inferior to the centre of the umbilicus, 2 points in all.

Indication　Infantile metopism, diarrhea, dysentery, borborygmus, abdominal pain and distension, edema, pain due to hernia.

Method　Acupuncture：the needle is inserted 0.5–1 cun perpendicularly, the acu-esthesia of soreness, distension and heaviness in the part will be obtained, and the feeling of twitching downwards may be sensed in Qixia point.

Moxibustion：moxibustion with 3–5 moxa cones or 3–9 cones of warm moxibustion with moxa roll is applied. Separated moxibustion up to one hundred cones may be applied to infants.

Note　This group of acupoints may be used separately, and the name is Qishang 0.5 cun or Qixia 0.5 cun.

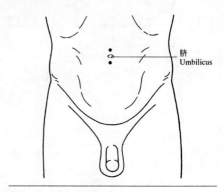

图2-98　脐上下0.5寸
Fig. 2-98　Qishangxia 0.5 cun

脐中四边
Qizhongsibian

组成　本穴组由脐中穴及上下左右各1寸四点共五点组合而成。

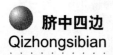

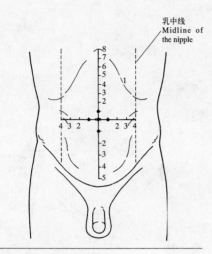

乳中线
Midline of the nipple

图 2-99 脐中四边
Fig. 2-99 Qizhongsibian

位置 腹中部，脐之中点一穴，上下左右各 1 寸处一穴。

主治 小儿暴痫，角弓反张，痉挛，肠鸣，腹痛，水肿，肠泻，疝痛，胃痛脘胀，消化不良。

操作 刺法：直刺 0.5～1 寸，局部酸胀沉重感觉，脐下 1 穴可有向下抽动感。

灸法 艾炷灸 3～5 壮，艾条温灸 3～9 壮。

按注 针刺时脐中穴不刺，灸之则可。

Composition This group of acupoints is composed of five points of Qizhong and four points 1 cun superior, inferior and lateral to Qizhong.

Location On the middle part of the abdomen, one point is in the centre of the umbilicus, the other four points are 1 cun superior, inferior and lateral to the centre of the umbilicus respectively.

Indications Infantile sudden epilepsy, opisthotonus, convulsion, borborygmus, abdominal pain, edema, diarrhea, pain due to hernia, epigastric pain and distension, indigestion.

Methods Acupuncture：the needle is inserted 0.5−1 cun perpendicularly, the acu-esthesia of soreness, distension and heaviness in the part will be obtained, and the feeling of twitching downwards may be sensed in Qixia point.

Moxibustion：moxibustion with 3−5 moxa cones or 3−9 cones of warm moxibustion with moxa roll is applied.

Note Moxibustion is applied to Qizhong instead of acupuncture.

 退蛔
Tuihui

组成 本穴组由右肋弓下缘的四个点组合而成。

位置 右侧肋弓下缘，从正中线开始沿右侧肋弓下缘 0.6 寸处为第一穴。依次沿肋弓下缘，向右下方每隔 0.6 寸为一穴。

主治 胆道蛔虫症。

操作 针 0.3～0.5 寸，针感局部酸、胀。

Composition This group of acupoints is composed of four points on the lower border of the right costal arch.

Location On the lower border of the right costal

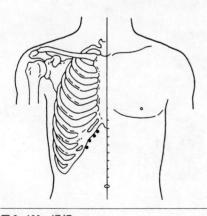

图 2-100 退蛔
Fig. 2-100 Tuihui

arch. The first point are 0.6 cun lateral to the anterior midline along the lower border of the right costal arch, then locate other points along the lower border of the costal arch in turn, each point is 0.6 cun inferior and lateral to the former point.

Indication   Biliary ascariasis.

Method   The needle is inserted 0.3−0.5 cun. The acu-esthesia of soreness and distension will be obtained.

风痱
Fengfei

组成   本穴组由上腹部的三个穴点组合而成。

位置   腹上部，胸膛窝下4.5寸，正中线上一穴；左右相平旁开各1.5寸处各一穴。或取中脘穴下0.5寸一穴，左右平开1.5寸二穴。

主治   风痱不能语，手足不遂。

操作   艾炷灸3～5壮，或累计灸百壮。

Composition   This group of acupoints is composed of three points on the upper abdomen.

Location   On the upper part of the abdomen, 4.5 cun below the depression of the chest, one point is on the anterior midline, the other two points are 1.5 cun lateral to it at the same level. This group of acupoints can also be located by selecting the point 0.5 cun below Zhongwan and two points 1.5 cun lateral to Zhongwan.

Indications   Aphasia due to rubella with pruritus, motor impairment of the four limbs.

Method   Moxibustion with 3−5 moxa cones or separated moxibustion up to one hundred cones is applied.

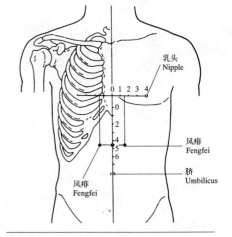

图2-101　风痱
Fig. 2-101　Fengfei

脐周三穴
Qizhousanxue

组成   本穴组由天枢、阴交、水分三穴组合而成。

位置   天枢：脐旁2寸。

阴交：脐下1寸。

水分：脐上1寸。

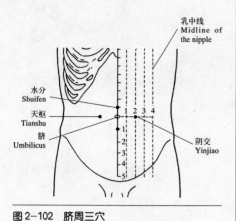

图 2-102 脐周三穴
Fig. 2-102 Qizhousanxue

主治 痹证，腹痛。

操作 针0.5～1寸，用捻提法，留15分钟、每1至2日1次。

Composition This group of acupoints is composed of Tianshu(ST25), Yinjiao(CV7) and Shuifen(CV9).

Location Tianshu：2 cun lateral to the centre of the umbilicus.

Yinjiao：1 cun below the centre of the umbilicus.

Shuifen：1 cun above the centre of the umbilicus.

Indication Bi-syndromes and abdominal pain.

Method The needle is inserted 0.5-1 cun. Rotating and lifting method is applied. Retain the needles for 15 minutes. Treat once every day or every other day.

● 篡刺术
Cuancishu

组成 本穴组由以会阴加中心左右上下各1寸共五穴点组合而成。

位置 会阴：男性在阴囊根部与肛门的中间，女性在大阴唇后联合与肛门的中间。

会阴上下左右四点：在会阴穴上下左右各1寸处为穴。

主治 痔疮，小便不利，遗精，月经不调，癫狂，昏厥。

操作 直刺0.5～1寸，酸胀感可向前阴后阴扩散。

Composition This group of acupoints is composed of five points of Huiyin and the four points 1 cun superior, inferior and lateral to it.

Location Huiyin：at the midpoint between the posterior border of the scrotum and anus in male, and between the posterior commissure of the large labia and anus in female.

Huiyinshangxiazuoyousidian：1 cun superior, inferior and lateral to Huiyin.

Indications Hemorrhoids, dysuria, seminal emission, irregular menstruation, mania and syncope.

Method The needle is inserted 0.5-1 cun perpendicularly. The acu-esthesia of soreness and distension may radiate to the pubes and anus.

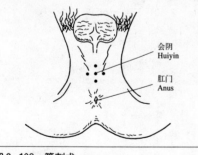

图 2-103 篡刺术
Fig. 2-103 Cuancishu

肛门四穴
Gangmensixue

组成　本穴组由肛门周围的四个刺激点组合而成。

位置　位于肛门上下左右各旁开0.5寸处是穴。

主治　截瘫引起的大便失禁。

操作　直刺1～2寸。

按注　本穴的截石位6点处一穴可治脑神经疾患；3与6点处二穴可治坐骨神经痛。

Composition　This group of acupoints is composed of four points around the anus.

Location　0.5 cun superior, inferior and lateral to the anus.

Indication　Encopresis due to paraplegia.

Method　The needle is inserted 1−2 cun perpendicularly.

Note　The point at six o'clock in lithotomy position of this group can be used to treat the diseases of cranial nerves. And the points at three and six o'clock can be used to treat sciatica.

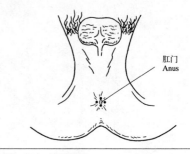

图2-104　肛门四穴
Fig. 2-104　Gangmensixue

膺中外俞
Yingzhongwaishu

组成　本穴组由中府、云门二穴组合而成。

位置　中府：胸前壁外上方，前正中线旁开6寸，平第一肋间隙。

云门：胸前壁外上方，距前正中线旁开6寸，当锁骨外端下缘凹陷中取穴。

主治　皮肤痛，寒热，上气喘，汗出，欬动肩背，胸中烦满，肩背痛。

操作　刺法：向外斜刺0.5～1寸。

灸法：艾炷灸1～3壮，或温灸5～10分钟。

Composition　This group of acupoints is composed of Zhongfu(LU1) and Yunmen(LU2).

Location　Zhongfu：in the superior lateral part of the anterior thoracic wall, 6 cun lateral to the anterior midline, at the level of the 1st intercostal space.

Yunmen：in the superior lateral part of the anterior

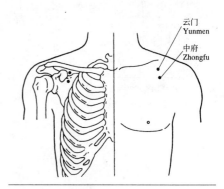

图2-105　膺中外俞
Fig. 2-105　Yingzhongwaishu

thoracic wall, 6 cun lateral to the anterior midline, in the depression below the lateral part of the clavicle.

Indications Skin pain, fever, asthma, sweating, severe cough, fullness and depression in the chest, pain in the shoulder and back.

Methods Acupuncture: the needle is inserted 0.5−1 cun outwards obliquely.

Moxibustion: moxibustion with 1−3 moxa cones or warm moxibustion for 5−10 minutes is applied.

肺募俞
Feimushu

组成 本穴组由中府、肺俞二穴组合而成。

位置 中府：胸前壁外上方，前正中线旁开6寸，平第一肋间隙。

肺俞：第三胸椎棘突下，旁开1.5寸。

主治 肺脏及呼吸系统病证，皮毛病证，鼻疾等。

操作 刺法：二穴斜刺0.5～0.8寸。中府穴不宜向内下方深刺，注意免伤肺脏。

灸法：艾炷灸5～9壮，或温灸10～20分钟。

按注 二穴不能深刺，以免刺伤肺脏，发生意外。

Composition This group of acupoints is composed of Zhongfu(LU1) and Feishu(BL13).

Location Zhongfu: in the superior lateral part of the anterior thoracic wall, 6 cun lateral to the anterior midline, at the level of the 1st intercostal space.

Feishu: 1.5 cun lateral to the point below the spinous process of the 3rd thoracic vertebra.

Indication Diseases of the lung and respiratory system, skin disease, nasal diseases, etc..

Method Acupuncture: the needle is inserted 0.5−0.8 cun obliquely. It is not advisable to puncture Zhongfu deeply inwards and downwards in case of lung injuries.

Moxibustion: moxibustion with 5−9 moxa cones, or warm moxibustion for 10−20 minutes is applied.

Note Both acupoints can't be punctured deeply in order to avoid injuring the lung.

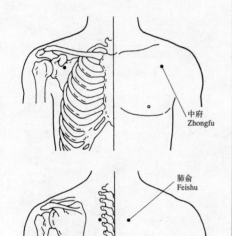

中府
Zhongfu

肺俞
Feishu

图 2-106 肺募俞
Fig. 2-106 Feimushu

心募俞
Xinmushu

组成　本穴组由巨阙、心俞二穴组合而成。

位置　巨阙：脐上6寸。

心俞：第五胸椎棘突下，旁开1.5寸。

主治　心脏病证，血脉病证，舌疾，胃疾。

操作　刺法：斜刺0.5～0.8寸。

灸法：艾炷灸5～9壮，或温灸10～20分钟。

按注　巨阙、心俞不能深刺，以防意外。

Composition　This group of acupoints is composed of Juque(CV14) and Xinshu(BL15).

Location　Juque：6 cun above the centre of the umbilicus.

Xinshu：1.5 cun lateral to the point below the spinous process of the 5th thoracic vertebra.

Indications　Heart diseases, blood vessel diseases, tongue diseases, gastric diseases.

Methods　Acupuncture：the needle is inserted 0.5−0.8 cun obliquely.

Moxibustion：moxibustion with 5−9 moxa cones, or warm moxibustion for 10−20 minutes is applied.

Note　These two points cannot be needled too deeply in case of accidents.

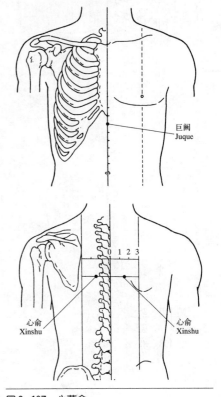

图2-107　心募俞
Fig. 2-107　Xinmushu

心包募俞
Xinbaomushu

组成　本穴组由膻中、厥阴俞二穴组合而成。

位置　膻中：前正中线，平第四肋间隙。

厥阴俞：第四胸椎棘突下，旁开1.5寸。

主治　心脏病证，神志病。

操作　刺法：膻中穴平刺0.5～1寸，厥阴俞斜刺0.5～0.8寸。

灸法：艾炷灸5～9壮，或温灸10～20分钟。

按注　厥阴俞禁直刺、深刺，以免伤内脏而发生意外。

Composition　This group of acupoints is composed of Danzhong (CV17) and Jueyinshu(BL14).

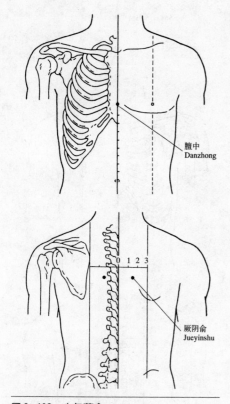

图 2-108　心包募俞
Fig. 2-108　Xinbaomushu

Location　Danzhong：on the anterior midline, at the level of the 4th intercostal space.

Jueyinshu：1.5 cun lateral to the point below the spinous process of the 4th thoracic vertebra.

Indications　Heart diseases and mental diseases.

Methods　Acupuncture：Danzhong is needled 0.5−1 cun horizontally, Jueyinshu is needles 0.5−0.8 cun obliquely.

Moxibustion：moxibustion with 5−9 moxa cones, or warm moxibustion for 10−20 minutes is applied.

Note　Jueyinshu is prohibited to be punctured perpendicularly or deeply in order to avoid injuring the viscera.

脾募俞
Pimushu

组成　本穴组由章门、脾俞二穴组合而成。
位置　章门：第十一肋端。
脾俞：第十一胸椎棘突下，旁开1.5寸。
主治　脾脏病证，肌病，口疾及肝病等。
操作　刺法：斜刺0.5～0.8寸。
灸法：艾炷灸5～9壮，或温灸10～20分钟。
按注　二穴不能深刺，以防刺伤内脏，发生意外事故。

Composition　This group of acupoints is composed of Zhangmen (LR13) and Pishu(BL20).

Location　Zhangmen：on the end of the 11th rib.

Pishu：1.5 cun lateral to the point below the spinous process of the 11th thoracic vertebra.

Indication　Spleen diseases, muscle diseases, mouth diseases and hepatic diseases, etc..

Method　Acupuncture：the needle is inserted 0.5−0.8 cun obliquely.

Moxibustion：moxibustion with 5−9 moxa cones, or warm moxibustion for 10−20 minutes is applied.

Note　Both acupoints can't be punctured deeply in order to avoid injuring the viscera.

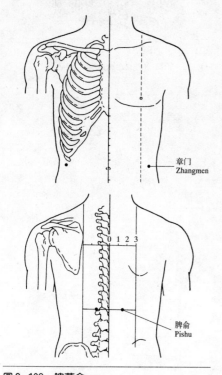

图 2-109　脾募俞
Fig. 2-109　Pimushu

胃募俞
Weimushu

组成　本穴组由中脘、胃俞二穴组合而成。

位置　中脘：脐上4寸。

胃俞：第十二胸椎棘突下，旁开1.5寸。

主治　胃腑病证，消化系统病证等。

操作　刺法：直刺0.5~1寸。

灸法：艾炷灸5~9壮，或温灸10~20分钟。

Composition　This group of acupoints is composed of Zhongwan (CV12) and Weishu(BL21).

Location　Zhongwan：4 cun above the centre of the umbilicus.

Weishu：1.5 cun lateral to the point below the spinous process of the 12th thoracic vertebra.

Indications　Gastric diseases, diseases of digestive system, etc..

Method　Acupuncture：the needle is inserted 0.5−1 cun.

Moxibustion：Moxibustion with 5−9 moxa cones, or warm moxibustion for 10−20 minutes is applied.

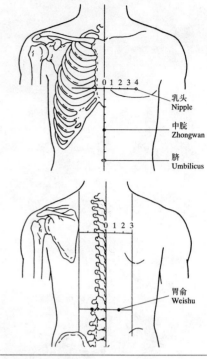

图2-110　胃募俞
Fig. 2-110　Weimushu

肝募俞
Ganmushu

组成　本穴组由期门、肝俞二穴组合而成。

位置　期门：乳头直下，第六肋间隙。

肝俞：第九胸椎棘突下，旁开1.5寸。

主治　肝脏病证，筋病，目疾，胃疾等。

操作　刺法：期门斜刺或平刺0.5~0.8寸，肝俞斜刺0.5~0.8寸。

灸法：艾炷灸5~9壮，或温灸10~20分钟。

按注　肝俞、期门二穴不能深刺，以防意外。

Composition　This group of acupoints is composed of Qimen (LR14) and Ganshu (BL18).

Location　Qimen：directly below the nipple, in the 6th intercostal space.

Ganshu：1.5 cun lateral to the point below the spinous

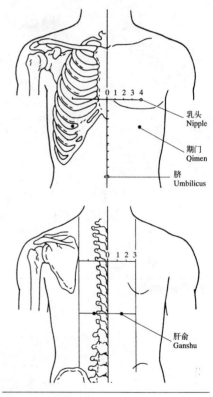

图2-111　肝募俞
Fig. 2-111　Ganmushu

process of the 9th thoracic vertebra.

Indications Hepatic diseases, tendon diseases, eye diseases, gastric diseases, etc..

Methods Acupuncture：Qimen is needled 0.5-0.8 cun obliquely or horizontally, Ganshu is needled 0.5-0.8 cun obliquely.

Moxibustion：moxibustion with 5-9 moxa cones, or warm moxibustion for 10-20 minutes is applied.

Note Ganshu and Qimen can't be punctured deeply in case of accidents.

● 胆募俞
Danmushu

组成 本穴组由日月、胆俞二穴组合而成。

位置 日月：乳头下方，第七肋间隙。

胆俞：第十胸椎棘突下，旁开1.5寸。

主治 胆、肝疾患，如季肋部痛，黄疸等。

操作 刺法：斜刺0.5～0.8寸，日月不宜深刺。

灸法：艾炷灸5～9壮，或温灸10～20分钟。

按注 不可深刺，以免伤及内脏发生意外。

Composition This group of acupoints is composed of Riyue (GB24) and Danshu (BL19).

Location Riyue：below the nipple, in the 7th inter-costal space.

Danshu：1.5 cun lateral to the point below the spinous process of the 10th thoracic vertebra.

Indications Diseases of the liver and gallbladder, such as pain in the hypochondriac region, jaundice,etc..

Methods Acupuncture：the needle is inserted 0.5-0.8 cun obliquely. Riyue can't be punctured deeply.

Moxibustion：moxibustion with 5-9 moxa cones, or warm moxibustion for 10-20 minutes is applied.

Note These points can't be punctured deeply in case of accidents.

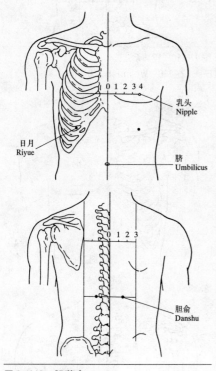

图2-112 胆募俞
Fig. 2-112 Danmushu

小肠募俞
Xiaochangmushu

组成　本穴组由关元、小肠俞二穴组合而成。

位置　关元：脐下3寸。

小肠俞：第一骶椎棘突下，旁开1.5寸。

主治　小肠膀胱病证及其他生殖、消化系统病证等。

操作　刺法：直刺1~1.5寸。

灸法：艾炷灸3~5壮，或温灸10~20分钟。

Composition　This group of acupoints is composed of Guanyuan (CV4) and Xiaochangshu (BL27).

Location　Guanyuan：3 cun below the centre of the umbilicus.

Xiaochangshu：1.5 cun lateral to the median sacral crest, on the level of the 1st posterior sacral foramen.

Indications　Small intestine, bladder diseases and other diseases of the genital, digestive systems.

Methods　Acupuncture：the needle is inserted 1-1.5 cun perpendicularly.

Moxibustion：moxibustion with 3-5 moxa cones, or warm moxibustion for 10-20 minutes is applied.

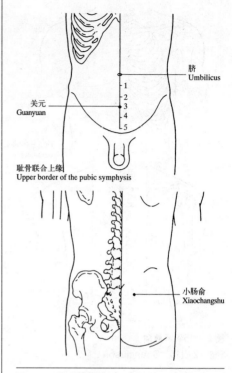

图2-113　小肠募俞
Fig. 2-113　Xiaochangmushu

大肠募俞
Dachangmushu

组成　本穴组由天枢、大肠俞二穴组合而成。

位置　天枢：脐旁2寸。

大肠俞：第四腰椎棘突下，旁开1.5寸。

主治　大肠病证及其他消化系统病证等。

操作　刺法：直刺1~1.5寸。

灸法：艾炷灸5~9壮，或温灸10~20分钟。

Composition　This group of acupoints is composed of Tianshu (ST25) and Dachangshu (BL25).

Location　Tianshu：2 cun lateral to the centre of the umbilicus.

Dachangshu：1.5 cun lateral to the spinous process of the 4th lumbar vertebra.

Indication　Large intestine diseases and other diseases

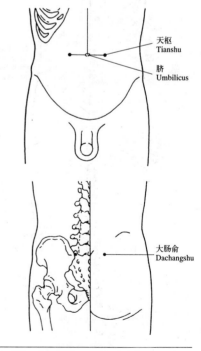

图2-114　大肠募俞
Fig. 2-114　Dachangmushu

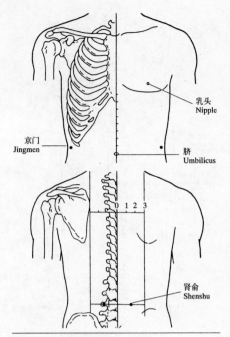

图2-115 肾募俞
Fig. 2-115 Shenmushu

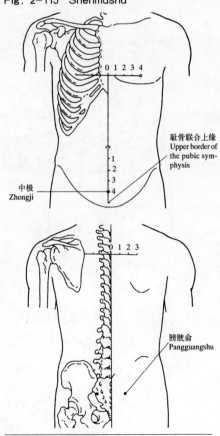

图2-116 膀胱募俞
Fig. 2-116 Pangguangmushu

126

汉 英 对 照

of the digestive system, etc..

Method Acupuncture: the needle is inserted 1-1.5 cun perpendicularly.

Moxibustion: moxibustion with 5-9 moxa cones, or warm moxibustion for 10-20 minutes is applied.

● 肾募俞
Shenmushu

组成 本穴组由京门、肾俞二穴组合而成。

位置 京门：第十二肋端。

肾俞：第二腰椎棘突下，旁开1.5寸。

主治 肾脏及生殖系统疾患，骨髓病证，耳疾等。

操作 刺法：肾俞直刺或斜刺0.5~1.2寸，京门穴斜刺0.5~0.8寸。

灸法：艾炷灸5~9壮，或温灸10~20分钟。

按注 京门禁深刺，以免伤及内脏，发生意外。

Composition This group of acupoints is composed of Jingmen (GB25) and Shenshu (BL23).

Location Jingmen: at the end of the 12th rib.

Shenshu: 1.5 cun lateral to the point below the spinous process of the 2nd lumbar vertebra.

Indications Kidney diseases and other diseases of the genital system, bone and marrow diseases, ear diseases, etc..

Methods Acupuncture: Shenshu is needled 0.5-1.2 cun perpendicularly or obliquely. Jingmen is inserted 0.5-0.8 cun obliquely.

Moxibustion: moxibustion with 5-9 moxa cones, or warm moxibustion for 10-20 minutes is applied.

Note Jingmen is prohibited to be punctured deeply in case of accidents of viscera injuries.

● 膀胱募俞
Pangguangmushu

组成 本穴组由中极、膀胱俞二穴组合而成。

位置 中极：脐下4寸。

膀胱俞：第二骶椎棘突下，旁开1.5寸。
主治　膀胱病证及其他泌尿生殖系统病证。
操作　刺法：直刺1～1.5寸。
灸法：艾炷灸5～9壮，或温灸10～20分钟。

Composition　This group of acupoints is composed of Zhongji (CV3) and Pangguangshu (BL28).

Location　Zhongji：4 cun below the centre of the umbilicus.

Pangguangshu：1.5 cun lateral to the sacral crest, at the level of the 2nd posterior sacral foramen.

Indication　Bladder diseases and other diseases of the urogenital system.

Method　Acupuncture：the needle is inserted 1−1.5 cun perpendicularly.

Moxibustion：moxibustion with 5−9 moxa cones, or warm moxibustion for 10−20 minutes is applied.

三焦募俞
Sanjiaomushu

组成　本穴组由石门、左右三焦俞共三穴组合而成。
位置　石门：脐下2寸。
三焦俞：第一腰椎棘突下，旁开1.5寸。
主治　三焦病证，水代谢障碍，如水肿、腹水、腹泄等。
操作　刺法：直刺1～1.5寸。
灸法：艾炷灸5～9壮，或温灸10～20分钟。

Composition　This group of acupoints is composed of Shimen (CV5) and Sanjiaoshu (BL22).

Location　Shimen：2 cun below the centre of the umbilicus.

Sanjiaoshu：1.5 cun lateral to the point below the spinous process of the 1st lumbar vertebra.

Indication　Sanjiao diseases, disorders of water metabolism, such as edema, ascites and diarrhea, etc..

Method　Acupuncture：the needle is inserted 1−1.5 cun perpendicularly.

Moxibustion：moxibustion with 5−9 moxa cones, or warm moxibustion for 10−20 minutes is applied.

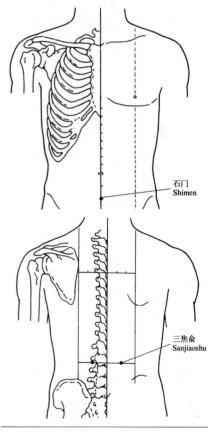

石门
Shimen

三焦俞
Sanjiaoshu

图 2-117　三焦募俞
Fig. 2-117　Sanjiaomushu

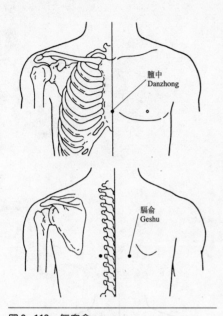

图2-118 气血会
Fig. 2-118 Qixuehui

气血会
Qixuehui

组成 本穴组由气会膻中、血会膈俞二穴组合而成。
位置 膻中：前正中线，平第四肋间隙。
膈俞：第七胸椎棘突下，旁开1.5寸。
主治 全身气血病证。
操作 刺法：斜刺0.5~0.8寸。
灸法：艾炷灸5~9壮，艾条温灸10~20分钟。

Composition This group of acupoints is composed of Danzhong (CV17), the Influential Point of Qi, and Geshu (BL17), the Influential Point of Blood.

Location Danzhong: on the anterior midline, at the level of the 4th intercostal space.

Geshu: 1.5 cun lateral to the point below the spinous process of the 7th thoracic vertebra.

Indication Diseases of Qi and blood of the whole body.

Method Acupuncture: the needle is inserted 0.5-0.8 cun obliquely.

Moxibustion: moxibustion with 5-9 moxa cones, or warm moxibustion with moxa roll for 10-20 minutes is applied.

脏腑会
Zangfuhui

组成 本穴组由脏会章门、腑会中脘二穴组合而成。
位置 章门：第十一肋端。
中脘：脐上4寸。
主治 一般脏腑病证。
操作 刺法：章门斜刺0.8~1寸。中脘直刺1~1.5寸。各以得气为度。
灸法：艾炷灸3-9壮，艾条温灸10~20分钟。

Composition This group of acupoints is composed of Zhangmen (LR13), the Influential Point of Zang-Organs, and Zhongwan (CV12), the Influential Point of Fu-Organs.

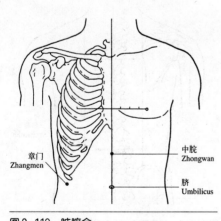

图2-119 脏腑会
Fig. 2-119 Zangfuhui

Location Zhangmen：at the end of the 11th rib.

Zhongwan：4 cun above the centre of the umbilicus.

Indication General diseases of Zang-Fu organs.

Methods Acupuncture：Zhangmen is inserted 0.8-1 cun obliquely.

Zhongwan is inserted 1-1.5 cun perpendicularly. Stop manipulating the needles till the acu-esthesia is obtained in both acupoints.

Moxibustion：moxibustion with 3-9 moxa cones, or warm moxibustion with moxa roll for 10-20 minutes is applied.

脏气会
Zangqihui

组成 本穴组由脏会章门、气会膻中二穴组合而成。

位置 章门：第十一肋端。

膻中：前正中线，平第四肋间隙。

主治 一般脏病。

操作 章门见"脏腑会"中章门穴操作。膻中见"气血会"中膻中穴操作。

Composition This group of acupoints is composed of Zhangmen (CV12), the Influential Point of Zang Organs, and Danzhong (CV17), the Influential Point of Qi.

Location Zhangmen：at the end of the 11th rib.

Danzhong：on the anterior midline, at the level of the 4th intercostal space.

Indications General diseases of Zang organs.

Method Zhangmen：See methods for Zhangmen in zangfuhui. Danzhong：See methods for Danzhong in Qixuehui.

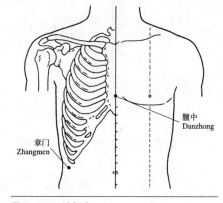

图 2-120 脏气会
Fig. 2-120 Zangqihui

脏血会
Zangxuehui

组成 本穴组由脏会章门、血会膈俞二穴组合而成。

位置 章门：第十一肋端。

膈俞：第七胸椎棘突下，旁开1.5寸。

主治　脏病血病及内脏血证。

操作　章门见"脏腑会"中章门穴操作。膈俞见"气血会"中膈俞穴操作。

Composition　This group of acupoints is composed of Zhangmen (LR13), the Influential Point of Zang Organs, and Geshu (BL17), the Influential Point of Blood.

Location　Zhangmen：at the end of the 11th rib.

Geshu：1.5 cun lateral to the point below the spinous process of the 7th thoracic vertebra.

Indication　Diseases of Zang organs, blood diseases, and blood syndromes of the visera.

Method　Zhangmen：See methods for Zhangmen in Zangfuhui. Geshu：See methods for Geshu in Qixuehui.

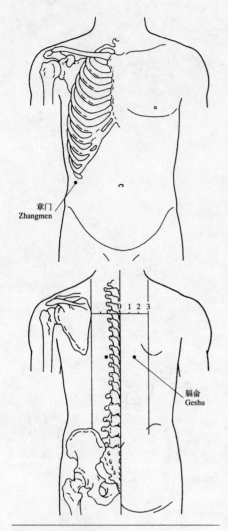

图 2-121　脏血会
Fig. 2-121　Zangxuehui

● 腑气会
Fuqihui

组成　本穴组由腑会中脘、气会膻中二穴组合而成。

位置　中脘：脐上 4 寸。

膻中：前正中线，平第四肋间隙。

主治　一般腑病，上中焦气机不利。

操作　中脘见"脏腑会"中中脘穴操作。膻中见"气血会"中膻中穴操作。

Composition　This group of acupoints is composed of Zhongwan (CV12), the Influential Point of Fu Organs, and Danzhong (CV17), the Influential Point of Qi.

Location　Zhongwan：4 cun above the centre of the umbilicus.

Danzhong：on the anterior midline, at the level of the 4th intercostal space.

Indication　Diseases of Fu organs, Qi disorders in upper and middle jiao.

Method　Zhongwan：See methods for zhongwan in Zangfuhui、Danzhong：See methods for Danzhong in Qixuehui.

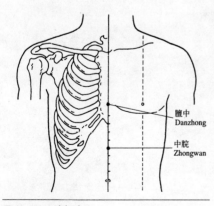

图 2-122　腑气会
Fig. 2-122　Fuqihui

腑血会
Fuxuehui

组成 本穴组由腑会中脘、血会膈俞二穴组合而成。

位置 中脘：脐上4寸。

膈俞：第七胸椎棘突下，旁开1.5寸。

主治 腑病，血病。

操作 中脘见"脏腑会"中中脘穴。膈俞见"气血会"中膈俞穴。

Composition This group of acupoints is composed of Zhongwan (CV12), the Influential Point of Fu Organs, and Geshu (GB17), the Influential Point of Blood.

Location Zhongwan：4 cun above the centre of the umbilicus.

Geshu：1.5 cun lateral to the point below the spinous process of the 7th thoracic vertebra.

Indication Diseases of Fu organs and blood diseases.

Method Zhongwan：See methods for zhongwan in Zangfuhui. Geshu：See methods for Geshu in Qixuehui.

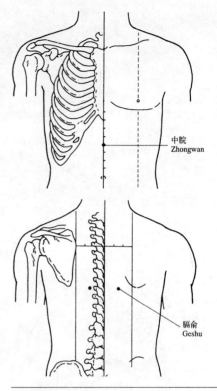

图2-123 腑血会
Fig. 2-123 Fuxuehui

气魄谚
Qipoyi

组成 本穴组由气舍、魄户、谚谵三穴组合而成。

位置 气舍：人迎直下、锁骨上缘，在胸锁乳突肌的胸骨头与锁骨头之间。

魄户：第三胸椎棘突下，旁开3寸。

谚谵：第六胸椎棘突下，旁开3寸。

主治 咳逆上气，胸部憋闷。

操作 刺法：针0.3~0.8寸，留针30分钟。

灸法：灸5~9壮，甚可则至15壮。

Composition This group of acupoints is composed of Qishe (ST11), Pohu (BL42) and Yixi (BL45).

Location Qishe：directly below Renying, on the upper border of the clavicle, between the sternal and clavicular heads of the sternocleidomastoid muscle.

Pohu：3 cun lateral to the point below the spinous process of the 3rd thoracic vertebra.

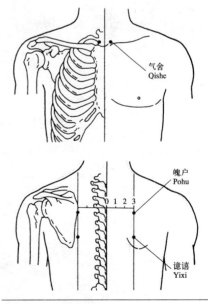

图2-124 气魄谚
Fig. 2-124 Qipoyi

Yixi: 3 cun lateral to the point below the spinous process of the 6th thoracic vertebra.

Indications Cough and reversed Qi, fullness in the chest.

Method Acupuncture: the needle is inserted 0.3-0.8 cun and retained for 30 minutes.

Moxibustion: 5-9 cones or even 15 cones of moxibustion can be applied.

⬤ 膻肺
Tanfei

组成 本穴组由膻中、肺俞二穴组合而成。
位置 膻中：前正中线，平第四肋间隙。
肺俞：第三胸椎棘突下，旁开1.5寸。
主治 哮喘。
操作 沿皮刺膻中1~1.5寸，再由上外方向下内方斜刺肺俞0.5~0.8寸，起针后于二穴止拔罐5~10分钟。

Composition This group of acupoints is composed of Danzhong (CV17) and Feishu (BL13).

Location Danzhong: on the anterior midline, at the level of the 4th intercostal space.

Feishu: 1.5 cun lateral to the point below the spinous process of the 3rd thoracic vertebra.

Indication Asthma.

Method Danzhong is needled 1-1.5 cun under the skin first, then Feishu is needled 0.5-0.8 cun downwards and inwards. Cupping for 5-10 minutes is applied after the withdrawal of needles.

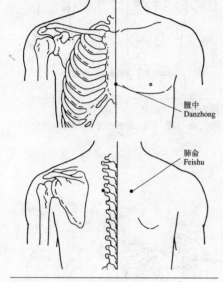

膻中
Danzhong

肺俞
Feishu

图2-125 膻肺
Fig. 2-125 Tanfei

⬤ 清胸热
Qingxiongre

组成 本穴组由大杼、背俞、中府三穴组合而成。
位置 大杼：第一胸椎棘突下，旁开1.5寸。
背俞：第二胸椎棘突下旁开1.5寸。
中府：胸前壁外上方，前正中线旁开6寸，平第一肋间隙处。

主治 胸肺热甚。

操作 先刺中府，再刺背俞、大杼，均用泻法，得气后留针15分钟，出针。缺盆用梅花针敲击稍见血。

Composition This group of acupoints is composed of Dazhu (BL11), Fengmen (BL12) and Zhongfu (LV1).

Location Dazhu：1.5 cun lateral to the point below the spinous process of thc 1st thoracic vertebra.

Fengmen：1.5 cun lateral to the point below the spinous process of the 2nd thoracic vertebra.

Zhongfu：on the superior and lateral part of the thoracic wall, 6 cun lateral to the anterior midline, at the level of the 1st intercostal space.

Indication Fever in the chest and lung.

Method Zhongfu is needles first, then Dazhu and Fengmen. Reducing method is applied to all points. Retain the needles for 15 minutes after the acu-esthesia is obtained. After the needles are withdrawn, Quepen is tapped to bleed slightly by the plum-blossom needle.

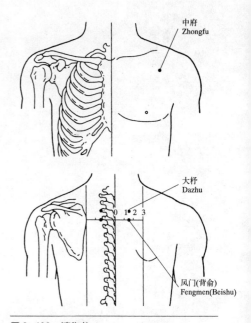

图2-126 清胸热
Fig. 2-126 Qingxiongre

咳喘
Kechuan

组成 本穴组由天突、膻中、肺俞、定喘四穴组合而成。
位置 天突：胸骨上窝正中。

膻中：前正中线，平第四肋间隙。

肺俞：第三胸椎棘突下，旁开1.5寸。

定喘：大椎穴旁开0.5寸。

主治 咳嗽，气喘。

操作 刺法：天突先直刺0.2寸，然后将针尖转向下方、紧靠胸骨后方刺入1~1.5寸，亦或向下斜刺0.3~0.5寸，得气为度。膻中平刺0.3~0.5寸。肺俞、定喘向脊椎方向斜刺0.5~0.8寸，得气为度。

灸法：艾炷灸5~9壮，温灸10~20分钟。

Composition This group of acupoints is composed of Tiantu (CV22), Danzhong (CV17), Feishu (BL13) and Dingchuan (EX-B1).

Location Tiantu：in the centre of the suprasternal fossa.

Danzhong：on the anterior midline, at the level of the 4th intercostal space.

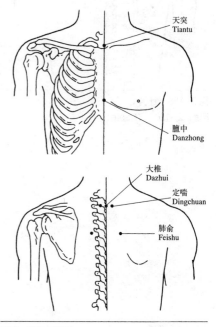

图2-127 咳喘
Fig. 2-127 Kechuan

Feishu：1.5 cun lateral to the point below the spinous process of the 3rd thoracic vertebra.

Dingchuang：0.5 cun lateral to Dazhui.

Indications　Cough and asthma.

Methods　Acupuncture：Tiantu：the needle is inserted 0.2 cun perpendicularly first, then it is inserted 1—1.5 cun downwards under sternum, or inserted 0.3—0.5 cun downwards obliquely, till the acu-esthesia is obtained. Danzhong：the needle is inserted 0.3—0.5 cun horizontally. Feishu, Dingchuan：the needle is inserted 0.5—0.8 cun obliquely towards the spine, till the acu-esthesia is obtained.

Moxibustion：moxibustion with 5—9 moxa cones, or warm moxibustion for 10—20 minutes is applied.

针劳
Zhenlao

组成　本穴组由膏肓、百劳二穴组合而成。
位置　膏肓：第四胸椎棘突下，旁开3寸。
百劳：第七颈椎棘突下的大椎穴直上2寸，再旁开1寸处。
主治　痨病。
操作　刺法：向脊椎方向斜刺0.5～0.8寸，百劳也可直刺1～1.5寸。
灸法：艾炷灸5～15壮，或累计灸百壮或百壮以上等。

Composition　This group of acupoints is composed of Gaohuang (BL43) and Bailao.

Location　Gaohuang：3 cun lateral to the point below the spinous process of the 4th thoracic vertebra.

Bailao：1 cun lateral to the point 2 cun directly above Dazhui which is below the spinous process of the 7th cervical vertebra.

Indication　Phthisis.

Methods　Acupuncture：the needle is inserted 0.5—0.8 cun obliquely towards the spine. Bailao can be needled 1—1.5 cun perpendicularly.

Moxibustion：moxibustion with 5—15 moxa cones, or separated moxibustion up to one hundred cones is applied.

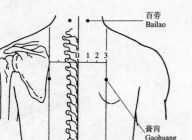

图2—128　针劳
Fig. 2—128　Zhenlao

里四灵
Lisiling

组成　本穴组由膏肓、里期门二穴组合而成。

位置　膏肓：第四胸椎棘突下，旁开3寸。

里期门：乳头直下第六肋间隙内侧0.5寸处。

主治　虚损，羸瘦。

操作　灸5～9壮，或可用累计灸百壮。

Composition　This group of acupoints is composed of Gaohuang (BL43) and Liqimen.

Location　Gaohuang：3 cun lateral to the point below the spinous process of the 4th thoracic vertebra.

Liqimen：0.5 cun medial to Qimen (LR14), in the 6th intercostal space.

Indications　Emaciation and weak constitution.

Method　5−9 cones of moxibustion or separated moxibustion up to one hundred cones is applied.

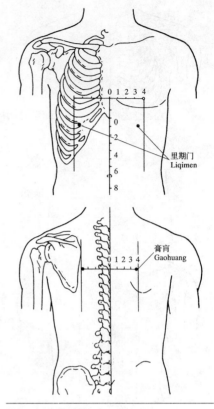

图2-129　里四灵
Fig. 2−129　Lisiling

驻泻
Zhuxie

组成　本穴组由神阙、关元、脾俞、大肠俞四穴组合而成。

位置　神阙：脐的中间。

关元：脐下3寸。

脾俞：第十一胸椎棘突下，旁开1.5寸。

大肠俞：第四腰椎棘突下，旁开1.5寸。

主治　老年人与体质虚弱者泄泻日久，大便时溏时泻，不思饮食，身倦乏力。

操作　先温灸关元30分钟，同时用隔盐灸神阙5～9壮。再温灸脾俞、大肠俞20分钟。

Composition　This group of acupoints is composed of Shenque (CV8), Guanyuan (CV4), Pishu (BL20) and Dachangshu (BL25).

Location　Shenque：in the centre of the umbilicus.

Guanyuan：3 cun below the centre of the umbilicus.

Pishu：1.5 cun lateral to the point below the spinous process of the 11th thoracic vertebra.

Dachangshu：1.5 cun lateral to the point below the

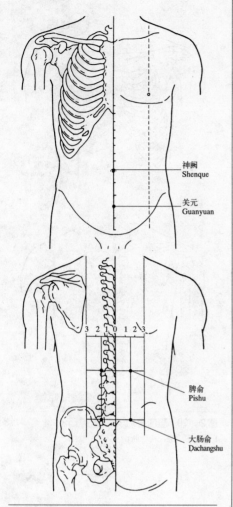

神阙
Shenque

关元
Guanyuan

脾俞
Pishu

大肠俞
Dachangshu

图2-130 驻泻
Fig. 2-130 Zhuxie

spinous process of the 4th lumbar vertebra.

Indications Loose stool, diarrhea, anorexia, fatigue in the elderly and the weak people who have prolonged diarrhea.

Method First warm moxibustion is applied to Guanyuan for 30 minutes, at the same time 5-9 cones of salt-cushioned moxibustion is applied to Shenque. Then warm moxibustion is applied to Pishu and Dachangshu for 20 minutes.

虚劳
Xulao

组成　本穴组由膈俞、胆俞、气海、长强四穴组合而成。

位置　膈俞：第七胸椎棘突下，旁开1.5寸。

胆俞：第十胸椎棘突下，旁开1.5寸。

气海：脐下1.5寸。

长强：尾骨尖下0.5寸，约当尾骨尖端与肛门的中点。

主治　五劳七伤，气血虚损，骨蒸潮热，咳嗽痰喘，五心烦热，四肢困倦，羸弱等。

操作　脊柱两旁的四穴同时灸，初灸7壮或14壮或21壮，以至百壮为妙。俟灸疮将瘥，或火疮发时，灸脊柱上两穴，一次灸3~5壮。

按注　不可多灸，多则恐人倦怠。凡此六穴，宜择离日火日灸之。灸后百日内宜慎房劳思虑，饮食应时，寒暑得中，将养调护，若疮愈后仍觉未瘥，依前法再灸，无不愈者。

Composition This group of acupoints is composed of Geshu, Danshu, Qihai (CV6) and Changqiang (CV1).

Location Geshu：which is 1.5 cun lateral to the point below the spinous process of the 7th thoracic vertebra.

Danshu：which is 1.5 cun lateral to the point below the spinous process of the 10th thoracic vertebra.

Qihai：1.5 cun below the centre of the umbilicus.

Changqiang：0.5 cun below the tip of the coccyx, at the midpoint of the line connecting the tip of the coccyx and anus.

Indications Phthisis, deficiency of Qi and blood, afternoon fever, cough, asthma, excessive heat in palms and soles, fatigue in the four limbs, emaciation, etc..

Method　Moxibustion is applied to the four points, 7 or 14, 21 cones or even one hundred cones are advisable. Moxibustion is applied to the two points on the spine when the scar is going to heal up, or when the blister is induced, 3—5 cones for each treatment.

Note　It's not appropriate to apply moxibustion excessively or else it will result in fatigue of the patient. It's advisable to apply moxibustion to the six points on Li day and Fire day. During one hundred days after the treatment, the patient should avoid the sexual intercourse and pensiveness. Pay attention to the cultivation of health, which contains appropriate food and environmental temperature. If the disease doesn't heal, the same method can be applied again, and the disease will be surely cured.

消痞
Xiaopi

组成　本穴组由中脘、章门、脊中三穴组合而成。

位置　中脘：脐上4寸。

章门：第十一肋端。

脊中：第十一胸椎棘突下。

主治　痰食凝结痞块。

操作　先取坐位针脊中，深0.3~0.5寸，得气后持续运针两分钟左右、出针；然后仰卧位针中脘0.5~1寸，使针感沿任脉向上、下放散；章门针0.5~0.7寸。诸穴得气后留针30分钟。

Composition　This group of acupoints is composed of Zhongwan (CV12), Zhangmen (LR13) and Jizhong(GV6).

Location　Zhongwan：4 cun above the centre of the umbilicus.

Zhangmen：at the end of the 11th rib.

Jizhong：below the spinous process of the 11th thoracic vertebra.

Indication　Abdominal masses due to phlegm or food.

Method　Jizhong is needled 0.3—0.5 cun first when the sitting position is selected, and keep on manipulating the needle for about 2 minutes after the acu-esthesia is

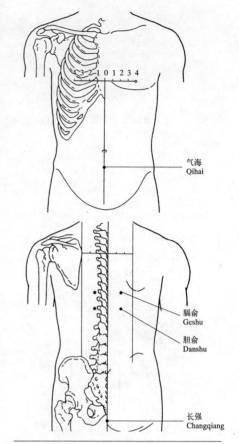

图 2-131　虚劳
Fig. 2-131　Xulao

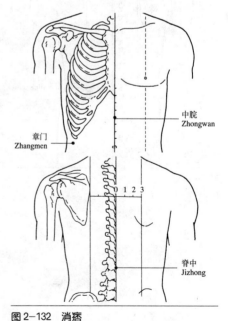

图 2-132　消痞
Fig. 2-132　Xiaopi

obtained. Withdraw the needle. The supine position is selected, Zhongwan is needled 0.5−1 cun and the acuesthesia should spread upwards and downwards along the Conception Vessel. Zhangmen is needled 0.5−0.7 cun. Retain the needles for 30 minutes after the acu−esthesia is obtained in all the points.

四神
Sishen

组成 本穴组由命门、天枢、气海、关元四穴组合而成。

位置 命门：第二腰椎棘突下。

天枢：脐旁2寸。

气海：脐下1.5寸。

关元：脐下3寸。

主治 脾肾阳虚，五更泻泄。

操作 先刺天枢、气海、关元，直刺1～1.5寸，针刺用补法，留针20分钟，同时加灸3～5壮；然后直刺命门1～1.2寸，针用补法，留针10分钟，同时加灸3～5壮。

Composition This group of acupoints is composed of Mingmen (GV4), Tianshu (ST25), Qihai (CV6) and Guanyuan (CV4).

Location Mingmen：below the spinous process of the 2nd lumbar vertebra.

Tianshu：2 cun lateral to the centre of the umbilicus.

Qihai：1.5 cun below the centre of the umbilicus.

Guanyuan：3 cun below the centre of the umbilicus.

Indication Yang deficiency of spleen and kidney, diarrhea at dawn.

Method Tianshu, Qihai and Guanyuan are needled 1−1.5 cun perpendicularly first, and the nourishing method is applied. Retain the needles for 20 minutes, and apply 3−5 cones of moxibustion at the same time. Then Mingmen is needled 1−1.2 cun perpendicularly, the reinforcing method is applied. Retain the needle for 10 minutes, apply 3−5 cones of moxibustion simultaneously.

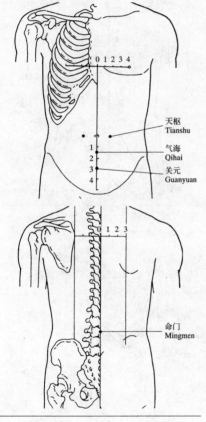

图2-133 四神
Fig. 2-133 Sishen

阳三针
Yangsanzhen

组成　本穴组由关元、气海、肾俞三穴组合而成。

位置　关元：脐下3寸。

气海：脐下1.5寸。

肾俞：第二腰椎棘突下，旁开1.5寸。

主治　阳痿，遗精，不育。

操作　关元、气海，直刺0.8~1寸，以向前阴放射为佳。

肾俞直刺1.2~1.5寸，得气为度。

Composition　This group of acupoints is composed of Guanyuan (CV4), Qihai (CV6) and Shenshu (BL23).

Location　Guanyuan：3 cun below the centre of the umbilicus.

Qihai：1.5 cun below the centre of the umbilicus.

Shenshu：1.5 cun lateral to the point below the spinous process of the 2nd lumbar vertebra.

Indication　Impotence, seminal emission and sterility.

Method　Guanyuan and Qihai are needled 0.8-1 cun perpendicularly. It will be better if the acu-esthesia radiates to the pubes. Shenshu is needled 1.2-1.5 cun perpendicularly till the acu-esthesia is obtained.

去相火
Quxianghuo

组成　本穴组由中极、曲骨、膏肓、肾俞四穴组合而成。

位置　中极：脐下4寸。

曲骨：耻骨联合上缘中点处。

膏肓：第四胸椎棘突下，旁开3寸。

肾俞：第二腰椎棘突下，旁开1.5寸。

主治　相火妄动之遗精，阳强易举，有梦而遗，或无梦滑泄。

操作　先针刺膏肓，深0.5~0.8寸；肾俞深1~1.5寸，得气后持续运针1分钟出针；再针刺中极、曲骨，得气后使针感传导放散至外生殖器，留针20~30分钟。

Composition　This group of acupoints is composed of Zhongji (CV3), Qugu (CV2), Gaohuang (BL43) and Shenshu

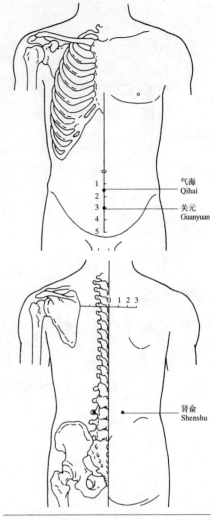

图2-134　阳三针
Fig. 2-134　Yangsanzhen

(BL23).

Location Zhongji：4 cun below the umbilicus.

Qugu：at the midpoint of the upper border of the pubic symphysis.

Gaohuang：3 cun lateral to the point below the spinous process of the 4th thoracic vertebra.

Shenshu：1.5 cun lateral to the point below the spinous process of the 2nd lumbar vertebra.

Indication Seminal emission due to hyperactive Xiang Fire, easy erection of the penis, nocturnal emission with dream, spermatorrhea without dream.

Method First, Gaohuang is needled 0.5−0.8 cun, Shenshu 1−1.5 cun. Withdraw the needles after manipulating them for 1 minute after the acu-esthesia is obtained. Then Zhongji and Qugu are needled, after the arrival of the acu-esthesia, manipulate the needles in order to induce the feeling to the pubes, retain the needles for 20−30 minutes.

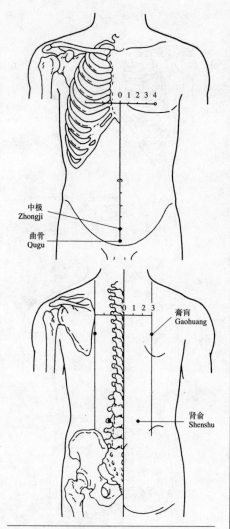

中极
Zhongji

曲骨
Qugu

膏肓
Gaohuang

肾俞
Shenshu

图 2-135 去相火
Fig. 2-135 Quxianghuo

止带
Zhidai

组成 本穴组由命门、神阙、中极三穴组合而成。

位置 命门：第二腰椎棘突下。

神阙：脐的中间。

中极：脐下 4 寸。

主治 寒湿型带下，量多，稀薄色白，无特殊气味，面色㿠白，肢体倦怠，腰酸腿软，头晕眼花，食欲不振。

操作 先取俯卧位针刺中极，使针感放散至阴部，留针20～30分钟，二穴均用平补平泻法；神阙穴隔姜灸5～7壮。

Composition This group of acupoints is composed of Mingmen (GV4), Shenque (CV8) and Zhongji (CV3).

Location Mingmen：below the spinous process of the 2nd lumbar vertebra.

Shenque：in the centre of the umbilicus.

Zhongji：4 cun below the centre of the umbilicus.

Indications Profuse thin and white leukorrhea due to cold and dampness without special smell, pale complexion, fatigue, aching and weak in the lower back and the lower limbs, dizziness, blurred vision, poor appetite.

Method Prone position is selected to puncture Zhongji, and the acu-esthesia should radiate to the pubes, retain the needle for 20−30 minutes. Even reinforcing-reducing techniques are applied to both points. 5−7 cones of ginger−cushioned moxibustion is applied to Shenque.

肝命
Ganming

组成　本穴组由肝俞、命门二穴组合而成。

位置　肝俞：第九胸椎棘突下，旁开1.5寸。

命门：第二腰椎棘突下。

主治　青盲，暴盲。

操作　肝俞向脊柱方向斜刺0.5～0.8寸。命门由下而上斜刺0.5～0.8寸，得气为度。

Composition This group of acupoints is composed of Ganshu (BL18) and Mingmen (GV4).

Location Ganshu：1.5 cun lateral to the point below the spinous process of the 9th thoracic vertebra.

Mingmen：below the spinous process of the 2nd lumbar vertebra.

Indication Glaucoma and sudden blindness.

Method Ganshu is needled 0.5−0.8 cun obliquely towards the spine.

Mingmen is needled 0.5−0.8 cun obliquely upwards till the acu-esthesia is obtained.

壮阳
Zhuangyang

组成　本穴组由命门、神阙二穴组合而成。

位置　命门：第二腰椎棘突下。

神阙：脐的中间。

主治　神昏肢逆，目合口开，手撒尿遗，鼻鼾或呼吸衰微，汗出痰壅等。

操作　命门用大艾炷灸，神阙用隔盐灸，不拘壮数。

Composition This group of acupoints is composed of

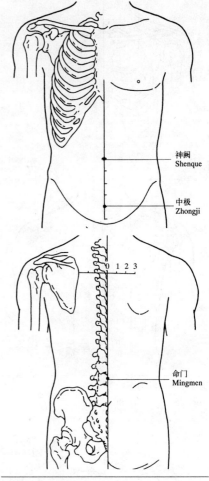

图 2-136　止带
Fig. 2-136　Zhidai

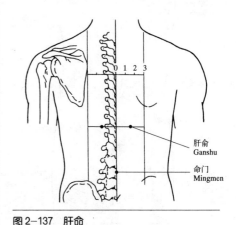

图 2-137　肝命
Fig. 2-137　Ganming

Mingmen (GV4) and Shenque (CV8).

Location Mingmen: below the spinous process of the 2nd lumbar vertebra.

Shenque: in the centre of the umbilicus.

Indications Loss of consciousness and cold limbs with closed eyes and open mouth, paralysis of limbs and incontinence of urine, feeble breathing, sweating and obstruction of the phlegm.

Method Moxibustion with big moxa cone is applied to Mingmen.

Salt-cushioned moxibustion is applied to Shenque without calculating the number of cones.

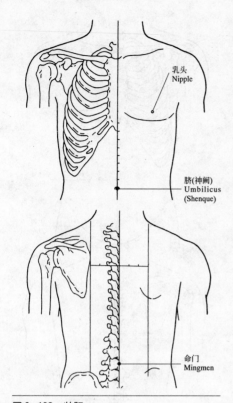

图2-138 壮阳
Fig. 2-138 Zhuangyang

● 四根岔
Sigencha

组成 本穴组由四根岔与环跳穴组成。

位置 四根岔：于肩前部，腋前皱襞直上1.5寸处。

环跳：股骨大转子高点与骶管裂孔连线处外1/3与内2/3交界处。

主治 瘫痪，肢痛。

操作 四根岔针1寸，环跳针2～3寸，针感分别向上肢下肢尖端放散。

Composition This group of acupoints is composed of Sigencha and Huantiao (GB30).

Location Sigencha: on the anterior part of the shoulder, 1.5 cun directly above the upper end of the anterior axillary fold.

Huantiao: at the junction of the lateral one-third and medial two-thirds of the line connecting the prominence of the great trochanter and the sacral hiatus.

Indication Paralysis and pain in the limbs.

Method Sigencha is needled 1 cun while Huantiao is needled 2-3 cun. The acu-esthesia will spread to the end of the upper and the lower limbs respectively.

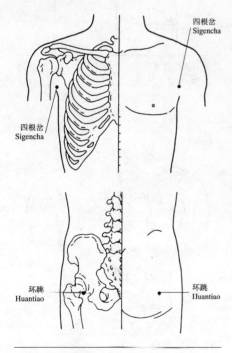

图2-139 四根岔
Fig. 2-139 Sigencha

四逆
Sini

组成　本穴组由气海、肾俞、肝俞三穴组合而成。

位置　气海：脐下1.5寸。

肾俞：第二腰椎棘突下，旁开1.5寸。

肝俞：第九胸椎棘突下，旁开1.5寸。

主治　四肢厥逆，面目清冷，蜷曲而卧，下利清谷，意识朦胧。

操作　先灸气海7~21壮，再灸肾俞、肝俞5~7壮。

Composition　This group of acupoints is composed of Qihai (CV6), Shenshu (BL23) and Ganshu (BL18).

Location　Qihai：1.5 cun below the centre of the umbilicus.

Shenshu：1.5 cun lateral to the point below the spinous process of the 2nd lumbar vertebra.

Ganshu：1.5 cun lateral to the point below the spinous process of the 9th thoracic vertebra.

Indication　Cold limbs and face, chills, dirrhea with undigested food, unconsciousness.

Method　7－21 cones of Moxibustion is applied to Qihai first, then 5－7 cones are applied to Shenshu and Ganshu respectively.

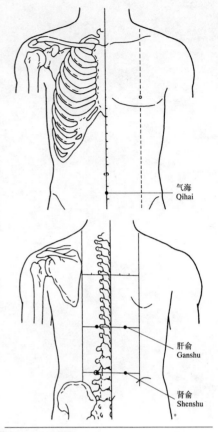

气海
Qihai

肝俞
Ganshu

肾俞
Shenshu

图2-140　四逆
Fig. 2-140　Sini

第三章　四肢部组合穴

CHAPTER 3 COMPOSED ACUPOINTS ON THE FOUR LIMBS

● 心原络
Xinyuanluo

组成　本穴组由神门和支正二穴组合而成。

位置　神门：腕横纹尺侧端，尺侧腕屈肌腱的桡侧凹陷中。

支正：阳谷穴与小海穴的连线上，阳谷穴上5寸。

主治　心脏及其经脉所属病证如心绞痛，心动过速，口干，目黄，上肢尺侧痛等。

操作　刺法：直刺或斜刺0.5～1寸。

灸法：麦粒灸1～3壮，或温灸5～10分钟。

Composition　This group of acupoints is composed of Shenmen (HT7) and Zhizheng (SI7).

Location　Shenmen：on the ulnar end of the palmar crease of the wrist, in the depression of the radial side of the tendon of the ulnar flexor muscle of the wrist.

Zhizheng：on the line connecting Yanggu (SI5) and Xiaohai (SI8), 5 cun above Yanggu.

Indication　Diseases of the heart and the Heart Meridian：angina, tachycardia, dryness of the mouth, yellowish sclera, pain in the ulnar side of the upper limbs, etc..

Method　Acupuncture：the needle is inserted 0.5-1 cun perpendicularly or obliquely.

Moxibustion：1-3 cones of moxibustion, or warm moxibustion for 5-10 wheat-sized moxa minutes is applied.

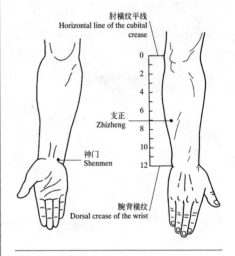

图3-1　心原络
Fig. 3-1　Xinyuanluo

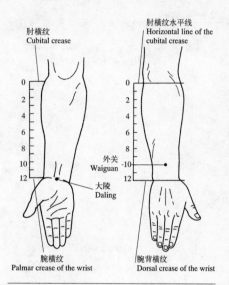

肘横纹
Cubital crease

肘横纹水平线
Horizontal line of the cubital crease

0
2
4
6
8
10
12

0
2
4
6
8
-10
12

外关
Waiguan

大陵
Daling

腕横纹
Palmar crease of the wrist

腕背横纹
Dorsal crease of the wrist

图3-2 心包原络
Fig. 3-2 Xinbaoyuanluo

心包原络
Xinbaoyuanluo

组成 本穴组由大陵、外关二穴组合而成。

位置 大陵: 腕横纹中央,掌长肌腱与桡侧腕屈肌腱之间。

外关: 腕背横纹上2寸,桡骨与尺骨之间。

主治 心包及其经脉所属病证,如前臂及手指痉挛,疼痛,胸胁痛,心悸,心烦,心区痛,掌心发热,喜笑不休等。

操作 刺法: 直刺0.5~1寸。

灸法: 麦粒灸3~5壮,或温灸5~10分钟。

Composition This group of acupoints is composed of Daling (PC7) and Waiguan (TE5).

Location Daling: at the midpoint of the palmar crease of the wrist, between the tendons of the long palmar muscle and radial flexor muscle of the wrist.

Waiguan: 2 cun above the dorsal crease of the wrist, between the radius and ulna.

Indication Diseases of the pericardium and the Pericardium Meridian: convulsion and pain of the forearm and the fingers, pain in the chest and hypochondriac region, palpitation, irritability, pain in the precardiac region, heat in the palms, manic, etc..

Method Acupuncture: the needle is inserted 0.5–1 cun perpendicularly.

Moxibustion: 3–5 wheat-sized moxa cones of moxibustion, or warm moxibustion for 5–10 minutes is applied.

肺原络
Feiyuanluo

组成 本穴组由太渊、偏历二穴组合而成。

位置 太渊: 掌后腕横纹桡侧端,桡动脉的桡侧凹陷中。

偏历: 在阳溪穴与曲池穴连线上,阳溪穴上3寸处。

主治 肺脏及其经脉所属病证,如气管炎,咽喉炎,气短,痰多,出汗,掌心发热,肩内侧痛,两乳痛等。

操作 刺法: 直刺或斜刺0.5~1寸。

灸法: 麦粒灸3~5壮,或温灸5~10分钟。

Composition This group of acupoints is composed of Taiyuan (LU9) and Pianli (LI6).

Location Taiyuan：at the radial end of the palmar crease of the wrist, in the depression of the radial side of the radial artery.

Pianli：on the line connecting Yangxi (LI5) and Quchi (LI11), 3 cun above Yangxi.

Indication Diseases of the lung and the Lung Meridian：tracheitis, faucitis, shortness of breath, profuse phlegm, sweating, heat in the palms, pain in the medial aspect of the shoulder, pain in the breasts, etc..

Method Acupuncture：the needle is inserted 0.5−1 cun perpendicularly or obliquely.

Moxibustion：3−5 cones of moxibustion, or warm moxibustion for 5−10 wheat-sized moxa minutes is applied.

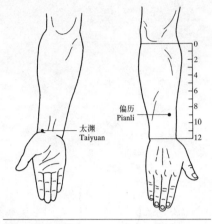

图 3−3　肺原络
Fig. 3−3　Feiyuanluo

 小肠原络
Xiaochangyuanluo

组成　本穴组由腕骨、通里二穴组合而成。

位置　腕骨：后溪穴直上，于第五掌骨基底与三角骨之间赤白肉际取之。

通里：腕横纹上1寸，尺侧腕屈肌腱的桡侧。

主治　小肠及其经脉所属病证，如下颌肿痛，肩痛，颈痛，耳聋，上肢外后侧痛等。

操作　刺法：直刺0.3～0.5寸。

灸法：麦粒灸3～5壮，或温灸5～10分钟。

Composition This group of acupoints is composed of Wangu (SI4) and Tongli (HT5).

Location Wangu：directly above Houxi (SI3), on the junction of the red and white skin between the basal part of the 5th metacarpal bone and triangular bone.

Tongli：1 cun above the palmar crease of the wrist, on the radial side of the tendon of the ulnar flexor muscle of the wrist.

Indication Diseases of the small intestine and the Small Intestine Meridian：swelling and pain of the jaw, pain in the shoulder and neck, deafness, pain in the lateral and posterior side of the upper limbs, etc..

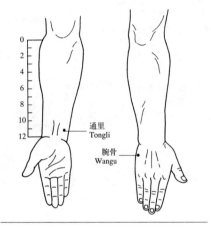

图 3−4　小肠原络
Fig. 3−4　Xiaochangyuanluo

Method Acupuncture: the needle is inserted 0.3−0.5 cun perpendicularly.

Moxibustion: 3−5 wheat−sized moxa cones of moxibustion, or warm moxibustion for 5−10 minutes is applied.

● 大肠原络
Dachangyuanluo

组成 本穴组由合谷、列缺二穴组合而成。

位置 合谷：手背，第一、第二掌骨之间，约平第二掌骨中点处。

列缺：桡骨茎突上方，腕横纹上1.5寸。

主治 大肠及其经脉所属病证，如齿龈炎，牙神经痛，颌下淋巴腺炎，腮腺炎，咽喉炎，口干，目黄，鼻流清涕，肩前侧痛等。

操作 刺法：合谷直刺0.5～1寸。列缺斜刺0.3～0.5寸。

灸法：麦粒灸3～5壮，或温灸5～10分钟。

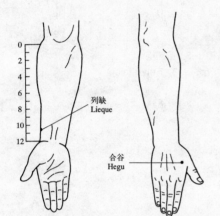

图3-5 大肠原络
Fig. 3-5 Dachangyuanluo

Composition This group of acupoints is composed of Hegu (LI4) and Lieque (LV7).

Location Hegu: on the dorsum of the hand, between the 1st and 2nd metacarpal bones, and near the midpoint of the 2nd metacarpal bone.

Lieque: on the styloid process of the radius, 1.5 cun above the palmar crease of the wrist.

Indication Diseases of the large intestine and the Large Intestine Meridian: gingivitis, toothache, sabmandibular lymphadenitis, parotitis, faucitis, dryness of the mouth, yellowish sclera, thin nasal discharge, pain in the anterior side of the shoulder, etc..

Method Acupuncture: Hegu is needled 0.5−1 cun perpendicularly, Lieque is needled 0.3−0.5 cun obliquely.

Moxibustion: 3−5 wheat−sized moxa cones of moxibustion, or warm moxibustion for 5−10 minutes is applied.

三焦原络
Sanjiaoyuanluo

组成 本穴组由阳池、内关二穴组合而成。

位置 阳池：腕背横纹中，指总伸肌腱尺侧缘凹陷中。

内关：腕横纹上2寸，掌长肌腱与桡侧腕屈肌腱之间。

主治 三焦及其经脉所属病证，如耳聋，咽喉炎，结膜炎，肩背痛，脊间痛，便秘，尿闭，遗尿等。

操作 刺法：直刺0.5~1寸。

灸法：麦粒灸3~5壮，或温灸5~10分钟。

Composition This group of acupoints is composed of Yangchi (TE4) and Neiguan (PC6).

Location Yangchi：at the midpoint of the dorsal crease of the wrist, in the depression on the ulnar side of the tendon of the extensor muscle of the fingers.

Neiguan：2 cun above the palmar crease of the wrist, between the tendons of the long palmar muscle and radial flexor muscle of the wrist.

Indication Diseases of Triple Energizer and the Triple Energizer Meridian：deafness, faucitis, conjunctivitis, pain in the shoulder and back, pain in the spine, constipation, retention of urine, enuresis, etc..

Method Acupuncture：the needle is inserted 0.5−1 cun perpendicularly.

Moxibustion：3−5 wheat-sized moxa cones of moxibustion, or warm moxibustion for 5−10 minutes is applied.

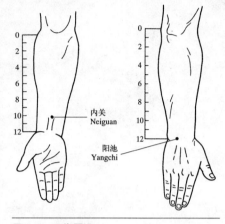

图3-6 三焦原络
Fig. 3-6 Sanjiaoyuanluo

心荥输
Xinyingshu

组成 本穴组由少府、神门二穴组合而成。

位置 少府：第四、第五掌骨之间，握拳，当小指端与环指端之间。

神门：腕横纹尺侧端，尺侧腕屈肌腱的桡侧凹陷中。

主治 心脑神志疾病等。

操作 针0.3~0.5寸，局部酸胀痛感。

Composition This group of acupoints is composed of

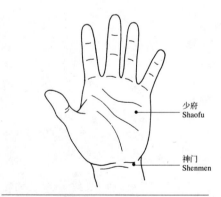

图3-7 心荥输
Fig. 3-7 Xinyingshu

Shaofu (HT8) and Shenmen (HT7).

Location　Shaofu：between the 4th and 5th metacarpal bones, i.e. between the tips of the ring finger and little finger.

Shenmen：on the ulnar end of the palmar crease of the wrist, in the depression of the radial side of the tendon of the ulnar flexor muscle of the wrist.

Indication　Diseases of the heart, brain and mind, etc..

Method　The needle is inserted 0.3—0.5 cun, the acuesthesia will be soreness, distension and pain in this part.

● 心包荥输
Xinbaoyingshu

组成　本穴组由劳宫、大陵二穴组合而成。
位置　劳宫：第二、第三掌骨之间，握拳，中指尖下是穴。
大陵：腕横纹中央，掌长肌腱与桡侧腕屈肌腱之间。
主治　心包病证，神志病，热病。
操作　针0.5~1寸，局部酸、麻、胀、痛感。

Composition　This group of acupoints is composed of Laogong (PC8) and Daling (PC7).

Location　Laogong：between the 2nd and 3rd metacarpal bones, where the tip of the middle finger reaches when a fist is made.

Daling：at the midpoint of the palmar crease of the wrist, between the tendons of the long palmar muscle and radial flexor muscle of the wrist.

Indication　Diseases of the pericardium, mind diseases, febrile diseases.

Method　The needle is inserted 0.5—1 cun. The acuesthesia of soreness, numbness, distension and pain will be obtained in this part.

● 肺荥输
Feiyingshu

组成　本穴组由鱼际、太渊二穴组合而成。

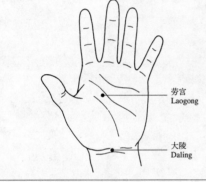

劳宫
Laogong

大陵
Daling

图3-8　心包荥输
Fig. 3-8　Xinbaoyingshu

位置　鱼际：第一掌骨中点，赤白肉际处。

太渊：掌后腕横纹桡侧端，桡动脉的桡侧凹陷中。

主治　呼吸系病证，如咳嗽喘息，咽痛等。

操作　针 0.3～0.5 寸，局部酸、胀痛感。

Composition　This group of acupoints is composed of Yuji (LU10) and Taiyuan (LU9).

Location　Yuji：at the midpoint of the 1st metacarpal bone, and on the junction of the red and white skin.

Taiyuan：at the radial end of the palmar crease of the wrist, in the depression on the radial side of the radial artery.

Indication　Diseases of the respiratory system, such as cough, asthma, sore throat, etc..

Method　The needle is inserted 0.3−0.5 cun, the acu-esthesia of soreness, distension and pain will be obtained in this part.

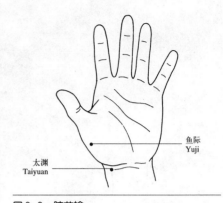

图 3-9　肺荥输

Fig. 3-9　Feiyingshu

手三原
Shousanyuan

组成　本穴组由太渊、大陵、神门三原穴组合而成。

位置　太渊：掌后腕横纹桡侧端，桡动脉的桡侧凹陷。

大陵：腕横纹中央，掌长肌腱与桡侧腕屈肌腱之间。

神门：腕横纹尺侧端，尺侧腕屈肌腱的桡侧凹陷中。

主治　上焦疾患，以心肺病及脑病为主。

操作　直刺或斜刺 0.3～0.5 寸。

Composition　This group of acupoints is composed of Taiyuan (LU9), Daling (PC7) and Shenmen (HT7).

Location　Taiyuan：at the radial end of the palmar crease of the wrist, in the depression on the radial side of the radial artery.

Daling：at the midpoint of the palmar crease of the wrist, between the tendons of the long palmar muscle and radial flexor muscle of the wrist.

Shenmen：on the ulnar end of the palmar crease of the wrist, in the depression of the radial side of the tendon of the ulnar flexor muscle of the wrist.

Indication　Diseases of the Upper Energizer，mainly the diseases of the heart, lung and brain.

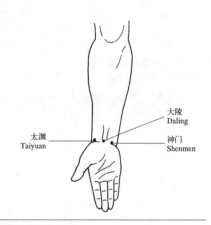

图 3-10　手三原

Fig. 3-10　Shousanyuan

Method　The needle is inserted 0.3—0.5 cun perpendicularly or obliquely.

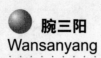

腕三阳
Wansanyang

组成　本穴组由阳溪、阳池、阳谷三穴组合而成。

位置　阳溪：腕背横纹桡侧端，拇短伸肌腱与拇长伸肌腱之间的凹陷中。

阳池：腕背横纹中，指总伸肌腱尺侧缘凹陷中。

阳谷：腕背横纹尺侧端，尺骨茎突前凹陷中。

主治　手腕痛，肩臂痛，耳鸣，耳聋。

操作　刺法：直刺0.3~0.5寸。

灸法：温灸5~10分钟。

Composition　This group of acupoints is composed of Yangxi (LI5), Yangchi (TE4) and Yanggu (SI5).

Location　Yangxi：at the radial end of the dorsal crease of the wrist, in the depression between the tendons of the short extensor and long extensor muscles of the thumb.

Yangchi：at the midpoint of the dorsal crease of the wrist, in the depression on the ulnar side of the tendon of the extensor muscle of the fingers.

Yanggu：at the ulnar end of the dorsal crease of the wrist, in the depression in the front of the styloid process of the ulna.

Indication　Pain in the wrist, pain in the shoulder and arm, tinnitus, deafness.

Method　Acupuncture：the needle is inserted 0.3—0.5 cun.

Moxibustion：warm moxibustion for 5—10 minutes is applied.

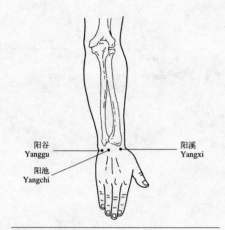

阳谷
Yanggu

阳池
Yangchi

阳溪
Yangxi

图3-11　腕三阳
Fig. 3-11　Wansanyang

肩三针
Jiansanzhen

组成　本穴组由肩髃、肩前、肩后三穴组合而成。

位置　肩髃：肩峰端下缘，当肩峰与肱骨大结节之间，三角肌上部中央。肩平举时，肩部出现两个凹陷，前方的凹陷中。

肩前：见肩内陵。

肩后：腋窝后皱襞尽端处。

主治 肩痛不举，肩关节周围软组织病变。

操作 刺法：直刺0.5～1.5寸，留5～10分钟。

灸法：艾炷灸3～5壮，或温灸5～15分钟。

按注 肩后亦称后腋。

Composition This group of acupoints is composed of Jianyu (LI15), Jianqian and Jianhou.

Location Jianyu：on the lower border of the acromial extremity of the clavicle, between the acromial extremity of the clavicle and the greater tuberosity of the humerus, on the midpoint of the upper part of the deltoid muscle. There will be two depressions on the shoulder when the arm is lifted abducently to the horizontal level, and Jianyu is in the anterior one.

Jianqian：See Jianneiling.

Jianhou：at the end of posterior axillary fold.

Indication Pain and motor impairment of the shoulder, periarthritis of the shoulder joint.

Method Acupuncture：the needle is inserted 0.5−1.5 cun and retained for 5−10 minutes.

Moxibustion：moxibustion with 3−5 cones, or warm moxibustion for 5−15 minutes is applied.

Note Jianhou is also called Houye.

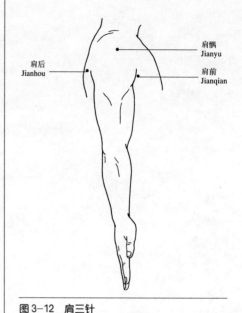

图 3−12 肩三针
Fig. 3−12 Jiansanzhen

新肩三针
Xinjiansanzhen

组成 本穴组由肩部的三个点组合而成。

位置 肩峰端下缘、当肩峰与肱骨大结节之间，三角肌上部中央取肩髃 、肩髃 直上0.5寸为一穴，以肩髃为中点，向腋前后水平方向各旁开2寸为第二穴，第三穴。

主治 肩痹(肩关节周围炎、肩颈综合征)，上肢瘫痪，肩不举。

操作 第一针向肩关节方向直刺或斜刺并可采取恢刺的方法改变角度和方向后再固定，深度为1.2～1.5寸。肩髃前后两针采用前后对刺，深度0.8～1.2寸。也可针尖与穴位成90°角，直刺0.8～1寸，注意不要刺入胸腔。

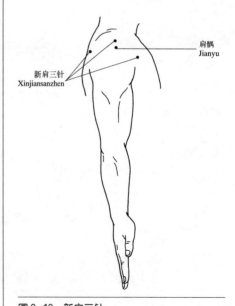

图 3−13 新肩三针
Fig. 3−13 Xinjiansanzhen

Composition   This group of acupoints is composed of three points in the shoulder region.

Location   Locate Jianyu on the lower border of the acromial extremity of the clavicle, between the acromial extremity of the clavicle and the greater tuberosity of the humerus, and on the midpoint of the upper part of the deltoid muscle. The first point is 0.5 cun directly above Jianyu. The 2nd and 3rd points are 2 cun lateral to the anterior and posterior of the axillary fold on the horizontal level, and Jianyu is the midpoint between them.

Indications   Bi-syndromes of the shoulder (periarthritis of the shoulder joint, syndromes of the neck and shoulder), paralysis of the upper limbs, motor impairment of the shoulder.

Methods   The first needle is inserted perpendicularly or obliquely towards the shoulder joint, and the needle may be fixed after changing the needling direction with Huici method, the depth is 1.2–1.5 cun. The two needles anterior and posterior to Jianyu are inserted oppositely from the anterior and the posterior, the depth is about 0.8–1.2 cun. The needle can also be inserted at the angle of 90° which is formed by the handle of the needle and the skin, that is, insert the needle 0.8–1 cun perpendicularly. Attention should be paid so as not to insert needles into the thorax.

三肩
Sanjian

组成   本穴组由肩髃、肩髎、肩内陵三穴组合而成。

位置   肩髃：肩峰端下缘，当肩峰与肱骨大结节之间，三角肌上部中央。肩平举时，肩部出现两个凹陷，前方的凹陷中。

肩髎：肩峰后下方，上臂外展，当肩髃穴后寸许的凹陷中。

肩内陵：腋前皱襞顶端与肩髃连线的中点(一说在腋前皱襞上1寸)。

主治   肩痛不举，臂痛，上肢瘫痪，以及肩关节周围软组织疾患。

操作   刺法：直刺1～1.5寸。

灸法：艾炷灸3～5壮，或温灸5～15分钟。

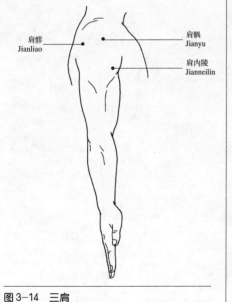

肩髎
Jianliao

肩髃
Jianyu

肩内陵
Jianneilin

图3-14 三肩
Fig. 3-14 Sanjian

汉 英 对 照

Composition This group of acupoints is composed of Jianyu (LI15), Jianliao (TE14) and Jianneiling.

Location Jianyu: on the lower border of the acromial extremity of the clavicle, between the acromial extremity of the clavicle and the greater tuberosity of the humerus, on the midpoint of the upper part of the deltoid muscle. There will be two depressions on the shoulder when the arm is lifted abducently to the horizontal level, and Jianyu is in the anterior one.

Jianliao: posterior and inferior to the acromion, in the depression 1 cun posterior to Jianyu when the arm is abducted.

Jianneiling: at the midpoint between the end of the anterior axillary fold and Jianyu (or, the point cun above the anterior axillary fold).

Indications Pain and motor impairment of the shoulder, pain in the arm, paralysis of the upper limbs and soft tissue injury of the shoulder joint.

Method Acupuncture: the needle is inserted 1−1.5 cun perpendicularly.

Moxibustion: moxibustion with 3−5 cones, or warm moxibustion for 5−15 minutes is applied.

臂丛
Bicong

组成 本穴组由臂丛1、臂丛2、臂丛3三穴组合而成。

位置 臂丛1穴：腋窝部，腋前皱襞与腋动脉交叉处。

臂丛2穴：臂丛1穴外侧0.5寸处。

臂丛3穴：位于臂丛1穴内侧0.5寸处。

主治 漏肩风，手痛麻，上肢痿痹。

操作 针0.5~1寸，针感麻、酸至手。

Composition This group of acupoints is composed of Bicong 1, Bicong 2 and Bicong 3.

Location Bicong1: in the axillary fossa, at the junction of the anterior axillary fold and axillary artery.

Bicong 2: 0.5 cun lateral to Bicong 1.

Bicong 3: 0.5 cun medial to Bicong 1.

Indication Periarthritis of the shoulder joint, pain

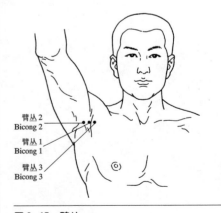

臂丛2
Bicong 2

臂丛1
Bicong 1

臂丛3
Bicong 3

图3−15 臂丛
Fig. 3−15 Bicong

and numbness of the hands, muscular atrophy and paralysis of the upper limbs.

Method   The needle is inserted 0.5–1 cun. The acuesthesia of numbness and soreness will radiate to the hand.

极泉中心
Jiquanzhongxin

组成　本穴组以极泉为中心上下左右1寸处各取一点，共五个穴点。

位置　极泉：腋窝正中，腋动脉搏动处。

极泉周四点：即在极泉上下左右各1寸处之四点。

主治　漏肩风，上肢痿痹不遂。

操作　从极泉由下向上直刺，再取其上下左右各1寸处选取四点，分别略向下向上、向左向右方向刺之，深0.5～1寸，针感酸麻感或触电状为度。

Composition   This group of acupoints is composed of Jiquan (HT1) and the four points 1 cun superior, inferior and lateral to Jiquan, five points in all.

Location   Jiquan：at the centre of the axillary fossa, where the axillary artery pulsates.

Jiquanzhousidian：the four points 1 cun superior, inferior and lateral to Jiquan.

Indication   Periarthritis of the shoulder joint, muscular atrophy and paralysis of the upper limbs.

Method   The needle is inserted perpendicularly upwards from the lower aspect of Jiquan. Then locate the four points 1 cun superior, inferior and lateral to it, the needles are inserted downwards, upwards and towards left and right slightly respectively, the depth is 0.5–1 cun till the acu-esthesia of soreness and numbness or electric shock sensation is obtained.

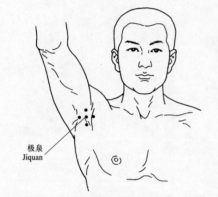

极泉
Jiquan

图3-16　极泉中心
Fig. 3-16　Jiquanzhongxin

上痿痹
Shangweibi

组成　本穴组由肩髃、曲池、合谷三穴组合而成。

位置　肩髃：肩峰端下缘，当肩峰与肱骨大结节之间，三角肌上部中央。肩平举时，肩部出现两个凹陷，前方的凹陷中。

曲池：屈肘，成直角，当肘横纹外端与肱骨外上髁连线的中点。

合谷：手背，第一、第二掌骨之间，约平第二掌骨中点处。

主治　上肢痿痹。

操作　刺法：直刺0.8～1寸，得气为度。

灸法：艾条灸10～20分钟。

按注　本穴组临床常加配颈1～胸1夹脊，则效更佳。

Composition　This group of acupoints is composed of Jianyu (LI15), Quchi (LI11) and Hegu (LI4).

Location　Jianyu：on the lower border of the acromial extremity of the clavicle, between the acromial extremity of the clavicle and the greater tuberosity of the humerus, on the midpoint of the upper part of the deltoid muscle. There will be two depressions on the shoulder when the arm is lifted abducently to the horizontal level, and Jianyu is in the anterior one.

Quchi：at the midpoint of the line between the radial end of the cubital crease and the external humeral epicondyle when the elbow is flexed at 90°.

Hegu：on the dorsum of the hand, between the 1st and 2nd metacarpal bones, and near the midpoint of the 2nd metacarpal bone.

Indication　Muscular atrophy and paralysis of the upper limbs.

Method　Acupuncture：the needle is inserted 0.8−1 cun till the acu-esthesia is obtained.

Moxibustion：moxibustion with moxa roll for 10−20 minutes is applied.

Note　The curative effect will be better if this group is combined with Jiaji from the 1st cervical vertebra to the 1st thoracic vertebra.

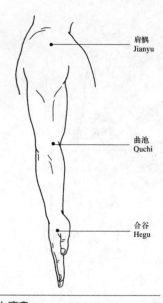

图3-17　上痿痹
Fig. 3-17　Shangweibi

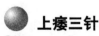

上痿三针
Shangweisanzhen

组成　本穴组由合谷、曲池、尺泽三穴组合而成。

位置　合谷：手背，第一、第二掌骨之间，约平第二掌骨中点处。

曲池：屈肘，成直角，当肘横纹外端与肱骨外上髁连线的中点。

尺泽：肘横纹中，肱二头肌腱桡侧缘。

主治 痿证（小儿麻痹症，脊髓炎，多发性神经炎，癔病性瘫痪等）。

操作 直刺1～1.5寸，局部酸、胀、重、麻等，得气为度。

Composition This group of acupoints is composed of Hegu (LI4), Quchi (LI11) and Chize (LU5).

Location Hegu：on the dorsum of the hand, between the 1st and 2nd metacarpal bones, and near the midpoint of the 2nd metacarpal bone.

Quchi：at the midpoint of the line between the radial end of the cubital crease and the external humeral epicondyle when the elbow is flexed at 90°.

Chize：in the cubital crease, on the radial side of the tendon of the biceps muscle of the arm.

Indication Flaccidity syndromes (infantile paralysis, myelitis, polyneuritis, paralysis due to hysteria).

Method The needle is inserted 1-1.5 cun perpendicularyly till the acu-esthesia of soreness, distension, heaviness and numbness is obtained.

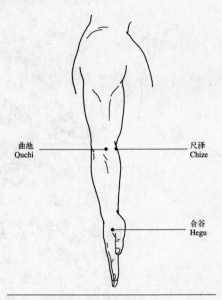

图3-18 上痿三针
Fig. 3-18 Shangweisanzhen

 窗会
Chuanghui

组成 本穴组由天窗、臑会二穴组合而成。

位置 天窗：喉结旁开3.5寸，在胸锁乳突肌之后缘。

臑会：在尺骨鹰嘴与肩髎穴连线上，肩髎穴下3寸，当三角肌的后缘。

主治 颈部漫肿或结块，皮色不变，不痛亦不溃烂，肿块多为圆形，可随吞咽动作而上下移动。实证兼见烦躁易怒，心悸，心烦，多汗，眼球突出，脉数有力等；虚证兼见食少，气短，乏力，心悸，失眠，脉细数无力等。

操作 先刺天窗，直刺0.5～1寸，据病证虚实用提插捻转法进行补泻，留针30分钟，行针2次，每次5分钟。后取臑会，直刺0.5～1寸，据病证虚实施以补泻法，留针30分钟。

Composition This group of acupoints is composed of Tianchuang (SI16) and Naohui (TE13).

Location Tianchuang：3.5 cun lateral to the laryngeal protuberance, posterior to the sternocleidomastoid

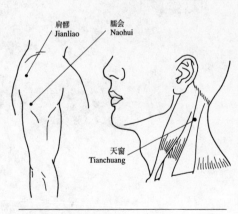

图3-19 窗会
Fig. 3-19 Chuanghui

muscle.

Naohui: on the line connecting the olecranon of the ulna and Jianliao, 3 cun below Jianliao, and on the posterior border of the deltoid muscle.

Indication Diffusive swelling or lumps in the neck with normal skin color, absence of pain or ulceration, the lumps are usually round, and can move up and down when swallowing. Palpitation, irritability, sweating, exophthalmos, rapid and forceful pulse may also be seen in the excessive type, while anorexia, shortness of breath, weakness, palpitation, insomnia, thin, rapid and weak pulse may be seen in the deficiency type.

Method Tianchuang is needled first. The needle is inserted 0.5−1 cun, and the reinforcing and reducing techniques by lifting and inserting or rotating needle can be used according to the deficiency or excessive type of the disease. Retain the needle for 30 minutes, and manipulate the needle twice during the period, 5 minutes each time. Then Naohui is needled 0.5−1 cun perpendicularly, and the reinforcing and reducing techniques can be applied according to the conditions of the disease. Retain the needle for 30 minutes.

 臂五
Biwu

组成 本穴组由臂臑、手五里二穴组合而成。

位置 臂臑：在曲池穴与肩髃穴连线上，曲池穴上7寸处，当三角肌下端。

手五里：在曲池穴与肩髃穴的连线上，曲池穴上3寸处。

主治 瘰疬。

操作 刺法：直刺1～1.5寸，得气为度。

灸法：艾炷灸5～9壮，艾条灸10～30分钟。

Composition This group of acupoints is composed of Binao (LI14) and Shouwuli (LI13).

Location Binao：on the line connecting Quchi and Jianyu, 7 cun above Quchi, on the lower border of the deltoid muscle.

Shouwuli：on the line connecting Quchi and Jianyu, 3

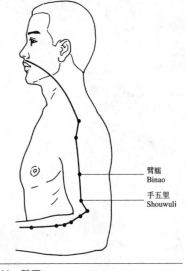

臂臑
Binao
手五里
Shouwuli

图3-20 臂五
Fig. 3-20 Biwu

cun above Quchi.

Indication Scrofula.

Method Acupuncture：the needle is inserted 1−1.5 cun till the acu-esthesia is obtained.

Moxibustion：moxibustion with 5−9 moxa cones, or moxibustion with moxa roll for 10−30 minutes is applied.

 三池
Sanchi

组成　本穴组由曲池穴及其上下各1寸处共三穴组合而成。

位置　曲池：屈肘，成直角，当肘横纹外端与肱骨外上髁连线的中点。

曲池上下点：曲池上下各1寸处。

主治　热病，鼻渊，肘臂酸痛，上肢不遂。

操作　刺法：直刺1~1.5寸。

灸法：艾炷灸1~3壮，或温灸5~10分钟。

Composition This group of acupoints is composed of Quchi (LI11) and two points 1 cun superior and inferior to Quchi, 3 points in all.

Location Quchi：at the midpoint of the line between the radial end of the cubital crease and the external humeral epicondyle when the elbow is flexed at 90°.

Quchishangxiadian：1 cun superior and inferior to Quchi respectively.

Indication Febrile diseases, rhinorrhea, soreness and pain in the elbow and arm, motor impairment of the upper limbs.

Method Acupuncture：the needle is inserted 1−1.5 cun vertically.

Moxibustion：moxibustion with 1−3 cones, or warm moxibustion for 5−10 minutes is applied.

 闪挫
Shancuo

组成　本穴组由挫闪、扭挫(挫闪1)、扭伤三穴组合而成。

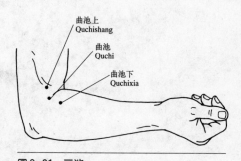

图3-21　三池
Fig. 3-21 Sanchi

曲池上 Quchishang
曲池 Quchi
曲池下 Quchixia

位置 挫闪：前臂伸侧，近端，鹰嘴突起与肱骨外上髁间凹陷下 1 寸处。

扭挫：前臂伸侧，近端鹰嘴突起与肱骨外上髁间凹陷下 3 寸处。

扭伤：前臂伸面桡侧，屈肘时肘横纹外凹陷下 3 寸处。

主治 闪腰，扭挫伤。

操作 挫闪、扭挫二穴针 0.3~0.5 寸，针感酸、麻至腕。扭伤穴针 0.8~1.2 寸，针感酸、麻至腕指，当捻针时一边嘱患者不断活动腰部或扭挫伤关节局部，至活动度加大、疼痛感轻时起针。

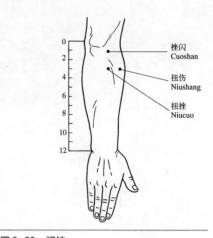

图 3-22 闪挫
Fig. 3-22 Shancuo

Composition This group of acupoints is composed of cuoshan, Niucuo (Cuoshan1) and Niushang.

Location Cuoshan: on the upper part of the lateral side of the forearm, 1 cun below the depression between the tip of the olecranon and the external humeral epicondyle.

Niucuo: on the upper part of the lateral side of the forearm, 3 cun below the depression between the tip of the olecranon and the external humeral epicondyle.

Niushang: on the radial side of the lateral side of the forearm, 3 cun below the depression lateral to the cubital crease when the elbow is flexed.

Indication Acute lumbar sprain, strained or sprained limbs or joints.

Method Cuoshan and Niucuo are needled 0.3−0.5 cun and the acu-esthesia of soreness and numbness will transmit to the wrist. Niushang is needled 0.8−1.2 cun and the acu-esthesia of soreness and numbness can racliate to the wrist and the fingers too. Ask the patient to move about the lumbar or the sprained joint when the needles are rotated. Withdraw the needles when the range of the movement is enlarged and the pain is relieved.

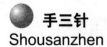

手三针
Shousanzhen

组成 本穴组由曲池、外关、合谷三穴组合而成。

位置 曲池：屈肘，成直角，当肘横纹外端与肱骨外上髁连线的中点。

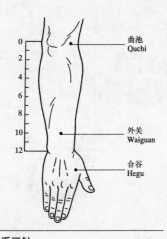

图3-23 手三针
Fig. 3-23 Shousanzhen

外关：腕背横纹上2寸，桡骨与尺骨之间。

合谷：手背，第一、第二掌骨之间，约平第二掌骨中点处。

主治 上肢痿痹，头、颈、肩、上肢疼痛症，外感发热，时行寒热及头面部疾病等。

操作 用捻转、提插法刺之，针0.8～1.2寸，得气为度。

Composition This group of acupoints is composed of Quchi (LI11), Waiguan (TE5) and Hegu (LI4).

Location Quchi：at the midpoint of the line between the radial end of the cubital crease and the external humeral epicondyle when the elbow is flexed at 90°.

Waiguan：2 cun above the dorsal crease of the wrist, between the radius and ulna.

Hegu：on the dorsum of the hand, between the 1st and 2nd metacarpal bones, and near the midpoint of the 2nd metacarpal bone.

Indication Muscular atrophy and paralysis of the upper limbs, pain in the head, neck, shoulder and upper limbs, fever due to invasion by exogenous factors, alternating chills and fever and the diseases of the head and face, etc..

Method The points are needled with rotating method or lifting and inserting method, the depth is 0.8–1.2 cun till the acu-esthesia is obtained.

手三关
Shousanguan

组成 本穴组由中关、尺关、桡关三穴组合而成。

位置 中关：前臂伸侧正中线、腕背横纹上1寸。

尺关：前臂伸侧正中线向尺侧旁开1寸，腕背横纹上1寸。

桡关：前臂正中线向桡侧旁开1寸，腕背横纹上1寸。

主治 上肢痿痹，伸肘，垂腕，手麻，指动不能，手足搐搦症、头痛、语謇、腰扭伤。

操作 三穴均沿皮下向上刺0.3～0.4寸，针感为肩和手指酸、麻、胀。

Composition This group of acupoints is composed of Zhongguan, Chiguan and Raoguan.

Location Zhongguan：on the midline of the lateral side of the forearm, 1 cun above the dorsal crease of the

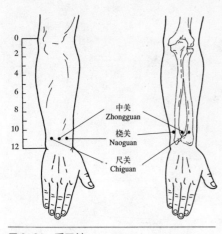

图3-24 手三关
Fig. 3-24 Shousanguan

wrist.

Chiguan: 1 cun lateral to the ulnar side of the midline of the forearm, 1 cun above the dorsal crease of the wrist.

Naoguan: 1 cun lateral to the radial side of the midline of the forearm, 1 cun above the dorsal crease of the wrist.

Indications Muscular atrophy and paralysis of the upper limbs, extended elbow, drooped wrist, incapability of the movement of the fingers, twitching hands and foots, headache, alalia, lumbar sprain.

Method The three points are all subcutaneously needled 0.3—0.4 cun upwards and the acu-esthesia of soreness, numbness and distension will be felt in the shoulder and fingers.

二白
Erbai

组成　本穴组由位于腕横纹上4寸处的二个点组合而成。

位置　腕横纹上4寸，桡侧腕屈肌腱两侧，一手两穴。

主治　痔疮，脱肛，前臂痛，胸胁痛。

操作　刺法：直刺0.5~1寸，局部酸麻胀感，或有麻电感传至腕部。

灸法：艾炷灸3~5壮，艾条灸5~10分钟。

Composition This group of acupoints is composed of two points 4 cun above the palmar crease of the wrist.

Location 4 cun above the palmar crease of the wrist, on each side of the tendon of the radial flexor muscle of the wrist, 2 points on each hand.

Indication Hemorrhoids, prolapse of the rectum, pain in the forearm, chest and hypochondriac region.

Method Acupuncture: the needle is inserted 0.5—1 cun perpendicularly. The acu-esthesia may be the feeling of soreness, numbness and distension in this part, or the feeling of electric shock radiates to the wrist.

Moxibustion: moxibustion with 3—5 moxa cones, or moxibustion with moxa roll for 5—10 minutes is applied.

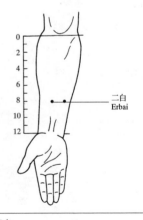

图3-25 二白
Fig. 3-25 Erbai

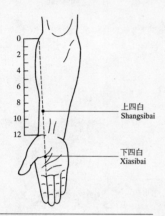

图 3-26　手四白
Fig. 3-26　Shousibai

手四白
Shousibai

组成　本穴组由上、下四白共二穴组合而成。

位置　上四白穴：位于前臂屈侧，由示指与中指缝向上划的直线上，腕横纹上3寸处。

下四白穴：位于手掌、示指与中指缝向上划的直线上，腕横纹下3寸处。

主治　脱肛，痔，夜尿频。

操作　针0.5~1寸，针感刺上四白时酸、麻、胀感，上传至肘，下传至手指；刺下四白时局部胀痛或示指麻胀。

Composition　This group of acupoints is composed of Shangsibai and Xiasibai.

Location　Shangsibai：on the medial side of the forearm, on the extended line of the margin between the index and the middle fingers, 3 cun above the palmar crease of the wrist.

Xiasibai：on the extended line of the margin between the index and the middle fingers, 3 cun below the palmar crease of the wrist.

Indication　Prolapse of the rectum, hemorrhoids, enuresis.

Method　The needle is inserted 0.5−1 cun. The acu-esthesia is soreness, numbness and distension which will radiate upwards to elbow and downwards to fingers when Shangsibai is needled. When Xiasibai is needled, the acu-esthesia will be the distension and pain in this part or the numbness and distension of the index finger.

定悸
Dingji

组成　本穴组由内关、阴郄、郄门三穴组合而成。

位置　内关：腕横纹上2寸，掌长肌腱与桡侧腕屈肌腱之间。

阴郄：腕横纹上0.5寸，尺侧腕屈肌腱的桡侧。

郄门：腕横纹上5寸，掌长肌腱与桡侧腕屈肌腱之间。

主治　心悸。

操作　刺法：内关、郄门直刺0.8~1.2寸。阴郄沿皮刺0.5~0.8寸，得气为度。

灸法：艾条温灸10~20分钟。

Composition　This group of acupoints is composed of Neiguan (PC6), Yinxi (HT6) and Ximen (PC4).

Location　Neiguan：2 cun above the palmar crease of the wrist, between the tendons of the long palmar muscle and radial flexor muscle of the wrist.

Yinxi：0.5 cun above the palmar crease of the wrist, on the radial side of the tendon of the ulnar flexor muscle of the wrist.

Ximen：5 cun above the palmar crease of the wrist, between the tendons of the long palmar muscle and radial flexor muscle of the wrist.

Indication　Palpitation.

Method　Acupuncture：Neiguan and Ximen are needled 0.8−1.2 cun perpendicularly. Yingxi is needled 0.5−0.8 cun subcutaneously till the acu-esthesia is obtained.

Moxibustion：warm moxibustion with moxa roll for 10−20 minutes is applied.

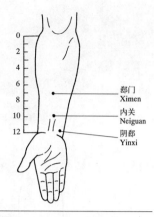

图3-27　定悸
Figl. 3-27　Dingji

宫陵
Gongling

组成　本穴组由劳宫、大陵二穴组合而成。

位置　劳宫：第二、第三掌骨之间，握拳，中指尖下是穴。

大陵：腕横纹中央，掌长肌腱与桡侧腕屈肌腱之间。

主治　心闷，疮痈。

操作　刺0.5~0.8寸，得气后行泻法，留针30分钟。

Composition　This group of acupoints is composed of Laogong (PC8) and Daling (PC7).

Location　Laogong：between the 2nd and 3rd metacarpal bones, where the tip of the middle finger reaches when a fist is made.

Daling：at the midpoint of the palmar crease of the wrist, between the tendons of the long palmar muscle and radial flexor muscle of the wrist.

Indication　Stuffy chest, sore and ulcer.

Method　The needle is inserted 0.5−0.8 cun. Reduc-

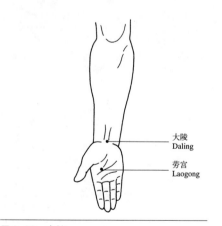

图3-28　宫陵
Fig. 3-28　Gongling

ing techniques are applied after the acu-esthesia is obtained. Retain the needles for 30 minutes.

● 手智三针
Shouzhisanzhen

组成　本穴组由内关、神门、劳宫三穴组合而成。

位置　内关：腕横纹上2寸，掌长肌腱与桡侧腕屈肌腱之间。

神门：腕横纹尺侧端，尺侧腕屈肌腱的桡侧凹陷中。

劳宫：第二、第三掌骨之间，握拳，中指尖下是穴。

主治　智力低下伴小儿多动症。

操作　内关穴直刺，针尖略向肘尖方向刺入0.8寸，使针感往上传，神门向间使方向斜刺0.8寸，劳宫以屈示、中二指时中指尖下是穴，直刺0.5寸。可用捻转补泻，以有较强烈得气感为佳。

按注　阳证、实证、热证用泻法，阴证、虚证、寒证用补法。

Composition　This group of acupoints is composed of Neiguan (PC6), Shenmen (HT7) and Laogong (PC8).

Location　Neiguan：2 cun above the palmar crease of the wrist, between the tendons of the long palmar muscle and radial flexor muscle of the wrist.

Shenmen：on the ulnar end of the palmar crease of the wrist, in the depression of the radial side of the tendon of the ulnar flexor muscle of the wrist.

Laogong：between the 2nd and 3rd metacarpal bones, where the tip of the middle finger reaches when a fist is made.

Indication　Hypophrenia combined with hyperkinesia.

Method　Neiguan is needled 0.8 cun pendicularly with the tip of the needle toward the tip of the elbow, so as to induce the upward transmission of the acu-esthesia. Shenmen is needled 0.8 cun obliquely towards Jianshi. Laogong is located where the tip of the middle finger reaches when the index and middle fingers are flexed, and it's needled 0.5 cun perpendicularly. Reinforcing and reducing techniques by rotation can be applied, and it's advisable to obtain the strong acu-esthesia.

Note　Reducing method is applied for Yang syndromes,

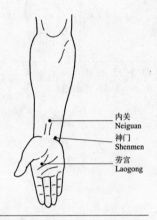

内关
Neiguan
神门
Shenmen
劳宫
Laogong

图3-29　手智三针
Fig. 3-29　Shouzhisanzhen

excessive syndromes and hot syndromes while reinforcing method is applied to Yin syndromes, deficiency syndromes and cold syndromes.

神安
Shenan

组成　本穴组由神门、大陵、内关三穴组合而成。

位置　神门：腕横纹尺侧端，尺侧腕屈肌腱的桡侧凹陷中。

大陵：腕横纹中央，掌长肌腱与桡侧腕屈肌腱之间。

内关：腕横纹上2寸，掌长肌腱与桡侧腕屈肌腱之间。

主治　多种病因所致之失眠症。

操作　仰卧位或坐位，内关直刺0.5~0.8寸，或艾条悬灸5~10分钟。大陵直刺0.3~0.5寸，或艾条悬灸3~5分钟。神门直刺0.3~0.5寸，或艾条悬灸3~5分钟。以上三穴若针刺得气后留针30分钟。

Composition　This group of acupoints is composed of Shenmen (HT7), Daling (PC7) and Neiguan (PC6).

Location　Shenmen：on the ulnar end of the palmar crease of the wrist, in the depression of the radial side of the tendon of the ulnar flexor muscle of the wrist.

Daling：at the midpoint of the crease of the wrist, between the tendons of the long palmar muscle and radial flexor muscle of the wrist.

Neiguan：2 cun above the crease of the wrist, between the tendons of the long palmar muscle and radial flexor muscle of the wrist.

Indication　Insomnia caused by various reasons.

Method　Supine or sitting posture is selected. Neiguan is needled 0.5−0.8 cun perpendicularly, or it can be treated with suspended moxibustion with moxa roll for 5−10 minutes; Daling is needled 0.3−0.5 cun, or it can be treated with suspended moxibustion with moxa roll for 3−5 minutes; Shenmen is needled 0.3−0.5 cun, or it can be treated with suspended moxibustion with moxa roll for 3−5 minutes. Retain the needles for 30 minutes after the acu-esthesia is obtained in above three points.

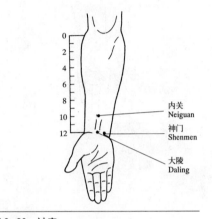

图 3-30　神安
Fig. 3-30　Shenan

渊缺
Yuanque

组成　本穴组由太渊、列缺二穴组合而成。

位置　太渊：掌后腕横纹桡侧端，桡动脉的桡侧凹陷中。

列缺：桡骨茎突上方，腕横纹上1.5寸。

主治　咳嗽风痰，寒痰，乳病。

操作　斜刺0.3～0.5寸，得气为度。

Composition　This group of acupoints is composed of Taiyuan (LU9) and Lieque (LU7).

Location　Taiyuan：at the radial end of the palmar crease of the wrist, in the depression of the radial side of the radial artery.

Lieque：superior to the styloid process of the radius, 1.5 cun above the palmar crease of the wrist.

Indication　Cough due to pathogenic wind, cold phlegm, breast diseases.

Method　The needle is inserted 0.3−0.5 cun obliquely till the acu-esthesia is obtained.

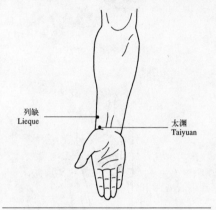

图3-31　渊缺
Fig. 3-31　Yuanque

扶关
Fuguan

组成　本穴组由扶突、内关二穴组合而成。

位置　扶突：喉结旁开3寸，当胸锁乳突肌的胸骨头与锁骨头之间。

内关：腕横纹上2寸，掌长肌腱与桡侧腕屈肌腱之间。

主治　呃逆。

操作　先向扶突直刺1寸，有触电感可传至肩和手时；内关刺0.5寸。得气后留针各5～10分钟。

Composition　This group of acupoints is composed of Futu (LI18) and Neiguan (PC6).

Location　Futu：3 cun lateral to the laryngeal protuberance, between the anterior and posterior heads of the sternocleidomastoid muscle.

Indication　Hiccup.

Method　First Futu is needled 1 cun perpendicularly. When the feeling of electric shock radiates to the shoul-

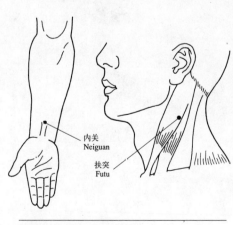

图3-32　扶关
Fig. 3-32　Fuguan

der and hand, Neiguan is needled 0.5 cun. Retain the needles for 5—10 minutes after the acu—esthesia is obtained.

鱼液
Yuye

组成　本穴组由鱼际、液门二穴组合而成。

位置　鱼际：第一掌骨中点，赤白肉际处。

液门：握拳，第四、第五指之间，指掌关节前凹陷中。

主治　喉痛。

操作　直刺0.5~0.8寸，局部酸胀痛感。

Composition　This group of acupoints is composed of Yuji (LU10) and Yemen (TE2).

Location　Yuji：at the midpoint of the 1st metacarpal bone, and on the junction of the red and white skin.

Yemen：between the 4th and 5th fingers, in the depression before the metacarpophalangeal joint when the fist is made.

Indication　Sore throat.

Method　The needle is inserted 0.5—0.8 cun perpendicularly. The acu-esthesia of soreness, distension and pain will be obtained in this part.

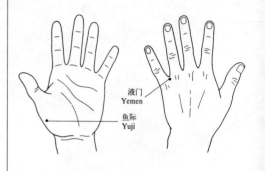

图3-33　鱼液
Fig. 3-33　Yuye

清咽
Qingyan

组成　本穴组由少商、内关、合谷三穴组合而成。

位置　少商：拇指桡侧指甲角旁约0.1寸。

内关：腕横纹上2寸，掌长肌腱与桡侧腕屈肌腱之间。

合谷：手背，第一、第二掌骨之间，约平第二掌骨中点处。

主治　咽喉肿痛。

操作　内关、合谷直刺0.5—1寸，得气为度。少商点刺出血。

Composition　This group of acupoints is composed of Shaoshang (LU11), Neiguan (PC6) and Hegu (LI4).

Location　Shaoshang：on the radial side of the thumb, 0.1 cun from the corner of the fingernail.

Neiguan：2 cun above the palmar crease of the wrist,

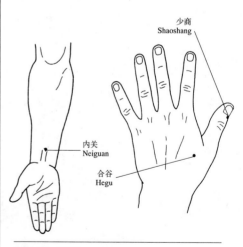

图3-34　清咽
Fig. 3-34　Qingyan

between the tendons of the long palmar muscle and radial flexor muscle of the wrist.

Hegu: on the dorsum of the hand, between the 1st and 2nd metacarpal bones, and near the midpoint of the 2nd metacarpal bone.

Indication Sore throat.

Method Neiguan and Hegu are needled 0.5—1 cun perpendicularly till the acu-esthesia is obtained.

Shaoshang is pricked to bleed.

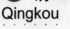

清口
Qingkou

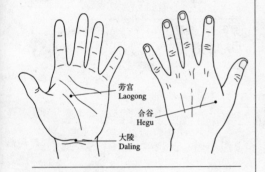

图 3-35 清口
Fig. 3-35 Qingkou

组成 本穴组由大陵、劳宫、合谷三穴组合而成。

位置 大陵: 腕横纹中央, 掌长肌腱与桡侧腕屈肌腱之间。

劳宫: 第二、第三掌骨之间, 握拳, 中指尖下是穴。

合谷: 手背, 第一、第二掌骨之间, 约平第二掌骨中点处。

主治 口臭。

操作 大陵直刺 0.5~1 寸。劳宫直刺 0.3~0.8 寸。合谷直刺 0.5~1 寸。各用提插捻转泻法, 留针 30 分钟。

Composition This group of acupoints is composed of Daling (PC7), Laogong (PC8) and Hegu (LI4).

Location Daling: at the midpoint of the palmar crease of the wrist, between the tendons of the long palmar muscle and radial flexor muscle of the wrist.

Laogong: between the 2nd and 3rd metacarpal bones, where the tip of the middle finger reaches when a fist is made.

Hegu: on the dorsum of the hand, between the 1st and 2nd metacarpal bones, and near the midpoint of the 2nd metacarpal bone.

Indication Halitosis.

Method Daling is needled 0.5—1 cun perpendicularly. Laogong is needled 0.3—0.8 cun perpendicularly. Hegu is needled 0.5—1 cun perpendicularly. Reducing technique by rotation is applied to each points, and retain the needles for 30 minutes.

陵门
Lingmen

组成　本穴组由大陵、郄门二穴组合而成。

位置　大陵：腕横纹中央，掌长肌腱与桡侧腕屈肌腱之间。

郄门：腕横纹上5寸，掌长肌腱与桡侧腕屈肌腱之间。

主治　心火亢盛之尿血症。

操作　大陵针0.3～0.4寸，灸3～5壮，或5～10分钟。郄门针0.5～0.8寸，灸3～7壮，或5～10分钟。得气后应使二穴针感放射至手指，留针20～30分钟。

Composition　This group of acupoints is composed of Daling (PC7) and Ximen (PC4).

Location　Daling：at the midpoint of the palmar crease of the wrist, between the tendons of the long palmar muscle and radial flexor muscle of the wrist.

Ximen：5 cun above the palmar crease of the wrist, between the tendons of the long palmar muscle and radial flexor muscle of the wrist.

Indication　Hematuria due to excessive heart fire.

Method　Daling is needled 0.3−0.4 cun, or it can be treated with 3−5 cones or 5−10 minutes' moxibustion. Ximen is needled 0.5−0.8 cun, or it can be treated with 3−7 cones or 5−10 minutes' moxibustion. The acuesthesia in both points should be induced to the fingers. Retain the needles for 20−30 minutes.

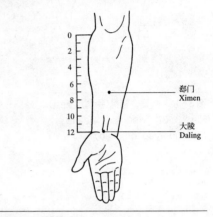

图3-36　陵门
Fig. 3-36　Lingmen

威灵，精灵(手背腰痛点)
Weiling, Jingling (Shoubeiyaotongdian)

组成　本穴组由手背骨间肌旁的二个穴点组合而成。

位置　威灵：伏掌，在手背第二、第三掌骨间中点，第二指伸肌腱桡侧凹陷处。

精灵：在手背第四、第五掌骨间中点，第四指伸肌腱尺侧凹陷处。

主治　急性腰扭伤，头痛，卒死，痰壅气促，小儿急、慢惊风，手背红肿疼痛。

操作　刺法：直刺0.3～0.5寸，局部酸麻感或向指尖传导。

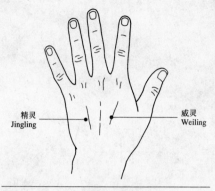

图 3-37 威灵，精灵(手背腰痛点)
Fig. 3-37 Weiling, Jingling
(Shoubeiyaotongdian)

灸法：麦粒灸1~3壮。

按注 本穴又名为手背腰痛点。

Composition This group of acupoints is composed of two points beside the muscles between the bones.

Location Palm facing downwards, on the dorsum of each hand, Weiling is at the midpoint between the 2nd and 3rd metacarpal bones, i.e. in the depression of the radial side of the tendon of the extensor muscle of the index finger. Jingling is at the midpoint between the 4th and 5th metacarpal bones, i.e. in the depression of the ulnar side of the tendon of the extensor muscle of the ring finger.

Indication Acute lumbar sprain, headache, sudden death, rapid breathing due to phlegm, acute and chronic infantile convulsions, redness, swelling and pain in the dorsum of the hand.

Method Acupuncture：the needle is inserted 0.3-0.5 cun perpendicularly. The acu-esthesia of soreness and numbness will be obtained in this part or radiate to the tip of the fingers.

Moxibustion：1-3 wheat-sized moxa cones of moxibustion is applied.

Note This acupoint is also called Shoubeiyaotongdian.

● 五虎
Wuhu

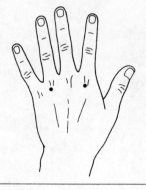

图 3-38 五虎
Fig. 3-38 Wuhu

组成 本穴组由手背第二、第四掌骨小头高点的二个点组合而成。

位置 于手背第二、第四掌骨小头高点。

主治 五指拘挛。

操作 刺法：浅刺0.3~0.5寸，局部胀痛或有麻感，也可点刺出血。

灸法：麦粒灸或温针灸3~5壮，艾条灸5~10分钟。

Composition This group of acupoints is composed of two points on the prominence of the heads of the 2nd and 4th metacarpal bones on the dorsum of the hand.

Location On the prominence of the heads of the 2nd and 4th metacarpal bones on the dorsum of the hand.

Indication Spasm and contracture of the fingers.

Methods Acupuncture：the needle is inserted 0.3—0.5 cun superficially, and the acu-esthesia of distension and pain or numbness will be obtained in this part. It can also be pricked to bleed.

Moxibustion：3—5 wheat-sized moxa cones of moxibustion or warm needle moxibustion, or moxibustion with moxa roll for 5—10 minutes is applied.

八邪
Baxie

组成 本穴组由手十指歧缝的四个点，双手计八个点组合而成。

位置 手十指，歧缝中。

主治 手背肿痛，手指麻木，头项强痛，咽痛，齿痛，目痛，烦热，毒蛇毒虫叮咬伤。

操作 针法：向上斜刺0.5~0.8寸，或点刺出血。

灸法：温针灸3~5壮，艾条温灸5~10分钟。

按注 本穴又名"八关"。

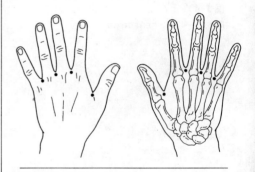

图3-39 八邪
Fig. 3-39 Baxie

Composition This group of acupoints is composed of four points in the web margins between each two fingers of each hand, and eight points on both hands.

Location In the web margins between each two fingers of each hand, and eight points on both hands.

Indication Swelling and pain of the dorsum of the hand, finger numbness, stiffness and pain of the head and nape, sore throat, toothache, ophthalmalgia, vexation, venomous snake or insect bite.

Method Acupuncture：the needle is inserted 0.5—0.8 cun upwards obliquely, or the points' can be pricked to bleed.

Moxibustion：3—5 cones of warm needle moxibustion, or warm moxibustion with moxa roll for 5—10 minutes is applied.

Note This group is also named Baguan.

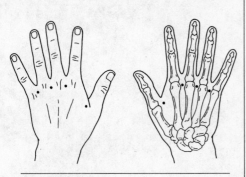

图3-40 上八邪
Fig. 3-40 Shangbaxie

● 上八邪
Shangbaxie

组成　本穴组由大都、中都、下都、上都四穴组合而成，左右手计八穴。

位置　位于手背，将手握起，每两个相邻掌骨小头之间点是穴。第一、第二掌骨小头间者又名大都；第二、第三掌骨小头间又名上都；第三、第四掌骨小头间又名中都；第四、第五掌骨小头间又名下都。

主治　头风，牙痛，手臂红肿、痹，头项强痛，咽痛齿痛，目痛，蛇虫叮咬伤。

操作　刺法：浅刺或向上斜刺0.3～0.5寸，局部胀痛或有麻感。也可点刺出血。

灸法：麦粒灸或温针灸3～5壮，艾条灸5～10分钟。

Composition　This group of acupoints is composed of Dadu, Zhongdu, Xiadu and Shangdu.

Location　On the dorsum of the hand, the points between each two heads of the adjacent metacarpal bones constitute this group. The point between the heads of the 1st and 2nd metacarpal bones is also called Dadu；and the point between the heads of the 2nd and 3rd metacarpal bones is Shangdu the point between the heads of the 3rd and 4th metacarpal bones is Zhongdu；the point between the heads of the 4th and 5th metacarpal bones is Xiadu.

Indication　Headache, toothache, redness ,swelling and paralysis of the arms, stiffness of the joints, sore throat, ophthalmalgia, venomous snake or insect bite.

Method　Acupuncture：the needle is inserted 0.3−0.5 cun superficially or upwards, the acu-esthesia of distension and pain or numbness will be obtained in this part. It can also be pricked to bleed.

Moxibustion：3−5 wheat-sized moxa cones of moxibustion or warm needle moxibustion, or moxibustion with moxa roll for 5−10 minutes is applied.

上邪
Shangxie

组成　本穴组由手背掌指关节后四个点组合而成。

位置　手背、每两个相邻掌指关节后1寸处，每手四个穴，左右计八穴。

主治　手指痉挛，麻木，疼痛。

操作　针0.3～0.5寸，针感麻、酸至指尖。

按注　本穴有书名为谓"痉挛刺激点"，止痉点，也有称为"上八邪"。

Composition　This group of acupoints is composed of four points posterior to the metacarpophalangeal joints on the dorsum of the hand.

Location　On the dorsum of the hand, 1 cun posterior to each two adjacent metacarpophalangeal joints, 4 points on each hand and 8 points on both hands.

Indication　Convulsion, numbness and pain of the fingers.

Method　The needle is inserted 0.3−0.5 cun, the acu−esthesia of numbness, soreness will transmit to the tips of the fingers.

Note　This group is also called "Jingluancijidian", "Zhijingdian" and "Shangbaxie" in some books.

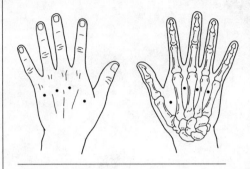

图3−41　上邪
Fig. 3−41　Shangxie

手四穴
Shousixue

组成　本穴组由大拇指、中指爪甲端的二个点组合而成。

位置　手拇指末端爪甲游离缘桡侧，距爪甲0.1寸处，左右二穴；又中指末端爪甲游离缘桡侧，距爪甲0.1寸处，左右二穴。共计四穴。

主治　食物中毒。

操作　三棱针速刺出血。

Composition　This group of acupoints is composed of two points on the tips of the fingernails of the thumb and the middle finger.

Location　On the radial side of the tip of the fingernail of the thumb, 0.1 cun lateral to the nail, 2 points

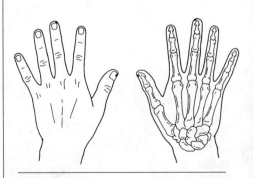

图3−42　手四穴
Fig. 3−42　Shousixue

on both hands; on the radial side of the fingernail of the middle finger, 0.1 cun lateral to the nail, 2 points on both hands. 4 points in all.

Indication   Food poisoning.

Method   The points are pricked to bleed by a three-edged needle.

五指节
Wuzhijie

组成   本穴组由五手指背侧之近节横纹中央的五个点组合而成。

位置   于手五指背侧，近侧指节横纹中点。

主治   腹痛，气血不畅，呼吸困难。

操作   提针圆针点按，或用拇示二指捻搓，局部酸痛感。

Composition   This group of acupoints is composed of five points at the midpoints of the proximal interphalangeal creases on the dorsum of the hand.

Location   On the dorsum of the hand, at the midpoints of the proximal interphalangeal creases.

Indication   Abdominal pain, stagnation of Qi and blood, dyspnea.

Method   The points are pressed by round-shaped tip needle, or kneaded by the thumb and the index finger. The feeling of soreness and pain will be sensed in this part.

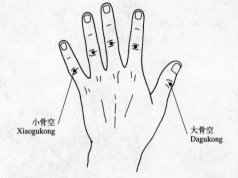

小骨空
Xiaogukong

大骨空
Dagukong

图 3-43   五指节
Fig. 3-43   Wuzhijie

大小骨空
Daxiaogukong

组成   本穴组由大骨空、小骨空二穴组合而成。

位置   大骨空：拇指背侧正中线，近侧指节骨与远侧指节骨关节之中点。

小骨空：小指背侧，远端指节骨与中指节骨关节之中点。

主治   眼眩溃烂，泪冷。

操作   麦粒灸3~5壮，艾条灸3~5分钟。

Composition   This group of acupoints is composed of Dagukong and Xiaogukong.

Location　Dagukong：on the midline of the dorsal side of the thumb, at the midpoint of the interphalangeal crease.

Xiaogukong：on the dorsal side of the little finger, at the midpoint of the distal interphalangeal crease.

Indication　Ulcerated eyelids, cold lacrimation.

Method　3—5 wheat-sized moxa cones of moxibustion, or moxibustion with moxa roll for 3—5 minutes is applied.

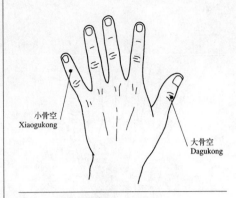

图 3-44　大小骨空
Fig. 3-44　Daxiaogukong

手鬼哭
Shouguiku

组成　本穴组由手拇指桡侧爪甲旁之二个点组合而成。

位置　位于手指背侧桡侧缘。左右拇指桡侧爪甲角各一穴。直对桡侧爪甲角处之皮肤部各一穴。

主治　癫，狂，痫，惊。

操作　麦粒灸3～5壮。

按注　本穴中一穴，实包括商穴。

Composition　This group of acupoints is composed of two points beside the radial side of the fingernail of the thumb.

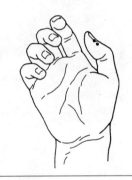

图 3-45　手鬼哭
Fig. 3-45　Shouguiku

Location　On the radial side of the dorsum of the hand, each point at the corner of the radial side of the fingernails of both hands, and each point on the skin opposite to the radial side of the corner of the fingernail.

Indication　Mania, epilepsy, epilepsy due to fright.

Method　3—5 wheat-sized moxa cones of moxibustion is applied.

Note　This group includes Laoshang actually.

五井
Wujing

组成　本穴组由少商、商阳、中冲、关冲、少泽五穴组合而成。

位置　少商：拇指桡侧指甲角旁约0.1寸。

商阳：示指桡侧指甲角旁约0.1寸。

中冲：中指尖端的中央。

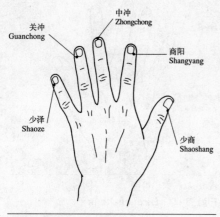

图 3-46　五井
Fig. 3-46　Wujing

关冲：第四指尺侧指甲角旁约 0.1 寸。

少泽：小指尺侧指甲角旁约 0.1 寸。

主治　壮热无汗，肌肤灼热，面红目赤，口唇干燥，烦渴、神昏，或中风闭证，痰涎壅盛，喉中痰鸣，舌红少津，苔黄，脉洪数或弦数。

操作　刺五井用泻法，留针 15 分钟，热甚则用三棱针点刺出血。

Composition　This group of acupoints is composed of Shaoshang (LU11), Shangyang (LI1), Zhongchong (PC9), Guanchong (TE1) and Shaoze (SI1).

Location　Shaoshang：0.1 cun lateral to the radial corner of the fingernail of the thumb.

Shangyang：0.1 cun lateral to the radial corner of the fingernail of the index finger.

Zhongchong：at the midpoint of the tip of the middle finger.

Guanchong：0.1 cun lateral to the ulnar corner of the fingernail of the ring finger.

Shaoze：0.1 cun lateral to the ulnar corner of the fingernail of the little finger.

Indication　High fever without sweating, heat in the skin, red face and eye, dryness of the mouth and lip, thirst and irritability, unconsciousness, or excess syndromes of apoplexy, obstruction of profuse phlegm, phlegm whooping in the throat, red tongue with little moisture, yellow coating, big and rapid pulse or wiry and rapid pulse.

Method　Wujing are needled with reducing techniques. Retain the needles for 15 minutes. If the fever is severe, these points can be pricked to bleed with a three-edged needle.

 十二井穴
Shierjingxue

组成　本穴组由手指端之少商、商阳、中冲、关冲、少冲和少泽六穴组合而成。

位置　少商：拇指桡侧指甲角旁约 0.1 寸。

商阳：示指桡侧指甲角旁约 0.1 寸。

中冲：中指尖端的中央。

关冲：第四指尺侧指甲角旁约 0.1 寸。

少冲：小指桡侧指甲角旁约 0.1 寸。

少泽：小指尺侧指甲角旁约 0.1 寸。

左右计十二穴。

主治　一切痧暑急症，高血压病。

操作　浅刺出血，或用三棱针点刺放血。

按注　有人认为十二井穴乃十二经之井穴组成，即由上之手六井穴加足六井穴即隐白、大敦、厉兑、窍阴、至阴和涌泉组成。

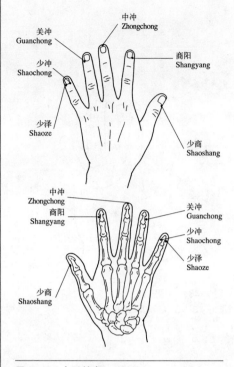

图 3-47　十二井穴
Fig. 3-47　Shierjingxue

Composition　This group of acupoints is composed of Shaoshang (LU11), Shangyang (LI1), Zhongchong (PC9), Guanchong (TE1), Shaochong (HT9) and Shaoze (SI1) which are at the tips of the fingers.

Location　Shaoshang：0.1 cun lateral to the radial corner of the fingernail of the thumb.

Shangyang：0.1 cun lateral to the radial corner of the fingernail of the index finger.

Zhongchong：at the midpoint of the tip of the middle finger.

Guanchong：0.1 cun lateral to the ulnar corner of the fingernail of the ring finger.

Shaochong：0.1 cun lateral to the radial corner of the fingernail of the little finger.

Shaoze：0.1 cun lateral to the ulnar corner of the fingernail of the little finger.

Indication　All acute diseases caused by summer-heat, hypertension.

Method　The points are pricked superficially to bleed, they can be pricked to bleed with a three-edged needle too.

Note　It is regarded by some people that Shierjingxue is composed of the Jing (well) points of the twelve meridians, i.e. the above six Jing (well) points plus the six Jing (well) points on the foot：Yinbai (SP1), Dadun (LR1), Lidui (ST45), Qiaoyin (GB44), Zhiyin (BL67) and Yongquan (KI1).

健理三针
Jianlisanzhen

组成　本穴组由手掌中央的三个点组合而成。

位置　手掌中央，第三、第四掌骨间隙之中点直后1寸处一穴，左右旁开0.5寸各一穴。

主治　肝、脾、胃病，头痛，眼病，咳嗽，哮喘，心悸，心力衰竭，水肿。

操作　直刺或向上斜刺0.5~1寸，针感手指麻、胀。

Composition　This group of acupoints is composed of three points in the center of the palm.

Location　In the centre of the palm, one point is 1 cun posterior to the midpoint of the 3rd and 4th metacarpal bones, the other two points are 0.5 cun lateral to above point.

Indication　Diseases of liver, spleen and stomach, headache, eye diseases, cough, asthma, palpitation, heart failure, edema.

Method　The needle is inserted 0.5−1 cun perpendicularly or upwards obliquely, the acu-esthesia of numbness and distension will be obtained in the fingers.

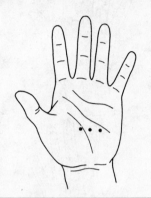

图3-48　健理三针
Fig. 3-48　Jianlisanzhen

 指根
Zhigen

组成　本穴组由位于手掌指侧缘的除大指外其余四指指根与掌相接之横纹中央的四穴组合而成。

位置　位于手掌指侧缘，第二、第三、第四、第五指指根与掌相接之横纹中央。

主治　手生痈疔，五指尽痛，解热，腹吐疼痛。

操作　刺法：点刺出血。

灸法：麦粒点3~5壮。

按注　疗痈、解热一般用灸之泻法。有书记"四横纹"穴与本穴位同，故合而为一穴。

Composition　This group of acupoints is composed of the points at the midpoints of the creases of the four metacarpophalangeal joints without the joint of the thumb on the palmar side of the hand.

Location　On the palmar side of the hand, at the

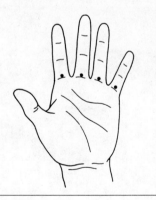

图3-49　指根
Fig. 3-49　Zhigen

midpoints of the creases of the 2nd, 3rd, 4th and 5th metacarpophalangeal joints.

Indication Furuncle and carbuncle on the hand, pain in the five fingers, fever, abdominal pain.

Method Acupuncture: the points are pricked to bleed.

Moxibustion: 3—5 wheat-sized moxa cones of moxibustion is applied.

Note The reducing method of moxibustion is used to treat furuncle and carbuncle. Sihengwen in some books are the same points as this group, and they're combined to one group.

四缝
Sifeng

组成 本穴组由第二、第三、第四、第五指掌面、近端指节纹中点的四个穴组合而成。

位置 第二、第三、第四、第五指掌面，近端指关节横纹中点。

主治 小儿疳积，百日咳，小儿食谷不化。

操作 点刺出血或挤出少许黄白色透明黏液。

按注 有书记有第二、第三、第四、第五指掌的远端指关节横纹中点名为"四缝"，今为区分，把此名为"前四缝"穴，其主治类同，其穴也不另列。

Composition This group of acupoints is composed of four points at the midpoints of the creases of the proximal interphalangeal joints of the 2nd, 3rd, 4th and 5th fingers on the palmar side.

Location On the palmar side of the 2nd, 3rd, 4th and 5th fingers, at the midpoints of the creases of the proximal interphalangeal joints.

Indication Malnutrition and indigestion syndrome in children, whooping cough, infantile indigestion.

Method The points are pricked to bleed or to squeeze out a small amount of yellowish viscous fluid.

Note In some books, Sifeng are the points at the midpoints of the creases of the distal insterphalangeal joins of the 2nd, 3rd, 4th and 5th fingers. These points are called Qiansifeng here in order to be distinguished

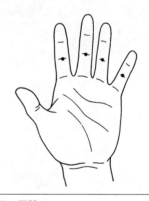

图 3—50 四缝
Fig. 3—50 Sifeng

from the Sifeng above, its indications are the same as Sifeng, and it won't be listed in this book.

● 六缝
Liufeng

组成　本穴组由四缝加拇指掌侧二节横纹中点的二个点计六个穴点组合而成。

位置　四缝：见四缝穴。

另一点在拇指掌侧近侧指节骨与远侧指节骨横纹中点一穴点。一点在拇指近侧指节骨与手掌间中点一穴点。

主治　疔疮，五脏六腑不和。

操作　点刺或挑刺0.1~0.2寸。

Composition　This group of acupoints is composed of six points including Sifeng and two points at the mid-point of the creases of the palmar side of the thumb.

Location　Sifeng：see Sifeng.

One point is at the midpoint of the crease between the proximal and distal phalanges of the palmar side of the thumb. The other point is at the midpoint of the crease between the proximal phalange and the palm.

Indication　Furuncle, disorders of five Zang and six Fu organs.

Method　The points can be spot-pricked or pricked 0.1−0.2 cun.

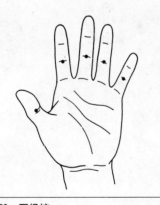

图3-51　六缝
Fig. 3-51　Liufeng

● 五经纹
Wujingwen

组成　本穴组由拇指指节横纹一穴点与其他四指近节横纹之四个点共五穴组合而成。

位置　位于手五指掌侧，拇指之指节横纹一穴。示、中、环、小指之近侧指节横纹四穴。

主治　五脏六腑气不和。

操作　针刺0.1~0.2寸，或点刺出黄白色液体。

按注　本穴包括在"六缝"穴中，本穴也即四缝穴加大指节横纹一穴共五穴之合称。

Composition　This group of acupoints is composed of

图3-52　五经纹
Fig. 3-52　Wujingwen

the point on the crease of the thumb and four points on the interphalangeal creases of the other four fingers.

Location On the palmar side of the hand, one point is on the interphalangeal crease of the thumb, the other four points are on the interphalangeal creases of the index, middle, ring and little fingers.

Indication Qi disorders of five Zang and six Fu organs.

Method The needle is inserted 0.1−0.2 cun, or the points can be pricked to squeeze some yellowish−whitish fluid.

Note This group is included in Liufeng. This group is also the collective name of the five points of Sifeng and the crease of the thumb.

手八掌
Shoubazhang

组成 本穴组由手掌部四个点组合而成。

位置 手掌部，第二、第三、第三、第四、第四、第五指蹼缘后0.2寸处各一穴，第五指掌关节横纹尺侧缘上0.2寸处一穴。左右计八穴。

主治 手掌红肿，手指不能屈伸，眼球胀痛，夜尿症。

操作 针0.3~0.5寸，手指有麻、胀感。

Composition This group of acupoints is composed of four points on the palm.

Location On the palm, 0.2 cun posterior to the web margin between 2nd and 3rd, 3rd and 4th, 4th and 5th fingers, and the point on the ulnar side of the 5th metacarpophalangeal crease, 8 points on both sides.

Indications Redness and swelling in the palm, motor impairment of the fingers, distension and pain in the eyesball, enuresis.

Method The needle is inserted 0.3−0.5 cun, and the acu-esthesia of numbness and distension will be obtained in the fingers.

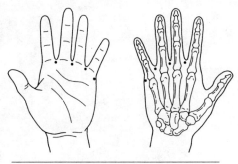

图3−53 手八掌
Fig. 3−53 Shoubazhang

十前
Shiqian

组成　本穴组由手指掌侧、每指远侧指节横纹二端之十个点组合而成。

位置　位于手指之掌侧，远侧指节横纹之两端，每指两穴。

主治　大骨节病，指关节末节疼痛。

操作　点刺0.1～0.2寸，局部疼痛感。

按注　本穴原书记为"四前"，应改名为十前为妥。

Composition　This group of acupoints is composed of ten points at both ends of each distal interphanlangeal crease on the palmar side of the fingers.

Location　On the palmar side of the fingers, at both ends of each distal interphanlangeal crease, 2 points on each fingers.

Indications　Kaschin-Beck disease, pain in the distal joints of the fingers.

Method　The points are punctured 0.1−0.2 cun, and the acu-esthesia of pain will be felt in this part.

Note　This group's original name is Siqian, but Shiqian is more proper for this group.

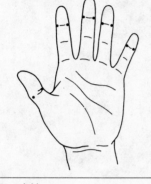

图3-54　十前
Fig. 3-54　Shiqian

十王
Shiwang

组成　本穴组由手十指掌侧爪甲后的十个点组合而成。

位置　位于手十指背侧，沿爪甲正中点向皮肤部约0.1寸处。

主治　卒死，痧症，中暑，霍乱，感冒。

操作　三棱针点刺出血各1～3滴。

Composition　This group of acupoints is composed of ten points posterior to the fingernails of ten fingers.

Location　On the dorsum of the ten fingers, 0.1 cun on the skin posterior to the midpoints of the fingernails.

Indication　Sudden death, sunstroke, cholera, common cold.

Method　The points are pricked to bleed 1−3 drops with a three-edged needle.

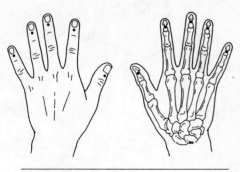

图3-55　十王
Fig. 3-55　Shiwang

十宣
Shixuan

组成　本穴组在手指头处十个穴点组合而成。

位置　在手十指头上，去爪甲0.1寸处约十个穴点。

主治　昏迷，晕厥，中暑，热病，小儿惊厥，咽喉肿痛，指端麻木。

操作　直刺0.1～0.2寸，或用三棱针点刺出血。

Composition　This group of acupoints is composed of ten points on the finger tips.

Location　On the tips of ten fingers, 0.1 cun from the corners of the fingernails.

Indication　Coma, syncope, sunstroke, febrile diseases, infantile convulsion, sore throat, numbness of the finger tips.

Method　The needle is inserted 0.1-0.2 cun perpendicularly, or the points can be pricked to bleed.

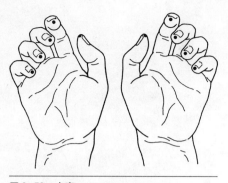

图3-56　十宣
Fig. 3-56　Shixuan

下痿痹
Xiaweibi

组成　本穴组由环跳、委中、阳陵泉、悬钟四穴组合而成。

位置　环跳：股骨大转子高点与骶管裂孔连线的外1/3与内2/3交界处。

阳陵泉：腓骨小头前下方凹陷中。

悬钟：外踝高点上3寸，腓骨后缘。

委中：腘横纹中央。

主治　下肢痿痹。

操作　刺法：环跳直刺2～3寸。委中刺0.5～1寸。悬钟刺0.5～1寸。阳陵泉直刺1～1.5寸。

得气为度。

灸法：艾条温灸10～20分钟。

按注　本穴组临床常加配腰3～骶1夹脊，则效更佳。

Composition　This group of acupoints is composed of Huantiao(GB30), Weizhong (BL40), Yanglingquan (GB34) and Xuanzhong (GB39).

Location　Huantiao：at the junction of the lateral 1/3 and medial 2/3 of the line connecting the prominence of

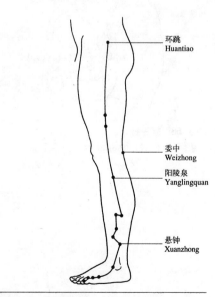

环跳
Huantiao

委中
Weizhong

阳陵泉
Yanglingquan

悬钟
Xuanzhong

图3-57　下痿痹
Fig. 3-57　Xiaweibi

the great trochanter and the sacral hiatus.

Yanglingquan: in the depression anterior and inferior to the head of the fibula.

Xuanzhong: 3 cun above the tip of the external malleolus, on the posterior border of the fibula.

Weizhong: at the midpoint of the popliteal crease.

Indication　Muscular atrophy and paralysis of the lower limbs.

Method　Acupuncture: Huantiao is needled 2—3 cun perpendicularly. Weizhong is needled 0.5—1 cun. Xuanzhong is needled 0.5—0.8 cun. Yanglingquan is needled 1—1.5 cun perpendicularly till the acu-esthesia is obtained.

Moxibustion: warm moxibustion with moxa roll for 10—20 minutes is applied.

Note　The curative effect will be better if this group is combined with Jiaji from the 1st lumbar vertebra to the 1st sacral vertebra.

髋三针
Kuansanzhen

组成　本穴组由秩边、居髎、环跳三穴组合而成。

位置　秩边：第四骶椎棘突下，旁开3寸。

居髎：髂前上棘与股骨大转子高点连线的中点。

环跳：股骨大转子高点与骶管裂孔连线的外1/3与内2/3交界处。

主治　下肢痿痹，半身不遂，腰胯疼痛，坐骨神经痛，小儿麻痹症，髋关节周围软组织疾患等。

操作　刺法：直刺1～3寸。

灸法：艾炷灸5～9壮，或温灸10～25分钟。

Composition　This group of acupoints is composed of Zhibian (BL54), Juliao (GB29) and Huantiao (GB30).

Location　Zhibian: below the 4th posterior sacral foramen and 3 cun lateral to the median sacral crest.

Juliao: at the midpoint of the line connecting the anteriosuperior iliac spine and the prominence of the great trochanter.

Huantiao: at the junction of the lateral 1/3 and me-

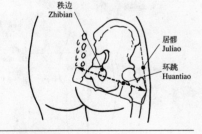

图 3-58　髋三针
Fig. 3-58　Kuansanzhen

dial 2/3 of the line connecting the prominence of the great trochanter and the sacral hiatus.

Indication　Muscular atrophy and paralysis of the lower limbs, hemiplegia, pain in the lower back, sciatica, infantile paralysis, diseases of the parenchyma of the coxa joint.

Method　Acupuncture：the needle is inserted 1−3 cun perpendicularly.

Moxibustion：moxibustion with 5−9 moxa cones, or warm moxibustion for 10−25 minutes is applied.

股三针
Gusanzhen

组成　本穴组由髀关、阴市、风市三穴组合而成。
位置　髀关：髂前上棘与髌骨外缘连线上，平臀沟处。
阴市：在髂前上棘与髌骨外缘连线上，髌骨外上缘上3寸。
风市：大腿外侧正中，腘横纹水平线上7寸。
主治　髀股痿痹，麻木，下肢不遂，股外侧皮神经炎。
操作　刺法：直刺0.5~1.5寸。
灸法：艾炷灸3~5壮，或温灸10~20分钟。

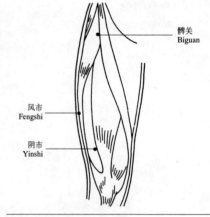

图3−59　股三针
Fig. 3−59　Gusanzhen

Composition　This group of acupoints is composed of Biguan (ST31), Yinshi (ST33) and Fengshi (GB31).

Location　Biguan：on the line connecting the anteriosuperior iliac spine and the lateral corner of the patella, on the level of the gluteal crease.

Yinshi：on the line connecting the anteriosuperior iliac spine and the lateral corner of the patella, 3 cun above the superiolateral border of the patella.

Fengshi：on the midline of the lateral side of the thigh, 7 cun above the popliteal crease.

Indication　Muscular atrophy and paralysis of the thigh, numbness and motor impairment of the lower limbs, and lateral femoral cutaneous neuritis.

Method　Acupuncture：the needle is inserted 0.5−1.5 cun perpendicularly.

Moxibustion：moxibustion with 3−5 moxa cones, or warm moxibustion for 10−20 minutes is applied.

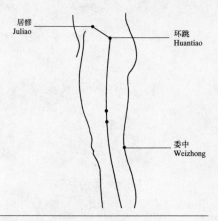

居髎
Juliao

环跳
Huantiao

委中
Weizhong

图3-60 腿风
Fig. 3-60 Tuifeng

腿风
Tuifeng

组成 本穴组由环跳、居髎、委中三穴组合而成。

位置 环跳：股骨大转子高点与骶管裂孔连线的外1/3与内2/3交界处。

居髎：髂前上棘与股骨大转子高点连线的中点。

委中：腘横纹中央。

主治 腿风湿痛。

操作 刺法：委中刺0.5～1寸，居髎直刺或斜刺1～2寸。各以得气为度。环跳：见悬跳。

灸法：居髎、环跳均可用，艾条灸10～20分钟。

Composition This group of acupoints is composed of Huantiao (GB30), Juliao (GB29) and Weizhong (BL40).

Location Huantiao：at the junction of the lateral 1/3 and medial 2/3 of the line connecting the prominence of the great trochanter and the sacral hiatus.

Juliao：at the midpoint of the line connecting the anteriosuperior iliac spine and the prominence of the great trochanter.

Weizhong：at the midpoint of the popliteal crease.

Indication Pain in the leg due to cold and dampness.

Method Acupuncture：Weizhong is needled 0.8-1 cun till the acu-esthesia is obtained. Juliao is needled 1-2 cun perpendicularly or obliquely till the acu-esthesia is obtained. Huantiao：see Xuantiao.

Moxibustion：moxibustion with moxa roll for 10-20 minutes can be applied to Juliao and Huantiao.

环陵
Huanling

组成 本穴组由环跳、阳陵泉二穴组合而成。

位置 环跳：股骨大转子高点与骶管裂孔连线的外1/3与内2/3交界处。

阳陵泉：腓骨小头前下方凹陷中。

主治 风冷湿痹，下肢痿痹。

操作 刺法：环跳见"悬跳"。阳陵泉直刺1～1.5寸，得

汉 英 对 照

气为度。

灸法：艾条灸10~20分钟。

Composition　This group of acupoints is composed of Huantiao (GB30) and Yanglingquan (GB34).

Location　Huantiao：at the junction of the lateral 1/3 and medial 2/3 of the line connecting the prominence of the great trochanter and the sacral hiatus.

Yanglingquan：in the depression anterior and inferior to the head of the fibula.

Indication　Bi-syndromes due to wind, cold or damp, muscular atrophy and paralysis of the lower limbs.

Method　Acupuncture：Huantiao：see Xuantiao. Yanglingquan is needled 1−1.5 cun perpendicularly till the acu-esthesia is obtained.

Moxibustion：moxibustion with moxa roll for 10−20 minutes is applied.

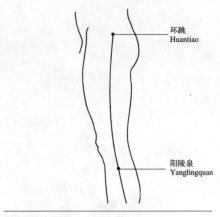

图3-61　环陵
Fig. 3-61　Huanling

悬跳
Xuantiao

组成　本穴组由悬钟、环跳二穴组合而成。

位置　悬钟：外踝高点上3寸，腓骨后缘。

环跳：股骨大转子高点与骶管裂孔连线的外1/3与内2/3交界处。

主治　躄足不能行。

操作　环跳针刺视臀部肌肉脂肪的厚度而定，一般刺2~3寸得气为度，针后拔罐则效更佳。悬钟直刺0.5~1寸，得气为度。

Composition　This group of acupoints is composed of Xuanzhong (GB39) and Huantiao (GB30).

Location　Xuanzhong：3 cun above the tip of the external malleolus, on the posterior border of the fibula.

Huantiao：at the junction of the lateral 1/3 and medial 2/3 of the line connecting the prominence of the great trochanter and the sacral hiatus.

Indication　Motor impairment of the lame leg.

Method　The insertion depth of Huantiao depends on the thickness of the muscle and fat of the buttocks. Usually the depth is 2−3 cun till the acu-esthesia is

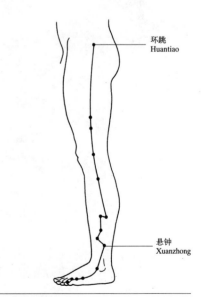

图3-62　悬跳
Fig. 3-62　Xuantiao

obtained. The curative effect will be better if cupping is applied after acupuncture. Xuanzhong is needled 0.5—1 cun till the acu-esthesia is obtained.

风市四穴
Fengshisixue

组成　本穴组由风市、风市上、上风市、前风市四穴组合而成。

位置　风市：大腿外侧正中，腘横纹水平线上7寸。

风市上：大腿外侧正中线，臀皱襞下2寸约当风市上5寸处。

上风市：大腿外侧正中线，腘窝横纹上8寸，约当风市上2寸处。

前风市：大腿外侧正中线，前方2寸，腘窝横纹上6寸，约当风市前2寸处。

主治　偏瘫，坐骨神经痛，下肢痿痹。

操作　刺法：针1～2寸，针感酸麻至腿膝。

灸法：灸3～5壮，艾条温灸10～20分钟。

Composition　This group of acupoints is composed of Fengshi (GB31), Fengshishang, Shangfengshi and Qianfengshi.

Location　Fengshi：on the midline of the lateral side of the thigh, 7 cun above the popliteal crease.

Fengshishang：on the midline of the lateral side of the thigh, 2 cun below the gluteal crease, i.e. 5 cun above Fengshi.

Shangfengshi：on the midline of the lateral side of the thigh, 8 cun above the popliteal crease, about 2 cun above Fengshi.

Qianfengshi：2 cun anterior to the midline of the lateral side of the thigh, 6 cun above the popliteal crease, about 2 cun anterior to Fengshi.

Indication　Hemiplegia, sciatica, muscular atrophy and paralysis of the lower limbs.

Method　Acupuncture：the needle is inserted 1—2 cun, and the acu-esthesia of soreness and numbness can radiate to the leg and the knee.

Moxibustion　3—5 cones of moxibustion, or warm moxibustion with moxa roll for 10—20 minutes is

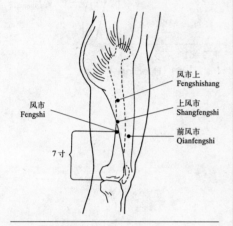

图3-63　风市四穴
Fig. 3-63　Fengshisixue

applied.

阴委
Yinwei

组成　本穴组由阴委1、阴委2、阴委3三穴组合而成。

位置　阴委1：大腿外侧，腘横纹端上1寸，股二头肌与髂胫束之间凹陷中。

阴委2：阴委1上1寸处。

阴委3：阴委1上2寸处。

主治　癫狂。

操作　直刺0.5~1寸，强刺激，得气感应强烈。

Composition　This group of acupoints is composed of Yinwei1, Yinwei2 and Yinwei3.

Location　Yinwei1：on the lateral side of the thigh, 1 cun above the popliteal crease, in the drepression between the biceps muscle of the thigh and the iliotibial tract.

Yingwei2：1 cun above Yinwei1.

Yinwei3：2 cun above Yinwei1.

Indication　Mania.

Method　The needle is inserted 0.5—1 cun. Strong stimulation is performed, and the acu-esthesia should be strong too.

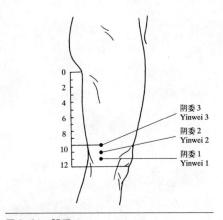

图3-64　阴委
Fig. 3-64　Yinwei

阳关三穴
Yangguansanxue

组成　本穴组由阳关、上阳关、后阳关三穴组合而成。

位置　阳关：阳陵泉穴上3寸，股骨外上髁上方的凹陷中。

上阳关：大腿外侧远端，股骨外上髁上方凹陷处直上1寸，约当阳关穴上1寸处。

后阳关：大腿外侧远端，股骨外上髁上方凹陷处平后方1寸处，约当阳关平后1寸处。

主治　膝痛，下肢痿痹。

操作　刺法：针0.5~1.5寸，针感酸麻至膝。

灸法：灸3~5壮，艾条温灸10~20分钟。

Composition　This group of acupoints is composed of

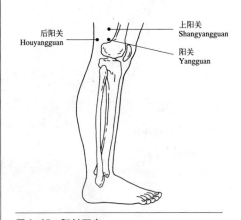

图3-65　阳关三穴
Fig. 3-65　Yangguansanxue

Yangguan, Shangyangguan and Houyangguan.

Location Yangguan: 3 cun above Yanglingquan, in the depression above the external epicondyle of the femur.

Shangyangguan: on the distal portion of the lateral side of the thigh, 1 cun above the external epicondyle of the femur, about 1 cun above Yangguan.

Houyangguan: on the distal portion of the lateral side of the thigh, 1 cun posterior to the depression above the external epicondyle of the femur, about 1 cun posterior to Yangguan.

Indications Pain in the knee, muscular atrophy and paralysis of the lower limbs.

Methods Acupuncture: the needle is inserted 0.5– 1.5 cun, and the acu-esthesia of soreness and numbness will radiate to the knee.

Moxibustion: 3–5 cones of moxibustion, or warm moxibustion with moxa roll for 10–20 minutes is applied.

双市
Shuangshi

组成　本穴组由风市、阴市二穴组合而成。

位置　风市：大腿外侧正中，腘横纹水平线上7寸。

阴市：在髂前上棘与髌骨外缘连线上，髌骨外上缘上3寸。

主治　腿脚乏力，疼痛。

操作　刺法：直刺1~1.5寸，得气为度。

灸法：艾条灸10~20分钟。

Composition This group of acupoints is composed of Fengshi (GB31) and Yinshi (ST33).

Location Fengshi: on the midline of the lateral side of the thigh, 7 cun above the popliteal crease.

Yinshi: on the line connecting the anteriosuperior iliac spine and the lateral corner of the patella, 3 cun above the superiolateral border of the patella.

Indication Weakness and pain of the leg and foot.

Method Acupuncture: the needle is inserted 1–1.5 cun till the acu-esthesia is obtained.

Moxibustion: moxibustion with moxa roll for 10–20 minutes is applied.

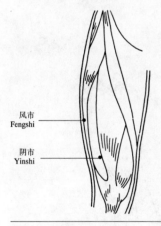

风市
Fengshi

阴市
Yinshi

图3-66　双市
Fig. 3-66　Shuangshi

髋骨
Kuangu

组成　本穴组由大腿伸侧远端之二个点组合而成。

位置　大腿伸侧远端，髌骨中线上3寸，股直肌外缘之点两侧各旁开1.5寸处。每侧两穴，左右计四穴。当"梁丘"穴两侧1.5寸处。

主治　股腿痛。

操作　刺法：直刺0.5~1寸，局部酸胀，并可向膝部扩散。

灸法：艾条或温针灸3~5壮，艾条灸5~10分钟。

Composition　This group of acupoints is composed of two points on the distal end of the anterior side of the thigh.

Location　On the distal end of the anterior side of the thigh, 1.5 cun lateral to the point which is 3 cun above the midline of the patella and on the lateral border of the straight muscle of the thigh. 2 points on each side, 4 points on both sides. i.e. 1.5 cun lateral to Liangqiu.

Indication　Pain in the thigh and leg.

Method　Acupuncture：the needle is inserted 0.5−1 cun perpendicularly, the acu-esthesia of soreness and distension will be obtained in the part and may radiate to the knee.

Moxibustion：3−5 cones of moxibustion with moxa cone or warm needle moxibustion is applied. Moxibustion with moxa roll for 5−10 minutes can be used too.

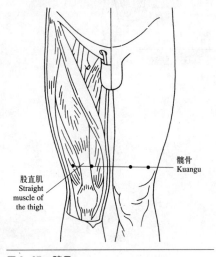

股直肌
Straight muscle of the thigh

髋骨
Kuangu

图3−67　髋骨
Fig. 3−67　Kuangu

 髓膏
Suigao

组成　本穴组由大腿伸侧远端之二个点组成，约近髋骨穴0.5寸处。

位置　大腿伸侧远端，髌骨中线上3寸，股直肌外缘之点，向两旁各平开1寸处。每侧两穴，左右计四穴。当"梁丘"穴两侧各1寸处。

主治　下股痿痹，膝痛，白虎历节风痛。

操作　刺法：直刺0.5~1寸，局部酸胀，或向膝部扩散。

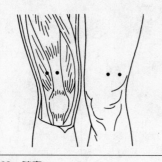

图 3-68 髓膏
Fig. 3-68 Suigao

灸法：艾粒灸温针灸 3～5 壮，艾条灸 5～10 分钟。

Composition   This group of acupoints is composed of two points on the distal end of the anterior side of the thigh, which are about 0.5 cun from Kuangu.

Location   On the distal end of the anterior side of the thigh, 1 cun lateral to the point which is 3 cun above the midline of the patella and on the lateral border of the straight muscle of the thigh. 2 points on each side, 4 points on both sides. i.e. 1 cun lateral to Liangqiu.

Indication   Muscular atrophy and paralysis of the lower limbs, pain in the knee, pain in the joints due to wind.

Method   Acupuncture：the needle is inserted 0.5−1 cun perpendicularly. The acu-esthesia of soreness and distension will be obtained in this part, or may transmit to the knee.

Moxibustion：3−5 cones of moxibustion or warm needle moxibustion is applied. Moxibustion with moxa roll for 5−10 minutes can be used too.

 ## 髋膝
Kuanxi

组成   本穴组由髋骨、膝关二穴组合而成。
位置   髋骨：即梁丘穴外开 1 寸处。
膝关：阴陵泉穴后 1 寸。
主治   腿痛步难。
操作   刺法：直刺 1～1.2 寸，得气为度。
灸法：温灸 10～20 分钟。

Composition   This group of acupoints is composed of Kuangu and Xiguan(LR7).

Location   Kuangu：1 cun lateral to Liangqiu.

Xiguan：1 cun posterior to Yinlingquan.

Indication   Pain and motor impairment of the leg.

Methods   Acupuncture：the needle is inserted 1−1.2 cun perpendicularly till the acu-esthesia is obtained.

Moxibustion：warm moxibustion for 10～20 minutes is applied.

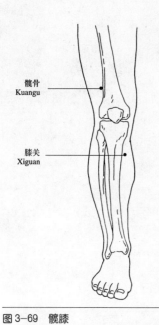

髋骨
Kuangu

膝关
Xiguan

图 3-69 髋膝
Fig. 3-69 Kuanxi

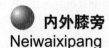

膝跟
Xigen

组成　本穴组由膝外侧的两个刺激点组合而成。

位置　位于膝关节外侧缘，犊鼻穴外侧的两个凹陷中。

主治　腿膝肿痛。

操作　刺法：直刺0.5～1寸。

灸法：温灸5～10分钟。

按注　近有人认为，膝跟即膝眼穴，跟与眼字形相近，似笔误所致。

Composition　This group of acupoints is composed of two stimulating points on the lateral side of the knee.

Location　On the lateral border of the knee joint, in the two depressions on the lateral side of Dubi.

Indication　Swelling and pain in the leg and pain.

Method　Acupuncture：the needle is inserted 0.5-1 cun perpendicularly.

Moxibustion：warm moxibustion for 5-10 minutes is applied.

Note　It is regarded by some people recently that Xigen is Xiyan practically. It may result from the similar font style of "跟" and "眼" in Chinese character.

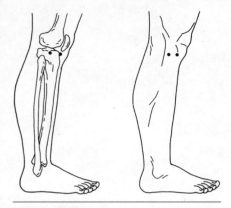

图3-70　膝跟
Fig. 3-70　Xigen

内外膝旁
Neiwaixipang

组成　本穴组由膝髌两旁之二个点组合而成。

位置　膝部，平髌骨中线，髌骨两旁之凹陷中各一穴，分别叫内外膝旁。左右计四穴，约当内外膝眼上1寸处。

主治　膝风湿，痹痛。

操作　刺法：斜向膝关节中央刺0.5～1.5寸，膝中酸胀沉重感。

灸法：温针灸3～5壮，艾条温灸5～10分钟。

Composition　This group of acupoints is composed of two points beside the patella.

Location　On the knee, at the midline of the patella, points in the two depressions beside the patella, and are called Neixipang and Waixipang respectively, 4 points on

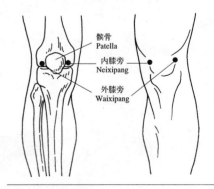

图3-71　内外膝旁
Fig. 3-71　Neiwaixipang

both sides. They are about 1 cun above Neixiyan and Waixiyan.

Indication   Pain and Bi-syndromes of the knee joint due to wind and dampness.

Method   Acupuncture：the needle is inserted 0.5–1.5 cun towards the centre of the knee obliquely, the acuesthesia of soreness, distension and heaviness will be felt in the knee.

Moxibustion：3–5 cones of warm needle moxibustion, or warm moxibustion with moxa roll for 5–10 minutes is applied.

● 膝旁
Xipang

组成   本穴组由腘窝部的两个刺激点组合而成。

位置   外侧一点：位于腘窝横纹外侧端(似与足太阳经的委阳穴同位)。

内侧一点：位于腘窝横纹内侧端(似与足少阴经的阴谷穴位同)。

主治   腰痛不能俯仰，脚酸不能久立。

操作   刺法：直刺0.5～1寸。

灸法：艾炷灸1～3壮，或温灸5～10分钟。

Composition   This group of acupoints is composed of two points in the popliteal fossa.

Location   The lateral point is at the lateral end of the popliteal crease (similar to Weiyang of the Meridian of Foot–Taiyang).

The medial point is at the medial end of the popliteal crease (similar to Yingu of the Meridian of Foot-Shaoyin).

Indication   Pain and motor impairment of the waist, aching and weakness of the feet.

Method   Acupuncture：the needle is inserted 0.5–1 cun perpendicularly.

Moxibustion：moxibustion with 1–3 cones, or warm moxibustion for 5–10 minutes is applied.

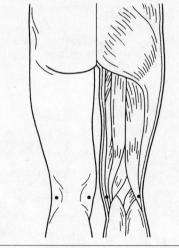

图3-72 膝旁
Fig. 3-72 Xipang

膝上二穴
Xishangerxue

组成　本穴组由膝关节上二个穴组合而成。

位置　膝关节部，平髌骨基底，股直肌腱两侧凹陷中。

主治　膝痛。

操作　刺法：直刺0.5~1寸，局部酸胀沉重感，或可向膝部扩散。

灸法：温针灸3~5壮，艾条温灸5~10分钟。

Composition　This group of acupoints is composed of two points on the knee joint.

Location　On the knee joint, at the level of the base of the patella, in the depressions besides the borders of the retus femoris.

Indication　Pain in the knee.

Method　Acupuncture：the needle is inserted 0.5–1 cun perpendicularly, the acu-esthesia of soreness, distension and heaviness will be obtained in this part, or may radiate to the knee.

Moxibustion：3–5 cones of warm needle moxibustion, or warm moxibustion with moxa roll for 5–10 minutes is applied.

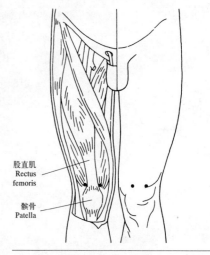

股直肌
Rectus
femoris

髌骨
Patella

图3-73　膝上二穴
Fig. 3-73　Xishangerxue

膝上三针
Xishangsanzhen

组成　本穴组由血海、梁丘、犊鼻三穴组合而成。

位置　血海：髌骨内上缘上2寸。

犊鼻：髌骨下缘，髌韧带外侧凹陷中。

梁丘：在髂前上棘与髌骨外缘连线上，髌骨外上缘上2寸。

主治　风湿性膝关节炎，类风湿性膝关节炎(历节风)，膝关节创伤性滑膜炎等所致的膝关节疼痛、无力等。

操作　犊鼻针尖向膝关节方向刺入0.8~1寸。血海、梁丘均直刺或斜刺0.8~1寸深。

Composition　This group of acupoints is composed of Xuehai(SP10) Liangqiu(ST34) and Dubi(ST35).

Location　Xuehai：2 cun above the superior medial corner of the patella.

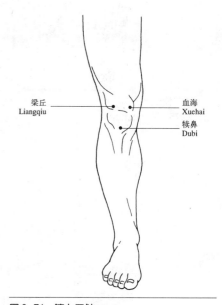

梁丘
Liangqiu

血海
Xuehai

犊鼻
Dubi

图3-74　膝上三针
Fig. 3-74　Xishangsanzhen

Dubi: on the lower border of the patella, in the depression lateral to the patellar ligament.

Liangqiu: on the line connecting the anteriosuperior iliac spine and the lateral corner of the patella, 2 cun above the superiolateral border of the patella.

Indication Rheumatic arthritis of the knee, post-traumatic synovitis of knee, pain and weakness of the knee joint.

Method Dubi is needled 0.8−1 cun with the tip of the needle towards the knee joint, Xuehai and Liangqiu are needled 0.8−1 cun perpendicularly or obliquely.

● 膝三针
Xisanzhen

组成　本穴组由阳陵泉穴与奇穴双膝眼三穴组合而成。

位置　阳陵泉：腓骨小头前下方凹陷中。

双膝眼穴：位于膝关节伸侧面，髌韧带两侧之凹陷中，屈膝取之。

主治　膝肿痛，脚气，膝关节炎。

操作　刺法：直刺或斜刺1～1.5寸。

灸法：温灸5～15分钟，阳陵泉可艾炷灸3～5壮。

Composition This group of acupoints is composed of Yanglingquan(GB34) and Shuanxiyan(EX).

Location Yanglingquan: in the depression anterior and inferior to the head of the fibula.

Shuangxiyan: when the knee is flexed, on the anterior side of the knee joint, in the depressions beside the borders of the patellar ligament.

Indication Swelling and pain in the knee, beriberi, arthritis of knee.

Method Acupuncture: the needle is inserted 1−1.5 cun perpendicularly or obliquely.

Moxibustion: warm moxibustion for 5−15 minutes is applied. Moxibustion with 3−5 cones can be applied at Yanglingquan.

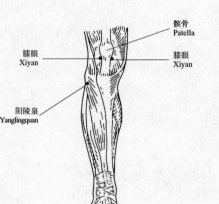

图3-75　膝三针
Fig. 3-75　Xisanzhen

汉 英 对 照

三膝穴
Sanxixue

组成　本穴组由犊鼻穴、内膝眼和膝下三穴组合而成。

位置　犊鼻：髌骨下缘，髌韧带外侧凹陷中。

内膝眼：位于髌骨下方，髌韧带内侧凹陷中。

膝下：位于髌骨下缘，髌韧带处。

三穴均屈膝取之。

主治　膝痹痛，鹤膝风，腿痛，脚气，转筋。

操作　刺法：向膝中斜刺1～1.5寸，双膝眼可对刺。

灸法：温灸5～10分钟。

按注　犊鼻、内膝眼又名膝眼，是临床治疗膝病之常用穴。

Composition　This group of acupoints is composed of Dubi(ST35), Neixiyan and Xixia.

Location　Dubi：on the lower border of the patella, in the depression lateral to the patellar ligament.

Neixiyan：inferior to the patella, in the depression on the medial side of the patellar ligament.

Xixia：on the lower border of the patella, on the patellar ligament.

All the three points are located when the knee is flexed.

Indications　Paralysis and pain of the knee, Bi-syndromes of the knee joint, pain in the leg, beriberi, cramp.

Method　Acupuncture：the needle is inserted 1－1.5 cun towards the centre of the knee. Both Xiyan can be needled oppositely.

Moxibustion：warm moxibustion for 5－10 minutes is applied.

Note　Dubi and Neixiyan is named Xiyan too, and is commonly used to treat the diseases of the knee.

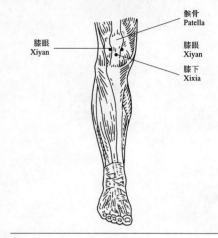

膝眼
Xiyan

髌骨
Patella

膝眼
Xiyan

膝下
Xixia

图3-76　三膝穴
Fig. 3-76　Sanxixue

鹤膝三穴
Hexisanxue

组成　本穴组由奇穴鹤顶、膝上三穴组合而成。

位置　鹤顶穴：位于髌骨上缘中点上之凹陷中。

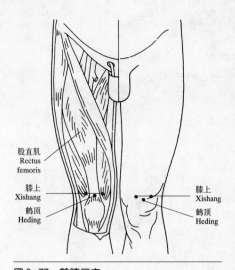

图 3-77 鹤膝三穴
Fig. 3-77 Hexisanxue

膝上穴：位于髌骨上缘、股直肌腱两侧凹陷中各一穴。
主治 鹤膝风，脚足无力，膝关节酸痛。
操作 刺法：直刺 0.5～1 寸。
灸法：艾炷灸 1～3 壮，或温灸 5～10 分钟。

Composition This group of acupoints is composed of Heding and Xishang.

Location Heding：in the depression of the midpoint of the upper border of the patella.

Xishang：on the upper border of the patella, each point in the depressions on both borders of the rectus femoris.

Indication Arthroncus of knee, weakness in the feet, and aching and pain of the knee joint.

Method Acupuncture：the needle is inserted 0.5−1 cun perpendicularly.

Moxibustion：moxibustion with 1−3 cones, or warm moxibustion for 5−10 minutes is applied.

● 膝眼
Xiyan

组成 本穴组由犊鼻、内膝眼二穴组合而成。
位置 犊鼻：髌骨下缘，髌韧带外侧凹陷中。
内膝眼：见三膝穴。
主治 膝关节酸痛，鹤膝风，脚气，腿痛。
操作 刺法：向膝中斜刺 0.5～1.2 寸，或透刺对侧膝眼。
灸法：艾条温灸 5～15 分钟。

Composition This group of acupoints is composed of Dubi(ST35) and Neixiyan.

Location Dubi：on the lower border of the patella, in the depression lateral to the patellar ligament.

Neixiyan：see Sanxi.

Indication Aching and pain in the knee joint, arthroncus of knee, beriberi, pain in the leg.

Method Acupuncture：the needle is inserted 0.5−1.2 cun towards the centre of the knee obliquely, or the needle can be penetrated to the Xiyan on the opposite side.

Moxibustion：warm moxibustion with moxa roll for 5−15 minutes is applied.

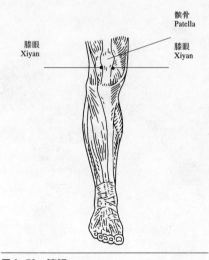

图 3-78 膝眼
Fig. 3-78 Xiyan

下痿三针
Xiaweisanzhen

组成　本穴组由足三里、三阴交、太溪三穴组合而成。

位置　足三里：犊鼻穴下3寸，胫骨前嵴外一横指处。

三阴交：内踝高点上3寸，胫骨内侧面后缘。

太溪：内踝高点与跟腱之间凹陷中。

主治　痿证(同上痿三针)。

操作　直刺1～1.5寸，针感酸、胀、重、麻等，得气为度。

Composition　This group of acupoints is composed of Zusanli(ST36), Sanyinjiao(SP6) and Taixi(KI3).

Location　Zusanli：3 cun below Dubi, one finger breadth from the anterior crest of the tibia.

Sanyinjiao：3 cun above the tip of the medial malleolus, on the posterior border of the medial side of the tibia.

Taixi：in the midpoint between the tip of the medial malleolus and Achilles's tendon.

Indication　Flaccidity syndromes (the same as Shangweisanzhen).

Method　The needle is inserted 1-1.5 cun perpendicularly till the acu-esthesia of soreness, distension, heaviness and numbness is obtained.

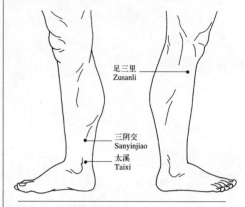

图3-79　下痿三针
Fig. 3-79　Xiaweisanzhen

足三针
Zusanzhen

组成　本穴组由足三里、三阴交、太冲三穴组合而成。

位置　足三里：犊鼻穴下3寸，胫骨前嵴外一横指处。

三阴交：内踝高点上3寸，胫骨内侧面后缘。

太冲：足背，第一、第二跖骨结合部之前凹陷中。

主治　胃腹疼痛，消化不良，泄泻，痢疾，失眠，健忘，肝痛，前阴病，妇科诸疾等。

操作　先取足三里，次取三阴交，后取太冲，深0.5～1.2寸，用捻转手法，得气为度。

Composition　This group of acupoints is composed of Zusanli(ST36), Sanyinjiao(SP6) and Taichong(LR3).

Location　Zusanli：3 cun below Dubi, one finger

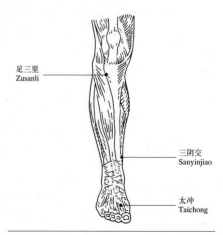

图3-80　足三针
Fig. 3-80　Zusanzhen

breadth from the anterior crest of the tibia.

Sanyinjiao：3 cun above the tip of the medial malleolus, on the posterior border of the medial side of the tibia.

Taichong：on the instep of the foot, in the depression anterior to the commissure of the 1st and 2nd metatarsal bones.

Indication　Gastric and abdominal pain, indigestion, diarrhea, dysentery, insomnia, poor memory, hepatic pain, diseases of external genitalia, women diseases.

Method　Zusanli is needled first, then Sanyinjiao and Taichong. The depth is 0.5-1.2 cun. Rotating techniques are applied till the acu-esthesia is obtained.

缓足
Huanzu

组成　本穴组由悬钟、条口、冲阳三穴组合而成。

位置　悬钟：外踝高点上3寸，腓骨后缘。

条口：上巨虚穴下2寸。

冲阳：足背在解溪穴下方，踇长伸肌腱和趾长伸肌腱之间，当第二、第三跖骨与楔状骨间。

主治　足缓不能收。

操作　刺法：悬钟直刺0.5～1寸。条口直刺1～1.5寸。冲阳斜刺0.3～0.5寸。得气为度。

灸法：麦粒灸3～5壮，艾条灸10～20分钟。

Composition　This group of acupoints is composed of Xuanzhong(GB39), Tiaokou(ST38) and Chongyang (ST42).

Location　Xuanzhong：3 cun above the tip of the external malleolus, on the posterior border of the fibula.

Tiaokou：2 cun below Shangjuxu.

Chongyang：inferior to Jiexi, between the tendons of the extensor hallucis longus and the extensor digitorum longus, on the instep of the foot.

Indication　Flaccid paralysis of the foot.

Method　Acupuncture：Xuanzhong is needled 0.5-1 cun perpendicularly. Tiaokou is needled 1-1.5 cun perpendicularly. Chongyang is needled 0.3-0.5 cun obliquely till the acu-esthesia is obtained.

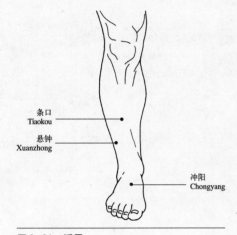

条口
Tiaokou

悬钟
Xuanzhong

冲阳
Chongyang

图3-81 缓足
Fig. 3-81 Huanzu

Moxibustion：3-5 wheat-sized moxa cones of moxibustion, or moxibustion with moxa roll for 10-20 minutes is applied.

降浊
Jiangzhuo

组成　本穴组由内庭、公孙、足三里三穴组合而成。

位置　内庭：足背第二、第三趾间缝纹端。

足三里：犊鼻穴下3寸，胫骨前嵴外一横指处。

公孙：第一跖骨基底部的前下缘，赤白肉际。

主治　脾虚腹胀，四肢倦怠，面黄便溏，纳呆乏力。

操作　内庭灸7~14壮。公孙、足三里各灸14~21壮。

Composition　This group of acupoints is composed of Neiting(ST44), Gongsun(SP4) and Zusanli(ST36).

Location　Neiting：at the end of the margin of the web between the 2nd and 3rd toes.

Zusanli：3 cun below Dubi, one finger breadth from the anterior crest of the tibia.

Gongsun：anterior and inferior to the base of the 1st metatarsal bone, on the junction of the red and white skin.

Indications　Abdominal distension due to deficiency of the Spleen, weakness of the four limbs, yellow complexion, loose stool, anorexia and weakness.

Methods　7-14 cones of moxibustion is applied to Neiting.14-21 cones of moxibustion is applied to Gongsun and Zusanli respectively.

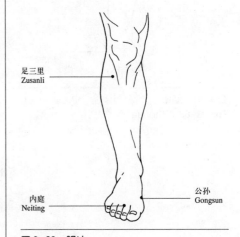

图3-82　降浊
Fig. 3-82　Jiangzhuo

助化
Zhuhua

组成　本穴组由足三里、公孙二穴组合而成。

位置　足三里：犊鼻穴下3寸，胫骨前嵴外一横指处。

公孙：第一跖骨基底部的前下缘，赤白肉际。

主治　消化不良。

操作　刺法：公孙直刺0.5~0.8寸。足三里直刺1~2寸，得气为度。

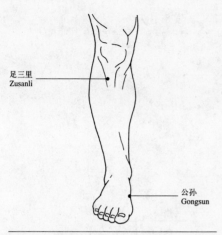

图3-83 助化
Fig. 3-83 Zhuhua

灸法：麦粒灸3～5壮，艾条灸10～20分钟。

Composition　This group of acupoints is composed of Zusanli(ST36) and Gongsun(SP4).

Location　Zusanli：3 cun below Dubi, one finger breadth from the anterior crest of the tibia.

Gongsun：anterior and inferior to the base of the 1st metatarsal bone, on the junction of the red and white skin.

Indication　Indigestion.

Method　Acupuncture：Gongsun is needled 0.5−0.8 cun perpendicularly. Zusanli is needled 1−2 cun perpendicularly till the acu-esthesia is obtained.

Moxibustion：3−5 wheat-sized moxa cones of moxibustion, or moxibustion with moxa roll for 10−20 minutes is applied.

● 运脾灸
Yunpijiu

组成　本穴组由大都、商丘、阴陵泉三穴组成。

位置　大都：踇趾内趾，第一跖趾关节前缘，赤白肉际。

商丘：内踝前下方凹陷中。

阴陵泉：胫骨内侧髁下缘凹陷中。

主治　脾胃虚弱，大便溏泄，饮食不消，形体瘦弱，胸脘痞满，四肢无力。

操作　艾炷灸大都、商丘、阴陵泉各7～14壮。

Composition　This group of acupoints is composed of Dadu(SP2), Shangqiu(SP5) and Yinlingquan(SP9).

Location　Dadu：on the medial side of the great toe, anterior and inferior to the 1st metatarsophalangeal joint, on the junction of the red and white skin.

Shangqiu：in the depression anterior and inferior to the medial malleolus.

Yinlingquan：in the depression below the medial condyle of the tibia.

Indication　Weakness of the Spleen and Stomach, loose stool, indigestion, emaciation, stuffy chest, weakness of the four limbs.

Method　7−14 cones of moxibustion is applied to

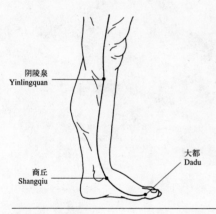

图3-84 运脾灸
Fig. 3-84 Yunpijiu

Dadu, Shangqiu and Yinlingquan respectively.

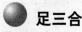

足三合
Zusanhe

组成 本穴组由足三里、上巨虚、下巨虚三个合穴组合而成。

位置 足三里：犊鼻穴下3寸，胫骨前嵴外一横指处。

上巨虚：足三里穴下3寸。

下巨虚：上巨虚穴下3寸。

主治 胃肠疾患，如胃痛，呕吐，腹胀，肠鸣，消化不良，泄泻，便秘，痢疾等。

操作 刺法：直刺1～1.5寸。

灸法：艾炷灸3～5壮，或温灸10～20分钟。

Composition This group of acupoints is composed of three He-Sea Points of Zusanli(ST36), Shangjuxu(ST37) and Xiajuxu(ST39).

Location Zusanli：3 cun below Dubi, one finger breadth from the anterior crest of the tibia.

Shangjuxu：3 cun below Zusanli.

Xiajuxu：3 cun below Shangjuxu.

Indications Diseases of the stomach and the intestine, such as stomachache, vomiting, abdominal distension, borborygmus, indigestion, diarrhea, constipation and dysentery, etc..

Methods Acupuncture：the needle is inserted 1-1.5 cun perpendicularly.

Moxibustion：moxibustion with 3-5 cones, or warm moxibustion for 10-20 minutes is applied.

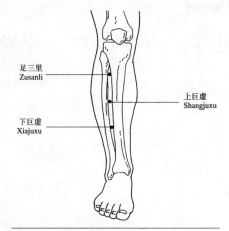

图 3-85 足三合
Fig. 3-85 Zusanhe

足三原
Zusanyuan

组成 本穴组由太溪、太白、太冲三原穴组合而成。

位置 太溪：内踝高点与跟腱之间凹陷中。

太白：第一跖骨小头后缘，赤白肉际。

太冲：足背，第一、第二跖骨结合部之前凹陷中。

主治 中下焦病证，以脾、肝、肾病为主。

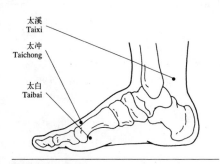

图 3-86 足三原
Fig. 3-86 Zusanyuan

操作　针0.5~1寸。

Composition　This group of acupoints is composed of three Yuan-Primary points of Taixi(KI3), Taibai(SP3) and Taichong(LR3).

Location　Taixi: in the midpoint between the tip of the medial malleolus and Achilles's tendon.

Taibai: posterior to the head of the 1st metatarsal bone, on the junction of the white and red skin.

Taichong: on the instep of the foot, in the depression anterior to the commissure of the 1st and 2nd metatarsal bones.

Indications　Diseases of Spleen, Liver and Kindey.

Methods　The needle is inserted 0.5-1 cun.

里白
Libai

组成　本穴组由足三里、隐白二穴组合而成。

位置　足三里：犊鼻穴下3寸，胫骨前嵴外一横指处。

隐白：踇趾内侧趾甲角旁约0.1寸。

主治　肠风下血，血色鲜红。

操作　先取足三里，灸5~9壮，或温灸10~15分钟，亦或用针法，针1~2寸，留针10~20分钟，使胀麻感沿经脉向下放射至足趾，向上放散至膝部或腹部；然后取隐白，针0.1~0.2寸，得气后局部有痛感，亦或灸2~3壮，或温灸5~10分钟。

Composition　This group of acupoints is composed of Zusanli(ST36) and Yinbai(SP1).

Location　Zusanli: 3 cun below Dubi, one finger breadth from the anterior crest of the tibia.

Yinbai: 0.1 cun from the corner of the toenail of the medial side of the great toe.

Indication　Brightly bloody stool.

Method　First, 5-9 cones of moxibustion, or 10-15 minutes' warm moxibustion is applied to Zusanli. Acupuncture can be used too. The depth is 1-2 cun, and the retention of the needle is 10-20 minutes. The acuesthesia of distension and numbness should be induced to the toes along the meridian, or to the knee or abdomen.

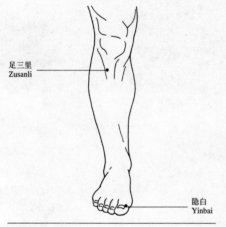

足三里
Zusanli

隐白
Yinbai

图3-87　里白
Fig. 3-87　Libai

Then Yinbai is needled 0.1—0.2 cun, pain can be sensed after the arrival of the acu-esthesia. 2—3 cones of moxibustion, or 5—10 minutes' warm moxibustion can be applied to Yinbai too.

⬤ 陵都
Lingdu

组成　本穴组由阳陵泉、中都二穴组合而成。

位置　阳陵泉：腓骨小头前下方凹陷中。

中都：内踝高点上7寸，胫骨内侧面的中央。

主治　肝病，筋病，肌病。

操作　针0.5～1.5寸。

Composition　This group of acupoints is composed of Yanglingquan(GB34) and Zhongdu(LR6).

Location　Yanglingquan：in the depression anterior and inferior to the head of the fibula.

Zhongdu：7 cun above the tip of the medial malleolus, in the centre of the medial surface of the tibia.

Indication　Hepatic diseases, diseases of tendon and muscle.

Method　The needle is inserted 0.5—1.5 cun.

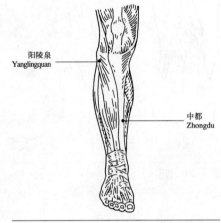

图3-88　陵都
Fig. 3-88　Lingdu

⬤ 陵丘
Lingqiu

组成　本穴组由阳陵泉、外丘二穴组合而成。

位置　阳陵泉：腓骨小头前下方凹陷中。

外丘：外踝高点上7寸，腓骨前缘。

主治　胆囊病证，胁肋疼痛。

操作　针1.0～1.5寸。

Composition　This group of acupoints is composed of Yanglingquan(GB34) and Waiqiu(GB36).

Location　Yanglingquan：in the depression anterior and inferior to the head of the fibula.

Waiqiu：7 cun above the tip of the external malleolus, on the anterior border of the fibula.

Indications　Diseases of the gallbladder, pain in the

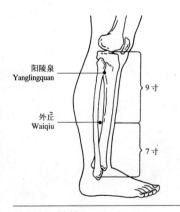

图3-89　陵丘
Fig. 3-89　Lingqiu

hypochondriac rib-side regions.

Method The needle is inserted 1–1.5 cun.

 谷里
Guli

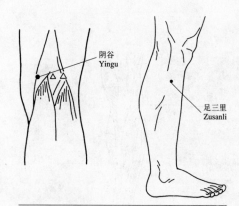

图3-90 谷里
Fig. 3-90 Guli

组成 本穴组由阴谷、足三里二穴组合而成。

位置 阴谷：屈膝，腘窝内侧，当半腱肌腱与半膜肌腱之间。

足三里：犊鼻穴下3寸，胫骨前嵴外一横指处。

主治 中邪霍乱。

操作 刺法：阴谷针0.5~1.2寸。足三里针1~1.5寸。得气为度，留针30~60分钟，留针期间可作多次运针手法。

灸法：足三里也可行艾炷灸5~9壮。两穴均可用艾条温灸10~20分钟。

Composition This group of acupoints is composed of Yingu(KI10) and Zusanli(ST36).

Location Yingu：when the knee is flexed, on the medial end of the popliteal fossa, in the depression between the tendons of the semitendinous and semimembranous muscles.

Zusanli：3 cun below Dubi, one finger breadth from the anterior crest of the tibia.

Indication Vomiting and diarrhea due to pathogenic factors.

Methods Acupuncture：Yingu is needled 0.8–1.2 cun, Zusanli is needled 1–1.5 cun till the acu-esthesia is obtained. Retain the needles for 30–60 minutes. Manipulating techniques can be performed repeatedly during the retention of the needles.

Moxibustion：5–9 cones of moxibustion may be applied to Zusanli. Warm moxibustion with moxa roll for 10–20 minutes can be applied to both points.

 然泉
Ranquan

组成 本穴组由然谷、阴陵泉二穴组合而成。

位置 然谷：足舟骨粗隆下缘凹陷中。

阴陵泉：胫骨内侧髁下缘凹陷中。

主治 肾精不足善恐，精神疲惫，心慌善恐，遗精盗汗，失眠虚烦。

操作 阴陵泉直刺0.5～1寸。然谷刺0.5～0.7寸，用补法得气。得气后二穴留针30分钟。

Composition This group of acupoints is composed of Rangu(KI2) and Yinlingquan(SP9).

Location Rangu：in the depression inferior to the tuberosity of the navicular bone.

Yinlingquan：in the depression below the medial condyle of the tibia.

Indication Deficiency of Kindey essence, timidity, fatigue, palpitation, seminal emission, night sweating, insomnia, irritability.

Method Yinlingquan is needled 0.5－1 cun perpendicularly, Rangu is needled 0.5－0.7 cun. Reinforcing techniques are performed to induce the acu-esthesia. Retain the needles for 30 minutes after the arrival of the acu-esthesia.

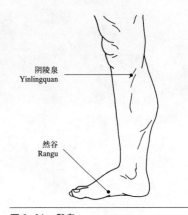

图3-91 然泉
Fig. 3-91 Ranquan

肝原络
Ganyuanluo

组成 本穴组由太冲、光明二穴组合而成。

位置 太冲：足背，第一、第二跖骨结合部之前凹陷中。

光明：外踝高点上5寸，腓骨前缘。

主治 肝脏及其经脉所属的病证，如睾丸炎，疝气痛，胸满，呕吐，腹痛，腹泻，尿闭，遗尿等。

操作 刺法：直刺0.5～1寸。

灸法：麦粒灸3～5壮，或温灸5～10分钟。

Composition This group of acupoints is composed of Taichong(LR3) and Guangming(GB37).

Location Taichong：on the instep of the foot, in the depression anterior to the commissure of the 1st and 2nd metatarsal bones.

Guangming：5 cun above the tip of the external malleolus, on the anterior border of the fibula.

Indications Diseases of the liver and the Liver Meridian,

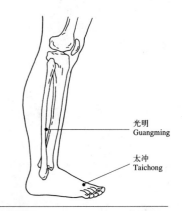

图3-92 肝原络
Fig. 3-92 Ganyuanluo

orchitis, pain due to hernia, stuffy chest, vomiting, abdominal pain, diarrhea, retention of urine and enuresis.

Methods Acupuncture：the needle is inserted 0.5—1 cun perpendicularly.

Moxibustion：3—5 wheat-sized moxa cones of moxibustion, or 5—10 minutes' warm moxibustion is applied.

脾原络
Piyuanluo

组成　本穴组由太白、丰隆二穴组合而成。

位置　太白：第一跖骨小头后缘，赤白肉际处。

丰隆：外踝高点上8寸，条口穴外1寸。

主治　脾脏及其经脉所属病证，如舌强，腹痛，呕吐，身体沉重无力，便秘，黄疸，下肢内侧痛等。

操作　刺法：直刺0.5～1.2寸。

灸法：麦粒灸3～5壮，或温灸5～10分钟。

Composition This group of acupoints is composed of Taibai(SP3) and Fenglong(ST40).

Location Taibai：posterior to the head of the 1st metatarsal bone, on the junction of the white and red skin.

Fenglong：8 cun above the tip of the external malleolus, 1 cun lateral to Tiaokou.

Indication Diseases of the spleen and the Spleen Meridian：stiff tongue, abdominal pain, vomiting, heavy feeling and weakness of the body, constipation, jaundice, pain in the medial side of the lower limbs.

Method Acupuncture：the needle is inserted 0.5—1.2 cun perpendicularly.

Moxibustion：3—5 wheat-sized moxa cones of moxibustion, or 5—10 minutes' warm moxibustion is applied.

肾原络
Shenyuanluo

组成　本穴组由太溪、飞扬二穴组合而成。

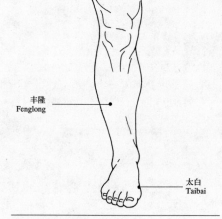

丰隆
Fenglong

太白
Taibai

图3-93　脾原络
Fig. 3-93　Piyuanluo

位置 太溪：内踝高点与跟腱之间凹陷中。

飞扬：昆仑穴直上7寸，承山穴外下方。

主治 肾脏及其经脉所属病证，如神经衰弱，精神不振，食欲不佳，视力减退，腰酸痛，下肢无力，面色灰黑等。

操作 刺法：直刺0.5～1寸。

灸法：麦粒灸3～5壮，或温灸5～10分钟。

Composition This group of acupoints is composed of Taixi(KI3) and Feiyang(BL58).

Location Taixi：in the midpoint between the tip of the medial malleolus and Achilles's tendon.

Feiyang：7 cun directly above Kunlun, lateral and inferior to Chengshan.

Indications Diseases of the kidney and the Kidney Meridian：neurasthenia, fatigue, anorexia, hypopsia, soreness and pain in the waist, weakness of the lower limbs, grey and dark complexion.

Methods Acupuncture：the needle is inserted 0.5－1 cun perpendicularly.

Moxibustion：3－5 wheat-sized moxa cones of moxibustion, or 5－10 minutes' warm moxibustion is applied.

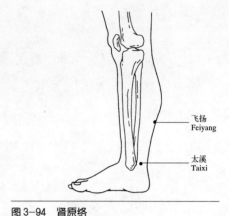

图3-94 肾原络
Fig. 3-94 Shenyuanluo

胆原络
Danyuanluo

组成 本穴组由丘墟、蠡沟二穴组合而成。

位置 丘墟：外踝前下方，趾长伸肌腱外侧凹陷中。

蠡沟：内踝高点上5寸，胫骨内侧面的中央。

主治 胆腑及其经脉所属病证，如胸肋痛，头痛，眼痛，颈淋巴腺结核，甲状腺肿等。

操作 刺法：直刺或斜刺0.5～1寸。

灸法：麦粒灸3～5壮，或温灸5～10分钟。

Composition This group of acupoints is composed of Qiuxu(GB40) and Ligou(LR5).

Location Qiuxu：anterior and inferior to the external malleolus, in the depression lateral to the tendon of the long extensor muscle of the toes.

Ligou：5 cun above the tip of the medial malleolus, in the centre of the medial aspect of the tibia.

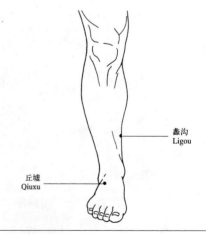

图3-95 胆原络
Fig. 3-95 Danyuanluo

Indication Diseases of the gallbladder and the Gall-bladder Meridian：pain in the hypochondriac region, headache, ophthalmalgia, scrofula in the neck and goiter, etc..

Method Acupuncture：the needle is inserted 0.5−1 cun perpendicularly or obliquely.

Moxibustion：3−5 wheat-sized moxa cones of moxibustion, or 5−10 minutes' warm moxibustion is applied.

胃原络
Weiyuanluo

组成 本穴组由冲阳、公孙二穴组合而成。

位置 冲阳：在解溪穴下方，姆长伸肌腱和趾长伸肌腱之间，当第二、第三跖骨与楔状骨间，足背。

公孙：第一跖骨基底部的前下缘，赤白肉际。

主治 胃腑及其经脉所属病证，如鼻出血，面神经麻痹，神经衰弱，下肢前侧痛，腹胀等。

操作 刺法：直刺0.3～0.8寸，刺冲阳须避开动脉。

灸法：麦粒灸3～5壮，或温灸5～10分钟。

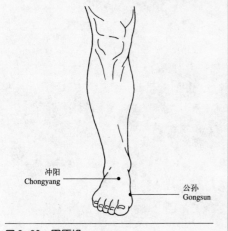

图3−96 胃原络
Fig. 3−96 Weiyuanluo

Composition This group of acupoints is composed of Chongyang(ST42) and Gongsun(SP3).

Location Chongyang：inferior to Jiexi, between the tendons of the long extensor muscle of the great toe and the long extensor muscle of the toes, on the instep of the foot.

Gongsun：anterior and inferior to the base of the 1st metatarsal bone, on the junction of the red and white skin.

Indication Diseases of the stomach and the Stomach Meridian：epistaxis, facial paralysis, neurasthenia, pain in the anterior side of the lower limbs, abdominal distension,etc..

Method Acupuncture：the needle is inserted 0.3−0.8 cun perpendicularly. Avoid puncturing the artery when Chongyang is needled.

Moxibustion：3−5 wheat-sized moxa cones of moxibustion, or 5−10 minutes' warm moxibustion is applied.

膀胱原络
Pangguangyuanluo

组成 本穴组由京骨、大钟二穴组合而成。

位置 京骨：第五跖骨粗隆下，赤白肉际。

大钟：太溪穴下0.5寸稍后，跟腱内缘。

主治 膀胱及其经脉所属病证，如眼痛，颈痛，腰背及下肢疼痛，癫痫，精神病角弓反张，眶上神经痛，鼻出血，脱肛，痔疾等。

操作 刺法：直刺0.3～0.5寸。

灸法：麦粒灸3～5壮，或温灸5～10分钟。

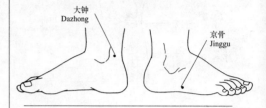

图3-97 膀胱原络
Fig. 3-97 Pangguangyuanluo

Composition This group of acupoints is composed of Jinggu(BL64) and Dazhong(KI4).

Location Jinggu：inferior to the tuberosity of the 5th metatarsal bone, at the junction of the red and white skin.

Dachong：0.5 cun slightly posterior to Taixi, on the medial side of the Achilles tendon.

Indication Diseases of the bladder and the Bladder Meridian：ophthalmalgia, pain in the neck, pain in the waist, back and lower limbs, epilepsy, psychosis, opisthotonus, supraorbital neuralgia, epistaxis, prolapse of the rectum and hemorrhoids,etc..

Method Acupuncture：the needle is inserted 0.3−0.5 cun perpendicularly.

Moxibustion：3−5 wheat-sized moxibustion cones of moxibustion, or 5−10 minutes' warm moxibustion is applied.

 脚气八处穴
Jiaoqibachuxue

组成 本穴组由风市、伏兔、犊鼻、内膝眼、足三里、上巨虚、下巨虚、悬钟八穴组合而成。

位置 风市：大腿外侧正中，腘横纹水平线上7寸。

伏兔：髂前上棘与髌骨外缘连线上，髌骨外上缘上6寸。

犊鼻：髌骨下缘，髌韧带外侧凹陷中。

足三里：犊鼻穴下3寸，胫骨前嵴外一横指处。

上巨虚：足三里穴下3寸。

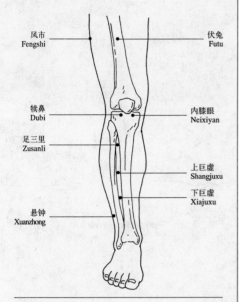

图3-98 脚气八处穴
Fig. 3-98 Jiaoqibachuxue

下巨虚：上巨虚穴下3寸。

内膝眼：髌韧带内侧与胫骨内侧髁所构成的凹陷中。

悬钟：外踝高点上3寸，腓骨后缘。

主治 脚气。

操作 灸20～30壮。

按注 《备急千金要方》云，"凡此诸穴，灸不必一顿灸尽壮数。可日日灸，灸之三日之中，灸令尽壮数为佳。"

Composition This group of acupoints is composed of Fengshi(GB31), Futu(ST32), Dubi(ST35), Neixiyan(EX), Zusanli(ST36), Shangjuxu(ST37), Xiajuxu(ST39) and Xuanzhong(GB39).

Location Fengshi：on the midline of the lateral side of the thigh, 7 cun above the popliteal crease.

Futu：on the line connecting the anteriosuperior iliac spine and the lateral corner of the patella, 7 cun above the superiolateral border of the patella.

Dubi：on the lower border of the patella, in the depression lateral to the patellar ligament.

Zusanli：3 cun below Dubi, one finger breadth from the anterior crest of the tibia.

Shangjuxu：3 cun below Zusanli.

Xiajuxu：3 cun below Shangjuxu.

Neixiyan：inferior to the patella, in the depression on the medial side of the patellar ligament.

Xuanzhong：3 cun above the tip of the external malleolus, on the posterior border of the fibula.

Indication Beriberi.

Method 20-30 cones of moxibustion is applied.

Note It is said in the book *Prescriptions Worth a Thousand Gold for Emergencies*："For all the points, it's not necessary to finish all the numbers of cone in a single treatment. Moxibustion can be applied to the points every day. But it is advisable to finish the numbers of cone in three days."

 脚气
Jiaoqi

组成 本穴组由悬钟、三阴交、足三里三穴组合而成。

位置　悬钟：外踝高点上3寸，腓骨后缘。

三阴交：内踝高点上3寸，胫骨内侧面后缘。

足三里：犊鼻穴下3寸，胫骨前嵴外一横指处。

主治　脚气。

操作　刺法：绝骨直刺0.5~1寸。三阴交、足三里直刺1~1.5寸。得气为度。

灸法：艾炷灸3~5壮，艾条灸10~20分钟。

Composition　This group of acupoints is composed of Xuanzhong(GB39), Sanyinjiao(SP6) and Zusanli(ST36).

Location　Juegu：3 cun above the tip of the external malleolus, on the posterior border of the fibula.

Sanyinjiao：3 cun above the tip of the medial malleolus, on the posterior border of the tibia.

Zusanli：3 cun below Dubi, one finger breadth from the anterior crest of the tibia.

Indication　Beriberi.

Method　Acupuncture：Juegu is needled 0.5−1 cun perpendicularly. Sanyinjiao and Zusanli are needled 1−1.5 cun till the acu-esthesia is obtained.

Moxibustion：moxibustion with 3−5 cones, or moxibustion with moxa roll for 10−20 minutes is applied.

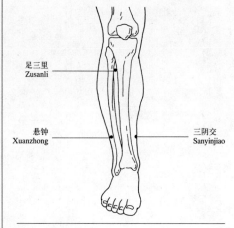

图3-99　脚气
Fig. 3-99　Jiaoqi

营池
Yingchi

组成　本穴组由内踝下缘前后凹处之二个点组合而成。

位置　位于足内踝下缘前后之凹陷处，每侧二穴。

主治　月经过多，漏下赤白，肠血，尿闭，跗肿痛。

操作　刺法：针0.3~0.5寸，可直刺斜刺，局部有酸痛感。

灸法：麦粒灸3~5壮，艾条温灸5~15分钟。

Composition　This group of acupoints is composed of two points in the depressions respectively anterior and posterior to the medial malleolus.

Location　In the depressions anterior and posterior to the medial malleolus, 2 points on each side.

Indication　Menorrhagia, morbid leukorrhea, bloody stool, retention of the urine, swelling and pain of the instep.

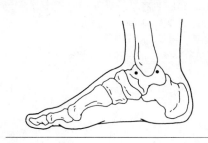

图3-100　营池
Fig. 3-100　Yingchi

Method Acupuncture：the needle is inserted 0.3−0.5 cun perpendicularly or obliquely. The acu-esthesia of soreness and pain will be obtained in this part.

Moxibustion：3−5 wheat-sized moxa cones of moxibustion, or 5−15 minutes' warm moxibustion with moxa roll is applied.

 机海

Jihai

组成　本穴组由地机、血海二穴组合而成。

位置　血海：髌骨内上缘上2寸。

地机：阴陵泉穴下3寸。

主治　月经不调。

操作　刺法：直刺1~1.5寸，得气为度。

灸法：艾炷灸3~5壮，艾条温灸5~15分钟。

Composition This group of acupoints is composed of Diji(SP8) and Xuehai(SP10).

Location Xuehai：2 cun above the superior medial corner of the patella.

Diji：3 cun below Yinlingquan.

Indication Irregular menstruation.

Method Acupuncture：the needle is inserted 1−1.5 cun till the acu-esthesia is obtained.

Moxibustion：moxibustion with 3−5 cones, or warm moxibustion with moxa roll for 5−15 minutes is applied.

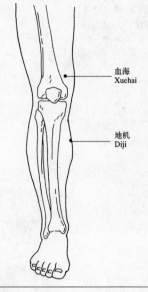

图3-101　机海

Fig. 3-101　Jihai

 信阳

Xinyang

组成　本穴组由交信、合阳二穴组合而成。

位置　交信：复溜穴前约0.5寸。

合阳：委中穴直下2寸。

主治　少气漏下。

操作　艾炷灸5~9壮，艾条灸5~15分钟。

Composition This group of acupoints is composed of Jiaoxin(KI8) and Heyang(BL55).

Location Jiaoxin：about 0.5 cun anterior to Fuliu.

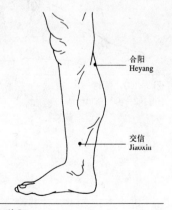

图3-102　信阳

Fig. 3-102　Xinyang

Heyang：2 cun directly below Weizhong.

Indication　Deficiency of Qi and uterine bleeding.

Method　Moxibustion with 5－9 cones, or moxibustion with moxa roll for 5－15 minutes is applied.

阴痒
Yinyang

组成　本穴组由蠡沟、太冲二穴组合而成。

位置　蠡沟：内踝高点上5寸，胫骨内侧面的中央。

太冲：足背，第一、第二跖骨结合部之前凹陷中。

主治　阴部瘙痒。

操作　蠡沟沿皮由下向上刺0.8~1.5寸，有针感向腿股阴行。太冲斜刺0.5~1寸，得气为度，留针30分钟，留针期间可运针一二次，并可用泻法。

Composition　This group of acupoints is composed of Ligou(LR5) and Taichong(LR3).

Location　Ligou：5 cun above the the tip of the medial malleolus, in the centre of the medial aspect of the tibia.

Taichong：on the instep of the foot, in the depression anterior to the commissure of the 1st and 2nd metatarsal bones.

Indication　Pruritus vulvae.

Method　Ligou is subcutaneously needled 0.8－1.5 cun upwards. The acu－esthesia will be induced to the leg and thigh.Taichong is needled 0.5－1 cun obliquely till the acu-esthesia is obtained. Retain the needles for 30 minutes. Manipulate the needles once or twice during the retention of the needles, and the reducing techniques can be applied.

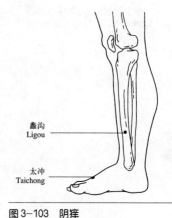

图3-103　阴痒
Fig. 3-103　Yinyang

兰门
Lanmen

组成　本穴组由腘窝内侧上下3寸之二个点组合而成。

位置　下肢胫侧正中线，腘窝横纹上下各3寸。左右计四穴，当曲泉穴上下各3寸。

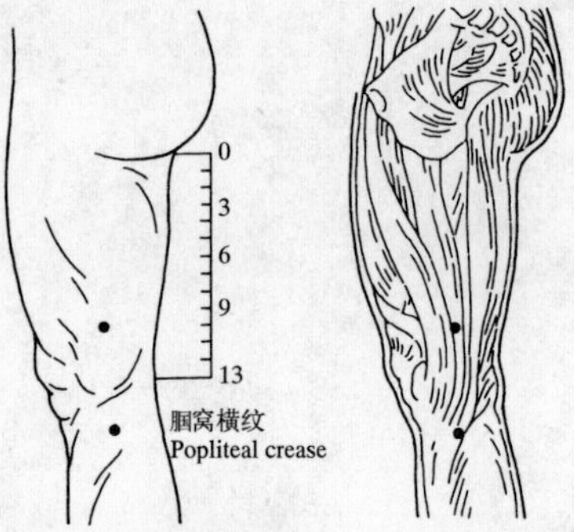

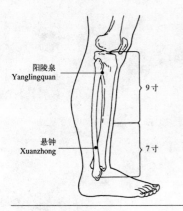

图3-104 兰门
Fig. 3-104 Lanmen

主治　疝气，奔豚气。

操作　刺法：直刺0.5～1寸。局部酸胀感，时或向膝部扩散。

灸法：艾炷灸温针灸5～9壮，艾条温灸5～15分钟。

Composition　This group of acupoints is composed of two points 3 cun superior and inferior to the medial end of the popliteal fossa.

Location　On the midline of the medial side of the lower limbs, 3 cun superior and inferior to the popliteal crease respectively, 4 points in all. i.e. 3 cun superior and inferior to Ququan(LR8).

Indication　Hernia, qi up-rushing syndrome.

Method　Acupuncture：the needle is inserted 0.5-1 cun perpendicularly. The acu-esthesia of soreness and distension will be obtained in this part, and it will radiate to the knee sometimes.

Moxibustion：5-9 cones of moxibustion or warm needle moxibustion, or 15 minutes' warm moxibustion with moxa roll is applied.

筋髓会
Jinsuihui

组成　本穴组由筋会阳陵泉、髓会悬钟二穴组合而成。

位置　阳陵泉：腓骨小头前下方凹陷中。

悬钟：外踝高点上3寸，腓骨后缘。

主治　全身筋、髓病证。

操作　刺法：针1～1.5寸。

灸法：麦粒灸5～9壮，温灸10～20分钟。

Composition　This group of acupoints is composed of Yanglingquan(GB34), the Influential Point of Tendon, and Xuanzhong(GB39), the Influential Point of Marrow.

Location　Yanglingquan：in the depression anterior and inferior to the head of the fibula.

Xuanzhong：3 cun above the tip of the external malleolus, on the posterior border of the fibula.

Indication　Diseases of the tendons and marrow of the whole body.

Method　Acupuncture：the needle is inserted 1-1.5

图3-105 筋髓会
Fig. 3-105 Jinsuihui

cun.

Moxibustion：5－9 cones of moxibustion, or 10－20 minutes' warm moxibustion is applied.

解痉
Jiejing

组成　本穴组由解痉1、解痉2二穴组合而成。

位置　解痉1：位于腘窝横纹近外侧端，股二头肌腱内侧，约当委中外侧处。

解痉2：位于腘窝横纹近内侧端，半腱肌的内侧，约当委中内侧处。

主治　外伤性截瘫，下肢痿痹。

操作　针0.5～1寸，针感酸麻至足。

Composition　This group of acupoints is composed of Jiejing 1 and Jiejing 2.

Location　Jiejing 1：on the lateral end of the popliteal crease, on the medial side of the biceps muscle of the thigh, lateral to Weizhong.

Jiejing 2：on the lateral end of the popliteal crease, on the medial side of the semitendious muscle, medial to Weizhong.

Indication　Traumatic paraplegia, muscular atrophy and paralysis of the lower limbs.

Method　The needle is inserted 0.5－1 cun. The acuesthesia of soreness and numbness will transmit to the foot.

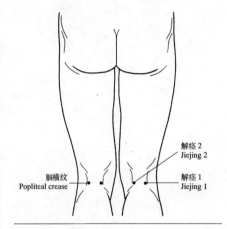

图3－106　解痉
Fig. 3－106　Jiejing

舒筋
Shujin

组成　本穴组由承山、阳陵泉二穴组合而成。

位置　承山：腓肠肌两肌腹之间凹陷的顶端。

阳陵泉：腓骨小头前下方凹陷中。

主治　小腿肌转筋。

操作　刺法：直刺1～1.5寸，得气为度。

灸法：艾炷灸3～5壮，艾条灸10～20分钟。

Composition　This group of acupoints is composed of

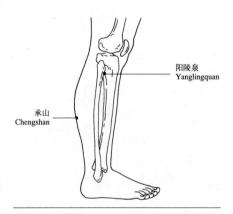

图3－107　舒筋
Fig. 3－107　Shujin

Chengshan(BL57) and Yanglingquan(GB34).

Location Chengshan：on the top of the depression below the belly of the gastrocnemius muscle.

Yanglingquan：in the depression anterior and inferior to the head of the fibula.

Indication Cramp in the gastrocnemius.

Methods Acupuncture：the needle is inserted 1−1.5 cun perpendicularly till the acu-esthesia is obtained.

Moxibustion：3−5 cones of moxibustion, or 10−20 minutes' moxibustion with moxa roll is applied.

转筋
Zhuanjin

组成 本穴组由承山、内踝尖二穴组合而成。

位置 承山：腓肠肌两肌腹之间凹陷的顶端。

内踝尖：内踝之高点上。

主治 小腿转筋。

操作 刺法：承山直刺1～2寸，得气为度。

灸法：内踝尖灸5壮。

Composition This group of acupoints is composed of Chengshan(BL57) and Neihuaijian.

Location Chengshan：on the top of the depression below the belly of the gastrocnemius muscle.

Neihuaijian：on the tip of the medial malleolus.

Indication Cramp in the leg.

Method Acupuncture：Chengshan is needled 1−2 cun perpendicularly till the acu-esthesia is obtained.

Moxibustion：5 cones of moxibustion is applied to Neihuaijian.

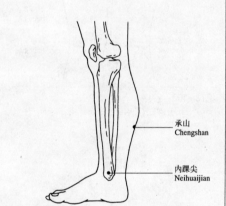

承山
Chengshan

内踝尖
Neihuaijian

图 3−108 转筋
Fig. 3−108 Zhuanjin

纠内翻
Jiuneifan

组成 本穴组由小腿腓侧之二个点组合而成。

位置 一穴：小腿近端腓侧、髌骨中线下4寸，胫骨与腓骨之间点外开1.5寸。另一穴：小腿远端腓侧，外踝上缘上4.5寸一穴。

左右计四穴。约当"足三里"穴外开1.5寸分处一穴。悬钟穴上1.5寸一穴。

主治　小儿麻痹后遗症。

操作　针0.5~1.5寸，针感外踝和足背酸、麻。

Composition　This group of acupoints is composed of two points on the lateral side of the leg.

Location　One point is on the upper part of the lateral side of the leg, 4 cun below the midline of the patella, 1.5 cun lateral to the point between the tibia and fibula.

The other point is on the lower part of the lateral side of the leg, 4.5 cun above the upper border of the external malleolus, 4 points on both sides. i.e. one point is 1.5 cun lateral to Zusanli and the other point 1.5 cun above Xuanzhong.

Indication　Sequela of poliomyelitis.

Method　The needle is inserted 0.5-1.5 cun. The acu-esthesia of soreness and numbness will be obtained in the external malleolus and instep.

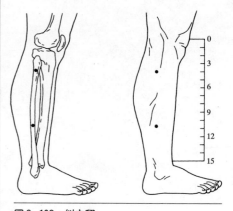

图3-109　纠内翻
Fig. 3-109　Jiuneifan

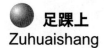 **足踝上**
Zuhuaishang

组成　本穴组由内外踝直上4寸之二个点组合而成。

位置　位于小腿部，在内踝上缘直上4寸处，和外踝上缘直上4寸处。左右计四穴，当三阴交穴上1寸和阳辅穴微后方。

主治　不热乳食，嗜睡眼不开，小儿重舌，脚转筋。

操作　刺法：直刺或斜刺1~1.5寸。

灸法：麦粒灸21壮(可日灸3次，每次7壮)，或温灸10~30分钟。

Composition　This group of acupoints is composed of two points 4 cun directy above the medial and external malleolus.

Location　On the leg, 4 cun directly above the medial malleolus, and 4 cun directly above the external malleolus, 4 points on both sides, i.e. the point 1 cun above Sanyinjiao and the point slightly posterior to Yangfu.

Indication　Anorexia, somnolence, infantile alalia, cramp in the feet.

Method　Acupuncture：the needle is inserted 1-1.5

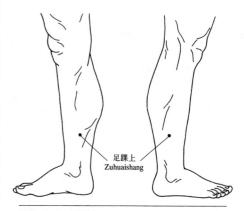

足踝上
Zuhuaishang

图3-110　足踝上
Fig. 3-110　Zuhuaishang

cun perpendicularly or obliquely.

Moxibustion: 21 wheat-sized moxa cones of moxibustion (7 cones each treatment and three treatments every day), or 10—30 minutes' warm moxibustion is applied.

瘰疬灸
Luolijiu

组成　本穴组由外踝尖直上3寸，再上下0.5寸之三个点组合而成。

位置　位于小腿腓侧远侧端，外踝尖(男左女右)正中直上2.5寸、3寸、3.5寸处。

主治　急性或慢性已溃或未溃瘰疬。

操作　灸3~5壮。

Composition　This group of acupoints is composed of three points of the point 3 cun directly above the external malleolus, and two points 0.5 cun respectively superior and inferior to above point.

Location　On the lower part of the lateral side of the leg, 2.5 cun, 3 cun, 3.5 cun directly above the centre of the tip of the external malleolus (For male, the points are on the left side, and for female, on the right side), 3 points in all.

Indication　Acute, chronic ulcerated or non-ulcerated scrofula.

Method　3—5 cones of moxibustion is applied.

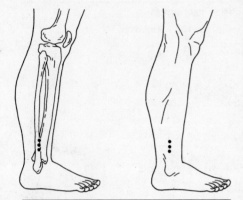

图 3-111　瘰疬灸
Fig. 3-111　Luolijiu

踝三针
Huaisanzhen

组成　本穴组由太溪、昆仑及解溪三穴组合而成。

位置　太溪：内踝高点与跟腱之间凹陷中。

昆仑：外踝高点与跟腱之间凹陷中。

解溪：足背踝关节横纹的中央，踇长伸肌腱与趾长伸肌腱之间。

主治　踝痛扭伤，足下垂。

操作　刺法：太溪穴和昆仑穴可针1~1.5寸，针感麻、胀

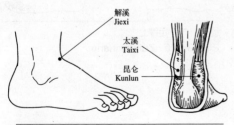

图 3-112　踝三针
Fig. 3-112　Huaisanzhen

至足跟。解溪穴针0.5寸,针感局部胀,放散至趾。

灸法:灸3~5壮,艾条灸5~10分钟。

Composition This group of acupoints is composed of Taixi(KI3), Kunlun(BL60) and Jiexi(ST41).

Location Taixi: in the midpoint between the tip of the medial malleolus and Achilles's tendon.

Kunlun: in the depression between the external malleolus and the heel tendon.

Jiexi: in the centre of the crease of the ankle joint on the instep, between the tendons of the long extensor muscle of the great toe and the long extensor muscle of the toes.

Indication Pain and sprain of the ankle and drooping foot.

Method Acupuncture: Taixi and Kunlun can be needled 1−1.5 cun. The acu-esthesia of numbness and distension will radiate to the heel.

Jiexi is needled 0.5 cun. The acu-esthesia of distension will radiate to the toes.

Moxibustion: 3−5 cones of moxibustion, or 5−10 minutes' moxibustion with moxa roll is applied.

内外昆仑(昆仑二穴)
Neiwaikunlun (Kunlunerxue)

组成 本穴组由昆仑穴、内昆仑二穴组合而成。

位置 昆仑穴:位于外踝与跟腱之间凹陷中。

内昆仑:位于内踝与跟腱之间凹陷中。

主治 足跟、足底痛,腰脊酸痛,眩晕,小儿阴肿。

操作 刺法:直刺0.5~1寸。

灸法:艾炷灸1~3壮,或温灸5~10分钟。

Composition This group of acupoints is composed of Kunlun(BL60) and Neikunlun.

Location Kunlun: in the depression between the external malleolus and the heel tendon.

Neikunlun: in the depression between the medial malleolus and the heel tendon.

Indication Pain in the heel and sole, aching and pain in the waist and spine, vertigo, swelling pubes of infants.

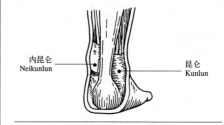

内昆仑
Neikunlun

昆仑
Kunlun

图3-113 内外昆仑(昆仑二穴)
Fig. 3-113 Neiwaikunlun (Kunlunerxue)

Method Acupuncture: the needle is inserted 0.5—1 cun perpendicularly.

Moxibustion: moxibustion with 1—3 moxa cones, or warm moxibustion for 5—10 minutes is applied.

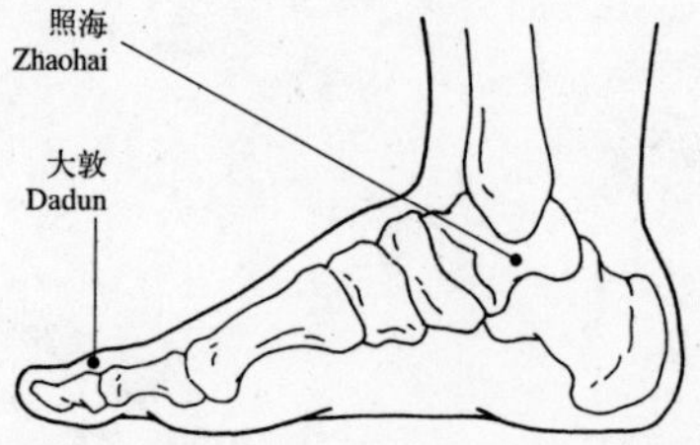

图 3—114 海敦
Fig. 3—114 Haidun

海敦
Haidun

组成 本穴组由照海、大敦二穴组合而成。

位置 照海：内踝下缘凹陷中。

大敦：踇趾外侧趾甲角旁约0.1寸。

主治 肝气郁结之癃证。

操作 照海针刺0.3~0.4寸。大敦针刺0.1~0.2寸，针毕两穴留针20~30分钟。如有血络郁结，当取肝肾二经之络穴大钟、蠡沟出血以去郁。

Composition This group of acupoints is composed of Zhaohai(KI6) and Dadun(LR1).

Location Zhaohai: in the depression on the lower border of the medial malleolus.

Dadun: 0.1 cun from the lateral corner of the toenail of the great toe.

Indication Retention of urine due to the depression of liver—qi.

Method Zhaohai is needled 0.3—0.4 cun, and Dadun 0.1—0.2 cun. Retain the needles for 20—30 minutes after the insertion. Dazhong and Ligou, the Luo-Connecting Points of the Liver and Kidney Meridians should be bled to release depression if there is the stagnation in the blood vein.

脾荥输
Piyingshu

组成 本穴组由大都、太白二穴组合而成。

位置 大都：踇趾内侧，第一跖趾关节前缘，赤白肉际。

太白：第一跖骨小头后缘，赤白肉际。

主治 脾病及消化系病证。

操作 针0.5~0.8寸，局部酸胀感。

Composition This group of acupoints is composed of Dadu(SP2) and Taibai(SP3).

Location Dadu：on the medial side of the great toe, anterior and inferior to the 1st metatarsophalangeal joint, on the junction of the red and white skin.

Taibai：posterior to the head of the 1st metatarsal bone, on the junction of the white and red skin.

Indication Diseases of the spleen and digestive system.

Method The needle is inserted 0.5—0.8 cun. The acu—esthesia of soreness and distension will be obtained in this part.

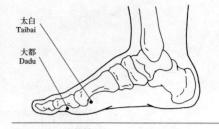

图3-115 脾荥输
Fig. 3-115 Piyingshu

肝荥输
Ganyingshu

组成 本穴组由行间、太冲组合而成。

位置 行间：足背，第一、第二趾间缝纹端。

太冲：足背，第一、第二跖骨结合部之前凹陷中。

主治 肝系病证，如肝炎，肝风，肝气，肝阳，目疾，筋病等。

操作 针0.5～1.2寸，局部酸胀麻痛。

Composition This group of acupoints is composed of Xingjian(LR2) and Taichong(LR3).

Location Xingjian：on the instep of the foot, on the end of the margin of the web between the 1st and 2nd toes.

Taichong：on the instep of the foot, in the depression anterior to the commissure of the 1st and 2nd metatarsal bones.

Indication Diseases of the hepatic system, such as hepatitis, liver wind, liver qi depression, liver yang hyperactivity, eye diseases, tendon diseases, etc..

Method The needle is inserted 0.5—1 cun. The acu-esthesia of soreness, distension, numbness and pain will be obtained in this part.

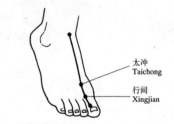

图3-116 肝荥输
Fig. 3-116 Ganyingshu

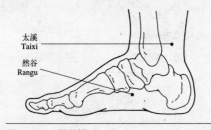

图 3-117 肾荥输
Fig. 3-117 Shenyingshu

肾荥输
Shenyingshu

组成　本穴组由然谷、太溪二穴组合而成。

位置　然谷：足舟骨粗隆下缘凹陷中。

太溪：内踝高点与跟腱之间凹陷中。

主治　肾病，泌尿生殖系病证。

操作　针0.5～1寸，局部酸、麻、胀、重、痛感。

Composition　This group of acupoints is composed of Rangu and Taixi.

Location　Rangu：in the depression inferior to the tuberosity of the navicular bone.

Taixi：in the midpoint between the tip of the medial malleolus and Achilles's tendon.

Indication　Kidney diseases, diseases of urogenital system.

Method　The needle is inserted 0.5-1 cun. The acu-esthesia of soreness, distension, heaviness and pain will be obtained in this part.

遗尿灸
Yiniaojiu

组成　本穴组由第一趾缝端两侧之二点组成。

位置　位于第一趾缝端两侧之二点。

主治　遗尿。

操作　灸5～9壮。

Composition　This group of acupoints is composed of two points on both sides of the margin of the web of the great toe.

Location　On both sides of the margin of the web of the great toe.

Indication　Enuresis.

Method　5-9 cones of moxibustion is applied.

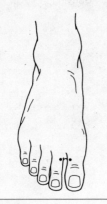

图 3-118 遗尿灸
Fig. 3-118 Yiniaojiu

趾平
Zhiping

组成　本穴组由足背各趾跟之中点穴组合而成。

位置　足背，各趾跟之中点，跖趾关节部。

主治　小儿麻痹后遗症，足下垂。

操作　刺法：针0.1～0.3寸，针感痛酸、麻至趾尖。

灸法：艾炷灸3～5壮，艾条灸5～10分钟。

Composition　This group of acupoints is composed of the midpoints of the toe roots on the instep.

Location　On the instep, at the midpoint of each toe root, where is the metatarsophalangeal joint.

Indications　Sequela of poliomyelitis, drooping foot.

Methods　Acupuncture：the needle is inserted 0.1–0.3 cun. The acu-esthesia of pain, soreness and numbness will radiate to the toes.

Moxibustion：moxibustion with 3–5 moxa cones, or moxibustion with moxa roll for 5–10 minutes is applied.

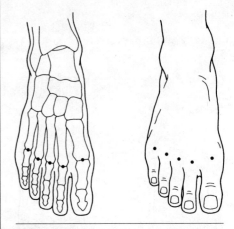

图3-119　趾平
Fig. 3–119　Zhiping

八风
Bafeng

组成　本穴组由各趾趾缝端凹处之四个点组合而成，二足共八点。

位置　足背各趾缝端凹陷中。

主治　脚气，趾痛，毒蛇咬伤足跗肿痛。

操作　刺法：斜刺0.5～0.8寸，或点刺出血。

灸法：温针灸3～5壮，艾条温灸5～10分钟。

Composition　This group of acupoints is composed of four points in the depression at the end of the margin of the webs between two neighbouring toes. 8 points on both feet.

Location　On the instep of both feet, in the depression at the end of the margin of the webs between any two neighbouring toes.

Indication　Beriberi, pain in the toes, swelling and pain in the instep due to venomous snake bite.

Method　Acupuncture：the needle is inserted 0.5–

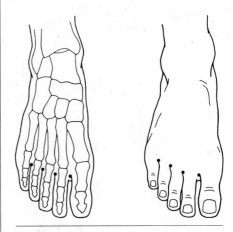

图3-120　八风
Fig. 3–120　Bafeng

0.8 cun obliquely, or the points can be pricked to bleed.

Moxibustion：3—5 cones of warm needle moxibustion, or warm moxibustion with moxa roll for 5—10 minutes is applied.

上八风
Shangbafeng

组成　本穴组由足部八风之上的四个点组合而成，双侧共八穴点。

位置　足背趾骨之间，当八风之上。

主治　脚气，趾痛，虫毒咬伤，足跗肿痛。

操作　针法：向上斜刺0.5～0.8寸，或点刺出血。

灸法：温针灸3～5壮，艾条温灸5～10分钟。

Composition　This group of acupoints is composed of four points superior to Bafeng on the feet, 8 points on both sides.

Location　On the instep of the foot, between the phalangeal bone, superior to Bafeng.

Indication　Beriberi, pain in the toes, venomous snake or insect bite, swelling and pain in the instep.

Method　Acupuncture：the needle is inserted 0.5—0.8 cun upwards obliquely, or the points can be pricked to bleed.

Moxibustion：3—5 cones of warm needle moxibustion, or 5—10 minutes' warm moxibustion with moxa roll is applied.

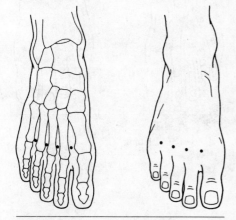

图3-121　上八风
Fig. 3-121　Shangbafeng

蛎兑（庭间）
Lidui (Tingjian)

组成　本穴组由行间、内庭二穴组合而成。

位置　行间：足背，第一、第二趾间缝纹端。

内庭：足背第二、第三趾间缝纹端。

主治　鼓胀、虚肿。

操作　针0.3～0.5寸。

Composition　This group of acupoints is composed of Xingjian(LR2) and Neiting(ST44).

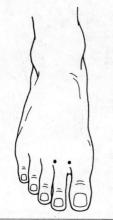

图3-122　蛎兑（庭间）
Fig. 3-122　Lidui(Tingjian)

Location Xingjian：on the instep of the foot, on the end of the margin of the web between the 1st and 2nd toes.

Neiting：at the end of the margin of the web between the 2nd and 3rd toes.

Indication Edema and flatulence of deficiency.

Method The needle is inserted 0.3—0.5 cun.

 白敦
Baidun

组成　本穴组由隐白、大敦二穴组合而成。

位置　隐白：踇趾内侧趾甲角旁约0.1寸。

大敦：踇趾外侧趾甲角旁约0.1寸。

主治　尸厥，死不知人，脉动如故。

操作　用三棱针刺放血。

Composition This group of acupoints is composed of Yinbai(SP1) and Dadun(LR1).

Location Yinbai：0.1 cun from the corner of the toenail of the medial side of the great toe.

Dadun：0.1 cun from the lateral corner of the toenail of the great toe.

Indication Syncope with normal pulsation, loss of consciousness.

Method The points are pricked to bleed with a three-edged needle.

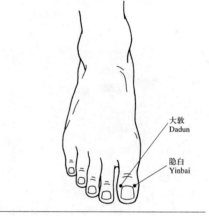

图 3—123　白敦
Fig. 3—123 Baidun

兑白
Duibai

组成　本穴组由厉兑、隐白二穴组合而成。

位置　厉兑：第二趾外侧趾甲角旁约0.1寸。

隐白：踇趾内侧趾甲角旁约0.1寸。

主治　梦魇不安。

操作　刺法：用三棱针点刺出血，或用皮内针埋针后胶布固定。

灸法：艾条温灸10～20分钟。

Composition This group of acupoints is composed of

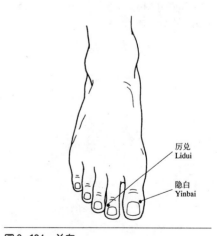

图 3—124　兑白
Fig. 3—124 Duibai

Lidui(ST45) and Yinbai(SP1).

Location Lidui: 0.1 cun from the lateral corner of the toenail of the 2nd toe.

Yinbai: 0.1 cun from the corner of the toenail of the medial side of the great toe.

Indication Nightmare-disturbed sleep.

Methods Acupuncture: the points can be pricked to bleed with a three-edged needle, or can be embedded with the intradermal needles.

Moxibustion: warm moxibustion with moxa roll for 10—20 minutes is applied.

● 足十甲
Zushijia

组成 本穴组由足十趾甲根部之五个点组合而成，两足共十个点。

位置 在足十趾爪甲根部，亦可取爪甲角处点刺或全刺。

主治 中暑，虚劳，哮喘，胁痛，干霍乱，腹痛，疳积，小儿夜啼，喉痛，齿痛，目赤肿痛。

操作 刺法：点刺0.1～0.2寸，局部有疼感。

灸法：麦粒灸3～5壮，艾条灸3～5分钟。

Composition This group of acupoints is composed of five points on the toenail roots of the toes, 10 points on both feet.

Location On the toenail roots of the ten toes. The corners of the toenail can also be pricked or needled.

Indication Sunstroke, emaciation, asthma, pain in the hypochondriac region, dry vomiting, abdominal pain, malnutrition and indigestion syndrome, infantile night crying, sore throat, toothache, redness, swelling and pain of the eye.

Method Acupuncture: the points are pricked 0.1— 0.2 cun, and the acu-esthesia of pain will be obtained.

Moxibustion: 3—5 wheat-sized moxa cones of moxibustion, or moxibustion with moxa roll for 3—5 minutes is applied.

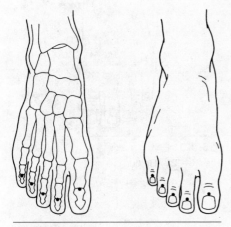

图3-125 足十甲
Fig. 3-125 Zushijia

气端
Qiduan

组成　本穴组由足十趾端之十个点组合而成。

位置　在足十趾尖端。

主治　中风急救，足趾麻木，脚背红肿，疼痛。

操作　刺法：直刺0.1～0.2寸。

灸法：麦粒灸3～5壮，艾条灸5～10分钟。

Composition　This group of acupoints is composed of ten points on the tips of the ten toes.

Location　On the tips of the ten toes.

Indication　First aid of apoplexy, numbness of the toes, redness, swelling, pain of the instep.

Method　Acupuncture：the needle is inserted 0.1－0.2 cun perpendicularly.

Moxibustion：3－5 wheat-sized moxa cones of moxibustion, or moxibustion with moxa roll for 5－10 minutes is applied.

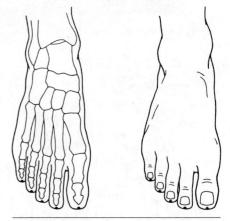

图3-126　气端
Fig. 3-126　Qiduan

足四白
Zusibai

组成　本穴组由前、后四白二穴组合而成。

位置　后四白：位于足跖正中线，从外踝高点与跟腱之间点引线，与足跖正中线交点处。左右计二穴。

前四白：位于后四白穴前三寸处。左右计二穴。

主治　脱肛，夜尿，头痛，小儿惊厥，偏瘫，脑膜炎，垂足，小儿吐乳。

操作　针0.5寸，针感局部胀、痛。

Composition　This group of acupoints is composed of Qiansibai and Housibai.

Location　Housibai：on the midline of the sole, at the junction of the line connecting the tip of the external malleolus and Achilles's tendon and the midline of the sole, 2 points on both sides.

Qiansibai：3 cun anterior to Housibai, 2 points on both sides.

Indication　Prolapse of the rectum, enuresis, headache,

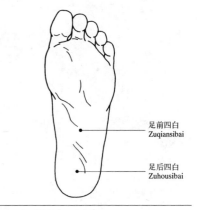

足前四白
Zuqiansibai

足后四白
Zuhousibai

图3-127　足四白
Fig. 3-127　Zusibai

infantile convulsion, hemiplegia, meningitis, droopint foot, infantile vomiting of milk.

Method The needle is inserted 0.5 cun, and the acu-esthesia of pain in this part will be obtained.

癌根
Aigen

组成 本穴组由癌根1、癌根2组合而成。

位置 癌根1：位于足跖部，第一跗跖关节向内过赤白肉际一横指、屈踇肌腱的外侧。

癌根2：位于足跖部，第一跖趾关节向后、向肉际一横指处。

主治 消化系统癌，慢性白血病等。

操作 刺法：针0.3～0.5寸，针感酸麻至趾。

灸法：麦粒灸3～9壮。

Composition This group of acupoints is composed of Aigen1 and Aigen2.

Location Aigen1：on the sole, one finger breadth from the red and white skin in the medial side of the 1st tarsometatarsal articulations, lateral to the tendon of the flexor muscle of the great toe.

Aigen2：on the sole, posterior to the 1st metatar-sophalangeal joint, one finger breadth from the red and white skin.

Indication Cancer of the digestive system, chronic leukemia, etc..

Method Acupuncture：the needle is inserted 0.3–0.5 cun, the acu-esthesia of soreness and numbness will radiate to the toes.

Moxibustion：3–9 wheat-sized moxa cones of moxibustion is applied.

前后隐珠
Qianhouyinzhu

组成 本穴组由足跖部涌泉前后的二个点组合而成。

位置 位于足跖部，涌泉穴前后各0.5寸处。

主治 腿部疔疮，下肢足跖挛痛，心悸怔忡，头痛，小儿

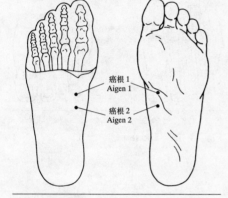

癌根1
Aigen 1

癌根2
Aigen 2

图3-128 癌根
Fig. 3-128 Aigen

搐搦。

操作　刺法：直刺0.3～0.5寸，局部痛感，有时可痛麻至趾尖。

灸法：艾条温灸5～15分钟(泻法)。

Composition　This group of acupoints is composed of two points respectively anterior and posterior to Yongquan (KI1).

Location　On the sole, 0.5 cun anterior and posterior to Yongquan respectively.

Indications　Furuncle on the leg, convulsion and pain of the sole and leg, palpitation, headache, infantile convulsion.

Method　Acupuncture：the needle is inserted 0.3-0.5 cun perpendicularly. The acu-esthesia is the pain in this part, and the pain or numbness will radiate to the tips of the toes.

Moxibustion：warm moxibustion with moxa roll for 5-15 minutes is applied with reducing methods.

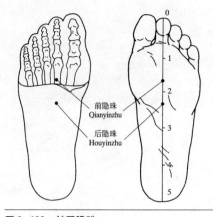

图3-129　前后隐珠
Fig. 3-129　Qianhouyinzhu

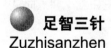 足智三针
Zuzhisanzhen

组成　本穴组由涌泉及左、右泉三穴组合而成。

位置　涌泉：于足底(去趾)前1/3处，足趾跖屈时呈凹陷处。

左泉：以涌泉穴与足跟连线的中点向外1寸处。

右泉：涌泉穴与足跟连线的中点向内1寸处。

主治　儿童智力低下，多动烦躁，巅顶头痛，高弓足、癫痫，昏迷，咽喉肿痛等。

操作　先针涌泉次针左右泉，以飞针法快速进针，并用捻转法进针0.5～0.8寸，针感放散至整个足底或局部胀痛。

Composition　This group of acupoints is composed of Yongquan(KI3), Zuoquan and Youquan.

Location　Yongquan：at the junction of the anterior one-third and middle one-third of the sole (the toes are not included), i.e. in the depression when the toes are extended downward.

Zuoquan：1 cun lateral to the midpoint of the line connecting Yongquan and the heel.

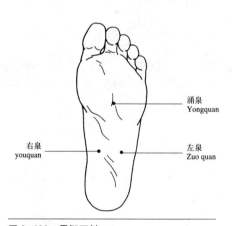

图3-130　足智三针
Fig. 3-130　Zuzhisanzhen

Youquan: 1 cun medial to the midpoint of the line connecting Yongquan and the heel.

Indication Infantile feeble-mindedness, hyperkinesis, irritability, pain in the vertex of the head, talipes cavus, epilepsy, coma, sore throat.

Method Yongquan is needled first and then Zuoquan and Youquan. The needle is inserted quickly with the flying method, and is inserted 0.5−0.8 cun more with rotation method. The acu-esthesia will radiate to the whole sole, or pain may sensed in this part.

● 足底曲泉
Zudiququan

组成 本穴组由足底内、外曲泉二穴组合而成。

位置 内曲泉：位于足跖胫侧缘，由外踝高点与跟腱之间点向足跖引线，与正中线之交点前3寸处，划一横线与足跖内侧缘之交点是穴。

外曲泉：位于足跖腓侧缘，由外踝高点与跟腱之间点向足跖引线与正中线之交点前3寸处，划一横线与足跖外侧缘之交点是穴。

主治 足内、外翻，下肢瘫痪。

操作 针0.5寸，针感局部胀、痛。

Composition This group of acupoints is composed of Neiququan and Waiququan on the sole.

Location Neiququan: on the medial side of the sole, locate a point which is 3 cun anterior to the junction of the line drawn from the point between the tip of the external malleolus and the Achilles's tendon towards the sole and the midline. Neiququan is at the junction of the transverse line through the above point and the medial border of the sole.

Waiququan: on the lateral side of the sole, locate a point which is 3 cun anterior to the junction of the line drawn from the point between the tip of the external malleolus and the Achilles's tendon towards the sole and the midline. Waiququan is at the junction of the transverse line through the above point and the lateral border of the sole.

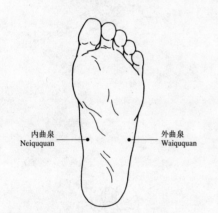

内曲泉
Neiququan

外曲泉
Waiququan

图3-131 足底曲泉
Fig. 3-131 Zudiququan

Indications Foot inversion, foot eversion, paralysis of the lower limbs.

Method The needle is inserted 0.5 cun. The acuesthesia of distension and pain will be obtained in this part.

炉底三针
Ludisanzhen

组成　本穴组由足底部三个点组合而成。

位置　足底部，由外踝高点与跟腱之间点引线与足底正中线之交点前1.5寸一穴，及左右旁开0.5寸二穴。

主治　高热，头痛，耳鸣，胃痛，肝、脾痛，便秘，鼓肠，泄泻，痢疾，腹水，浮肿，痈，瘫痪。

操作　针1~1.5寸，足趾胀、痛感。

Composition This group of acupoints is composed of three points on the sole.

Location On the sole, the point 1.5 cun anterior to the junction of the line drawn from the tip of the external malleolus and the Achilles's tendon and the midline of the sole, and the two points 0.5 cun lateral to the above point each.

Indication High fever, headache, tinnitus, stomachache, pain in the liver and spleen, constipation, distenstion in the intestine, diarrhea, dysentery, ascites, edema, carbuncle and paralysis.

Method The needle is inserted 1—1.5 cun, distension and pain will appear in the toes.

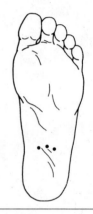

图3-132　炉底三针
Fig. 3-132 Ludisanzhen

通冲维
Tongchongwei

组成　本穴组由公孙、内关二穴组合而成。

位置　公孙：第一跖骨基底部的前下缘，赤白肉际。

内关：腕横纹上2寸，掌长肌腱与桡侧腕屈肌腱之间。

主治　心、胸、胃病证。

操作　刺法：直刺0.5~1寸。

灸法：艾炷灸3~5壮，或温灸5~10分钟。

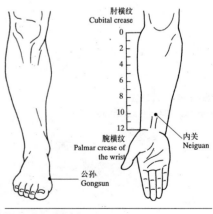

图3-133　通冲维
Fig. 3-133 Tongchongwei

Composition This group of acupoints is composed of Gongsun(SP3) and Neiguan(PC6).

Location Gongsun：anterior and inferior to the base of the 1st metatarsal bone, on the junction of the red and white skin.

Neiguan：2 cun above the crease of the wrist, between the tendons of the long palmar muscle and radial flexor muscle of the wrist.

Indication Diseases of the heart, chest and stomach.

Method Acupuncture：the needle is inserted 0.5—1 cun perpendicularly.

Moxibustion：moxibustion with 3—5 moxa cones, or warm moxibustion for 5—10 minutes is applied.

通督蹻
Tongduqiao

组成 本穴组由后溪、申脉二穴组合而成。
位置 后溪：握拳,第五指掌关节后尺侧,横纹头赤白肉际。
申脉：外踝下缘凹陷中。
主治 目内眦、颈项、耳、肩部病证。
操作 刺法：直刺0.5~1寸。
灸法：艾炷灸3~5壮,或温灸5~10分钟。

Composition This group of acupoints is composed of Houxi(SI3) and Shenmai(BL62).

Location Houxi：on the ulnar side of the proximal end of the 5th metacarpal bone, at the end of the palmar crease on the red and white skin when a fist is made.

Shenmai：in the depression on the lower border of the external malleolus.

Indication Diseases of the inner canthus, neck and nape, ear and shoulder.

Method Acupuncture：the needle is inserted 0.5—1 cun perpendicularly.

Moxibustion：moxibustion with 3—5 moxa cones, or warm moxibustion for 5—10 minutes is applied.

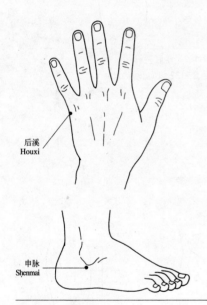

后溪
Houxi

申脉
Shenmai

图3-134 通督蹻
Fig. 3-134 Tongduqiao

通带维
Tongdaiwei

组成　本穴组由足临泣、外关二穴组合而成。

位置　足临泣：在第四、第五跖骨结合部前方，小趾伸肌腱外侧凹陷中。

外关：腕背横纹上2寸，桡骨与尺骨之间。

主治　目锐眦、耳后、颊、颈、肩部病证。

操作　刺法：直刺0.5~1寸。

灸法：艾炷灸3~5壮，或温灸5~10分钟。

Composition　This group of acupoints is composed of Zulinqi(GB41) and Waiguan(TE5).

Location　Zulinqi：anterior to the junction of the 4th and 5th metatarsal bone, in the depression lateral to the tendon of the extensor muscle of the littel toe.

Waiguan：2 cun above the dorsal crease of the wrist, between the radius and ulna.

Indication　Diseases of the outer canthus, posterior side of the ear, cheek, neck and shoulder.

Method　Acupuncture：the needle is inserted 0.5−1 cun perpendicularly.

Moxibustion：moxibustion with 3−5 moxa cones, or warm moxibustion for 5−10 minutes is applied.

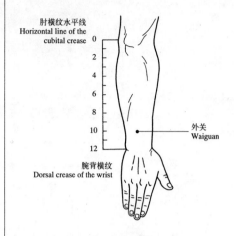

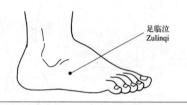

图3-135　通带维
Fig. 3-135　Tongdaiwei

通任蹻
Tongrenqiao

组成　本穴组由列缺、照海二穴组合而成。

位置　列缺：桡骨茎突上方，腕横纹上1.5寸。

照海：内踝下缘凹陷中。

主治　肺系、咽喉、胸膈部病证。

操作　刺法：直刺或斜刺0.3~0.8寸。

灸法：艾炷灸3~5壮，或温灸5~10分钟。

Composition　This group of acupoints is composed of Lieque(LU7) and Zhaohai(KI6).

Location　Lieque：on the styloid process of the radius, 1.5 cun above the palmar crease of the wrist.

Zhaohai：in the depression on the lower border of the

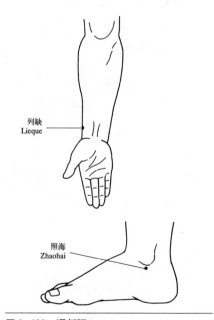

图3-136　通任蹻
Fig. 3-136　Tongrenqiao

medial malleolus.

Indication Diseases of the lung system, throat, chest and diaphragm.

Method Acupuncture：the needle is inserted 0.3−0.8 cun perpendicularly or obliquely.

Moxibustion：moxibustion with 3−5 moxa cones, or warm moxibustion for 5−10 minutes is applied.

脂三针
Zhisanzhen

组成　本穴组由内关、足三里、三阴交三穴组合而成。
位置　内关：腕横纹上2寸，掌长肌腱与桡侧腕屈肌腱之间。
足三里：犊鼻穴下3寸，胫骨前嵴外一横指处。
三阴交：内踝高点上3寸，胫骨内侧面后缘。
主治　胆固醇增高，高脂血症，动脉硬化，冠心病，中风后遗症。
操作　内关直刺0.5～1寸。足三里、三阴交直刺1～1.5寸，得气为度。

Composition This group of acupoints is composed of Neiguan(PC6), Zusanli(ST36) and Sanyinjiao(SP6).

Location Neiguan：2 cun above the palmar crease of the wrist, between the tendons of the long palmar muscle and radial flexor muscle of the wrist.

Zusanli：3 cun below Dubi, one finger breadth from the anterior crest of the tibia.

Sanyinjiao：3 cun above the tip of the medial malleolus, on the posterior border of the medial side of the tibia.

Indication Hypercholesterinemia, hyperlipaemia, arteriosclerosis, coronary heart disease, sequela of apoplexy.

Method Neiguan is needled 0.5−1 cun. Zusanli and Sanyinjiao are needled 1−1.5 cun perpenticularly till the acu-esthesia is obtained.

曲陵
Quling

组成　本穴组由曲池、阳陵泉二穴组合而成。

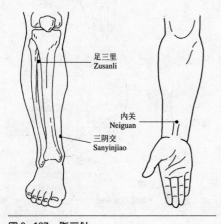

图3−137　脂三针
Fig. 3−137　Zhisanzhen

足三里
Zusanli

内关
Neiguan

三阴交
Sanyinjiao

位置　曲池：屈肘，成直角，当肘横纹外端与肱骨外上髁连线的中点。

阳陵泉：腓骨小头前下方凹陷中。

主治　中风半身不遂。

操作　刺法：直刺1~1.5寸，得气为度。

灸法：艾条温灸10~20分钟。

Composition　This group of acupoints is composed of Quchi(LI11) and Yanglingquan(GB34).

Location　Quchi：at the midpoint of the line between the radial end of the cubital crease and the external humeral epicondyle when the elbow is flexed at 90°.

Yanglingquan：in the depression anterior and inferior to the head of the fibula.

Indication　Hemiplegia due to apoplexy.

Method　Acupuncture：the needle is inserted 1-1.5 cun perpendicularly till the acu-esthesia is obtained.

Moxibustion：warm moxibustion with moxa roll for 10-20 minutes is applied.

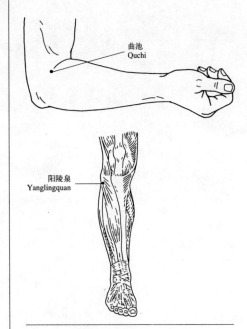

图3-138　曲陵
Fig. 3-138　Quling

 ## 沟溪谷
Gouxigu

组成　本穴组由支沟、太溪、然谷三穴组合而成。

位置　支沟：腕背横纹上3寸，桡骨与尺骨之间。

太溪：内踝高点与跟腱之间凹陷中。

然谷：足舟骨粗隆下缘凹陷中。

主治　心痛如针锥刺，疼痛甚剧，伴心悸，气短，胸脘痞满，腹胀，纳呆，四肢倦怠。

操作　先针太溪0.3~0.5寸，或灸3~5壮，留5~10分钟；然谷针0.3~0.4寸，或灸3~5壮，留5~10分钟；针支沟深0.5~0.8寸。得气后诸穴均行提插捻转之泻法，留针30分钟。

Composition　This group of acupoints is composed of Zhigou(TE6), Taixi(KI3) and Rangu(KI3).

Location　Zhigou：3 cun above the dorsal crease of the wrist, between the radius and ulna.

Taixi：in the midpoint between the tip of the medial malleolus and Achilles's tendon.

Rangu：in the depression inferior to the tuberosity of

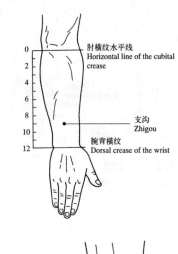

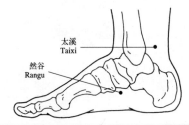

图3-139　沟溪谷
Fig. 3-139　Gouxigu

the navicular bone.

Indication   Sharp and piercing pain in the heart, accompanied by palpitation, shortness of breath, stuffy chest, abdominal distention, anorexia and weakness in the four limbs.

Method   Taixi is needled 0.3−0.5 cun first, 3−5 cones or 5−10 minutes' moxibustion can be applied too. Rangu is needled 0.3−0.4 cun, 3−5 cones or 5−10 minutes' moxibustion can be applied too. Then Zhigou is needled 0.5−0.8 cun. Reducing techniques by lifting, inserting and rotating the needles are applied to the above points after the acu-esthesia is obtained. Retain the needles for 30 minutes.

 郄陵
Xiling

组成   本穴组由阳陵泉、郄门二穴组合而成。

位置   阳陵泉：腓骨小头前下方凹陷中。

郄门：腕横纹上5寸，掌长肌腱与桡侧腕屈肌腱之间。

主治   心胸胁肋部病证和心肝之疾。

操作   针1~1.5寸。

Composition   This group of acupoints is composed of Yanglingquan(GB34) and Ximen(PC4).

Location   Yanglingquan：in the depression anterior and inferior to the head of the fibula.

Ximen：5 cun above the palmar crease of the wrist, between the tendons of the long palmar muscle and radial flexor muscle of the wrist.

Indication   Diseases of the heart, chest and hypochondriac region, diseases of the liver.

Method   The needle is inserted 1−1.5 cun.

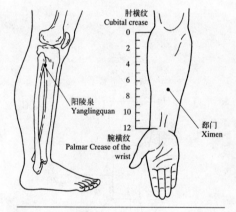

肘横纹
Cubital crease

阳陵泉
Yanglingquan

郄门
Ximen

腕横纹
Palmar Crease of the wrist

图3−140 郄陵
Fig. 3−140 Xiling

 神钟
Shenzhong

组成   本穴组由神门、大钟二穴组合而成。

位置   神门：腕横纹尺侧端，尺侧腕屈肌腱的桡侧凹陷中。

大钟：太溪穴下0.5寸稍后，跟腱内缘。

主治　呆痴。

操作　斜刺0.5～0.8寸，得气为度。

Composition　This group of acupoints is composed of Shenmen(HT7) and Dazhong(KI4).

Location　Shenmen：on the ulnar end of the palmar crease of the wrist, in the depression of the radial side of the tendon of the ulnar flexor muscle of the wrist.

Dazhong：slightly poseterior to the point 0.5 cun below Taixi, in the medial side of the the Achille's tendon.

Indication　Dementia.

Method　The needle is inserted 0.5—0.8 cun obliquely till the acu-esthesia is obtained.

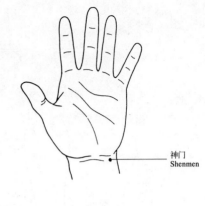
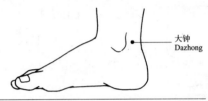

图3-141　神钟
Fig. 3-141　Shenzhong

 神溪
Shenxi

组成　本穴组由神门、太溪二穴组合而成。

位置　神门：腕横纹尺侧端，尺侧腕屈肌腱的桡侧凹陷中。

太溪：内踝高点与跟腱之间凹陷中。

主治　失眠。

操作　神门斜刺0.3～0.5寸。太溪直刺0.5～1寸，得气为度。

Composition　This group of acupoints is composed of Shenmen(HT7) and Taixi(KI3).

Location　Shenmen：on the ulnar end of the palmar crease of the wrist, in the depression of the radial side of the tendon of the ulnar flexor muscle of the wrist.

Taixi：in the midpoint between the tip of the medial malleolus and Achilles's tendon.

Indication　Insomnia.

Method　Shenmen is needled 0.3—0.5 cun obliquely.

Taixi is needled 0.5—1 cun till the acu-esthesia is obtained.

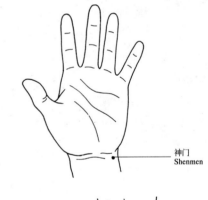
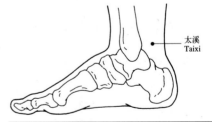

图3-142　神溪
Fig. 3-142　Shenxi

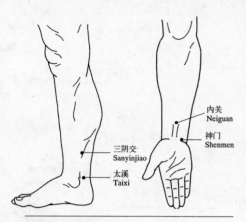

图3-143　眠宁
Fig. 3-143　Mianning

● 眠宁
Mianning

组成　本穴组由神门、三阴交、太溪、内关四穴组合而成。

位置　神门：腕横纹尺侧端，尺侧腕屈肌腱的桡侧凹陷中。

三阴交：内踝高点上3寸，胫骨内侧面后缘。

太溪：内踝高点与跟腱之间凹陷中。

内关：腕横纹上2寸，掌长肌腱与桡侧腕屈肌腱之间。

主治　失眠。

操作　刺法：神门斜刺0.5～0.8寸。余皆直刺0.5～1寸，得气为度。

灸法：艾条灸10～20分钟。

Composition　This group of acupoints is composed of Shenmen(HT7), Sanyinjiao(SP6), Taixi(KI3) and Neiguan (PC6).

Location　Shenmen：on the ulnar end of the palmar crease of the wrist, in the depression of the radial side of the tendon of the ulnar flexor muscle of the wrist.

Sanyinjiao：3 cun above the tip of the medial malleolus, on the posterior border of the medial side of the tibia.

Taixi：in the midpoint between the tip of the medial malleolus and Achilles's tendon.

Neiguan：2 cun above the palmar crease of the wrist, between the tendons of the long palmar muscle and radial flexor muscle of the wrist.

Indication　Insomnia.

Method　Acupuncture：Shenmen is needled 0.5-0.8 cun obliquely. Taixi is needled 0.5-1 cun perpendicularly till the acu-esthesia is obtained.

Moxibustion：moxibustion with moxa roll for 10-20 minutes is applied.

● 通钟
Tongzhong

组成　本穴组由通里、大钟二穴组合而成。

位置　通里：腕横纹上1寸，尺侧腕屈肌腱的桡侧。

大钟：太溪穴下0.5寸稍后，跟腱内缘。

主治　倦言，嗜卧。

操作　斜刺0.5～0.8寸，得气为度。

Composition　This group of acupoints is composed of Tongli(HT5) and Dazhong(KI4).

Location　Tongli：1 cun above the palmar crease of the wrist, in the depression of the radial side of the tendon of the ulnar flexor muscle of the wrist.

Dazhong：slightly poseterior to the point 0.5 cun below Taixi, in the medial side of the the Achille's tendon.

Indication　Lassitude, somnolence.

Method　The needle is inserted 0.5-0.8 cun till the acu-esthesia is obtained.

海海谷
Haihaigu

组成　本穴组由血海、照海、合谷三穴组合而成。

位置　血海：髌骨内上缘上2寸。

照海：内踝下缘凹陷中。

合谷：手背，第一、第二掌骨之间，约平第二掌骨中点处。

主治　嗜睡。

操作　血海直刺1～1.5寸。照海刺0.3～0.5寸。合谷直刺0.5～1寸，得气为度。或用皮内针埋照海、血海，胶布固定。

Composition　This group of acupoints is composed of Xuehai(SP10), Zhaohai(KI6) and Hegu(LI4).

Location　Xuehai：2 cun above the superior medial corner of the patellla.

Zhaohai：in the depression on the lower border of the medial malleolus.

Hegu：on the dorsum of the hand, between the 1st and 2nd metacarpal bones, and near the midpoint of the 2nd metacarpal bone.

Indication　Somnolence.

Method　Xuehai is needled 1-1.5 cun perpendicularly. Zhaohai is needled 0.3-0.5 cun. Hegu is needled 0.5-1 cun perpendicularly till the acu-esthesia is obtained. Zhaohai, Xuehai can be embedded with the intradermal

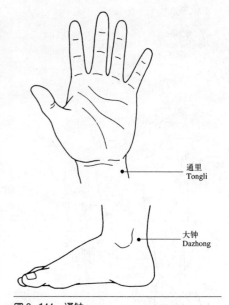

图3-144　通钟
Fig. 3-144　Tongzhong

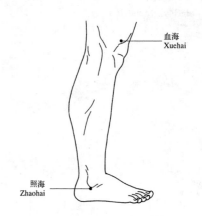

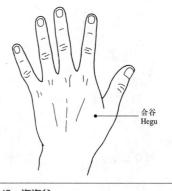

图3-145　海海谷
Fig. 3-145　Haihaigu

needles, fixed with plaster.

脉髓会
Maisuihui

组成　本穴组由脉会太渊、髓会悬钟二穴组合而成。

位置　太渊：掌后腕横纹桡侧端，桡动脉的桡侧凹陷中。

悬钟：外踝高点上3寸，腓骨后缘。

主治　血液病，脉骨病证。

操作　太渊：见"肺原络"中太渊穴操作。

悬钟：直刺0.8～1.2寸。

Composition　This group of acupoints is composed of Taiyuan(LU9), the Influential Point of Vessels, and Xuanzhong(GB39), the Influential Point of Marrow.

Location　Taiyuan：at the radial end of the palmar crease of the wrist, in the depression of the radial side of the radial artery.

Xuanzhong：3 cun above the tip of the external malleolus, on the posterior border of the fibula.

Indication　Diseases of blood, vessel and bone.

Method　Taiyuan see methods for Taiyuan in Feiyuanluo. Xuanzhong is inserted 0.8-1.2 cun perperdiculariy.

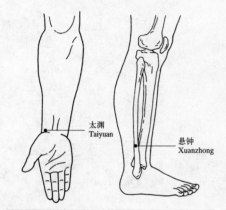

图3-146　脉髓会

Fig. 3-146　Maisuihui

郄丘陵
Xiqiuling

组成　本穴组由郄门、梁丘、阳陵泉三穴组合而成。

位置　郄门：腕横纹上5寸，掌长肌腱与桡侧腕屈肌腱之间。

梁丘：在髂前上棘与髌骨外缘连线上，髌骨外上缘上2寸。

阳陵泉：腓骨小头前下方凹陷中。

主治　吐血。

操作　直刺0.5～1.2寸，得气后施以泻法。

Composition　This group of acupoints is composed of Ximen(PC4), Liangqiu(ST34) and Yanglingquan (GB34).

Location　Ximen：5 cun above the palmar crease of the wrist, between the tendons of the long palmar muscle

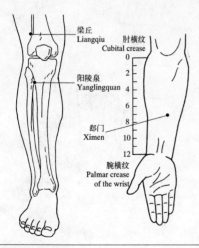

图3-147　郄丘陵

Fig. 3-147　Xiqiuling

and radial flexor muscle of the wrist.

Liangqiu: on the line connecting the anteriosuperior iliac spine and the lateral corner of the patella, 2 cun above the superiolateral border of the patella.

Yanglingquan: in the depression anterior and inferior to the head of the fibula.

Indication   Haematemesis.

Method   The needle is inserted 0.5−1.2 cun perpendicularly. Reducing techniques are applied after the acu−esthesia is obtained.

 ## 郄溪
Xixi

组成   本穴组由郄门、太溪二穴组合而成。

位置   郄门：腕横纹上5寸，掌长肌腱与桡侧腕屈肌腱之间。

太溪：内踝高点与跟腱之间凹陷中。

主治   咯血。

操作   直刺0.5~1寸，得气后施以泻法。

Composition   This group of acupoints is composed of Ximen(PC4) and Taixi(KI3).

Location   Ximen：5 cun above the palmar crease of the wrist, between the tendons of the long palmar muscle and radial flexor muscle of the wrist.

Taixi：in the midpoint between the tip of the medial malleolus and Achilles's tendon.

Indication   Emptysis.

Method   The needle is inserted 0.5−1 cun perpendicularly. Reducing techniques are applied after the acu−esthesia is obtained.

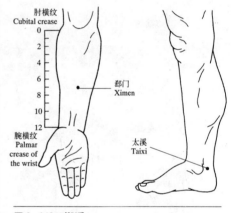

图3−148　郄溪
Fig. 3−148　Xixi

 ## 筋脉会
Jinmaihui

组成   本穴组由筋会阳陵泉、脉会太渊二穴组合而成。

位置   阳陵泉：腓骨小头前下方凹陷中。

太渊：掌后腕横纹桡侧端，桡动脉的桡侧凹陷中。

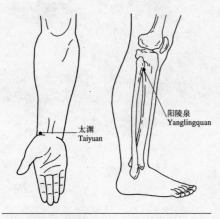

图 3-149　筋脉会
Fig. 3-149　Jinmaihui

主治　全身筋脉病。
操作　阳陵泉：直刺1～1.5寸。
太渊：见"肺原络"中太渊穴操作。

Composition　This group of acupoints is composed of Yanglingquan(GB34), the Influential Point of Tendon, and Taiyuan(CU9), the Influential Point of Vessel.

Location　Yanglingquan：in the depression anterior and inferior to the head of the fibula.

Taiyuan：at the radial end of the palmar crease of the wrist, in the depression of the radial side of the radial artery.

Indication　Diseases of the tendons and vessels of the whole body.

Method　Yanglingquan is inserted 1-1.5 cun perpendicularly.

Taiyuan：See method for Taiyuan in Feiyuanluo.

● 陵老
Linglao

组成　本穴组由阳陵泉、养老二穴组合而成。
位置　阳陵泉：腓骨小头前下方凹陷中。
养老：以掌向胸，当尺骨茎突桡侧缘凹陷中。
主治　筋病，肌病，颈椎腰椎病证。
操作　针0.5～1寸。

Composition　This group of acupoints is composed of Yanglingquan(GB34) and Yanglao(SI6).

Location　Yanglingquan：in the depression anterior and inferior to the head of the fibula.

Yanglao：in the depression on the radial side of the styloid process of the ulna when the hand faces the chest.

Indications　Diseases of the tendons, muscles, cervical and lumbar vertebrae.

Method　The needle is inserted 0.5-1 cun.

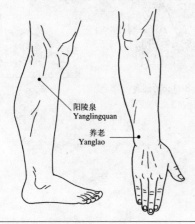

图 3-150　陵老
Fig. 3-150　Linglao

三合
Sanhe

组成　本穴组由尺泽、曲泽、委中三个合穴组合而成。
位置　尺泽：肘横纹中，肱二头肌腱桡侧缘。
曲泽：肘横纹中，肱二头肌腱尺侧。
委中：腘横纹中央。
主治　小儿急惊风。
操作　点刺出血。

Composition　This group of acupoints is composed of three He-sea points of Chize(LU5), Quze(PC3) and Weizhong(BL40).

Location　Chize：in the cubital crease, on the radial side of the tendon of the biceps muscle of the arm.

Quze：in the cubital crease, on the ulnar side of the tendon of the biceps muscle of the arm.

Weizhong：at the midpoint of the popliteal crease.

Indication　Acute infantile convulsions.

Method　The points are pricked to bleed.

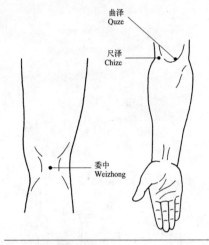

图 3-151　三合
Fig. 3-151　Sanhe

痫三针
Xiansanzhen

组成　本穴组由内关、申脉、照海三穴组合而成。
位置　内关：腕横纹上2寸，掌长肌腱与桡侧腕屈肌腱之间。
申脉：外踝下缘凹陷中。
照海：内踝下缘凹陷中。
主治　癫痫，足内、外翻。
操作　申脉、照海直刺0.5～0.8寸。内关直刺0.5～1寸。得气为度。

Composition　This group of acupoints is composed of Neiguan(PC6), Shenmai(BL62) and Zhaohai(KI6).

Location　Neiguan：2 cun above the palmar crease of the wrist, between the tendons of the long palmar muscle and radial flexor muscle of the wrist.

Shenmai：in the depression on the lower border of the external malleolus.

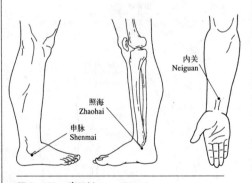

图 3-152　痫三针
Fig. 3-152　Xiansanzhen

Zhaohai: in the depression on the lower border of the medial malleolus.

Indication Epilepsy, foot inversion and eversion.

Method Shenmai and Zhaohai are needled 0.5-0.8 cun perpendicularly. Neiguan is needled 0.5-1 cun perpendicularly. Stop manipulating the needles after the acu-esthesia is obtained in all points.

● 痰咳
Tanke

组成 本穴组由丰隆、尺泽二穴组合而成。

位置 丰隆：外踝高点上8寸，条口穴外1寸。

尺泽：肘横纹中，肱二头肌腱桡侧缘。

主治 痰多咳嗽。

操作 直刺0.5～1寸，得气为度。

Composition This group of acupoints is composed of Fenglong(ST40) and Chize(LU5).

Location Fenglong：8 cun above the tip of the external malleolus, 1 cun lateral to Tiaokou.

Chize：in the cubital crease, on the radial side of the tendon of the biceps muscle of the arm.

Indication Productive cough.

Method The needle is inserted 0.5-1 cun perpendicularly till the acu-esthesia is obtained.

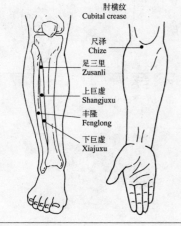

图3-153 痰咳

Fig. 3-153 Tanke

● 疏肝胁
Shuganxie

组成 本穴组由支沟、阳陵泉二穴组合而成。

位置 支沟：腕背横纹上3寸，桡骨与尺骨之间。

阳陵泉：腓骨小头前下方凹陷中。

主治 胁肋痛。

操作 直刺1～1.5寸得气后，一面活动胸胁如扩胸运动，一面深呼吸等可加强治疗效果。

Composition This group of acupoints is composed of Zhigou(TE6) and Yanglingquan(GB34).

Location Zhigou：3 cun above the dorsal crease of

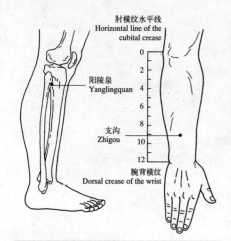

图3-154 疏肝胁

Fig. 3-154 Shuganxie

the wrist, between the radius and ulna.

Yanglingquan: in the depression anterior and inferior to the head of the fibula.

Indication Pain in the hypochondriac region.

Method The needle is inserted 1−1.5 cun. After the arrival of the acu-esthesia, the curative effect will be better if the patient breathes deeply and do some exercises for the chest and the hypochondriac region such as expanding the chest.

⬤ 三里二穴
Sanlierxue

组成 本穴组由手足阳明经的手、足三里二穴组合而成。

位置 手三里：在阳溪穴与曲池穴连线上，曲池穴下2寸处。

足三里：犊鼻穴下3寸，胫骨前嵴外一横指处。

主治 胃痛，腹胀，吐泻，食痞气块，中风偏瘫。

操作 刺法：直刺0.5～1.5寸。

灸法：艾炷灸5～9壮，或温灸10～30分钟。

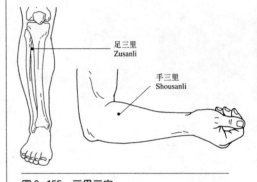

图3-155 三里二穴

Fig. 3-155 Sanlierxue

Composition This group of acupoints is composed of Shousanli(LI10) and Zusanli(ST36) of the Hand Yangmin and Foot Yangming Meridians.

Location Shousanli：on the line connecting Yangxi and Quchi, 2 cun below Quchi.

Zusanli：3 cun below Dubi, one finger breadth from the anterior crest of the tibia.

Indication Stomachache, abdominal distension, vomiting and diarrhea, abdominal flatulence, hemiplegia due to apoplexy.

Method Acupuncture：the needle is inserted 0.5−1.5 cun perpendicularly.

Moxibustion：moxibustion with 5−9 moxa cones, or warm moxibustion for 10−30 minutes is applied.

⬤ 退余热
Tuiyure

组成 本穴组由曲池、合谷、足三里三穴组合而成。

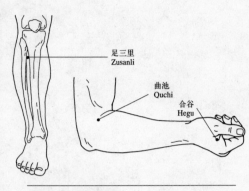

图 3-156 退余热
Fig. 3-156 Tuiyure

位置 曲池：屈肘，成直角，当肘横纹外端与肱骨外上髁连线的中点。

合谷：手背，第一、第二掌骨之间，约平第二掌骨中点处。

足三里：犊鼻穴下3寸，胫骨前嵴外一横指处。

主治 伤寒数日，余热不退。

操作 先针曲池、合谷，针用泻法，行针1～2分钟，留针20分钟；后针足三里，针用补法，留针30分钟。

Composition This group of acupoints is composed of Quchi(LI11), Hegu(LI4) and Zusanli(ST36).

Location Quchi：at the midpoint of the line between the radial end of the cubital crease and the external humeral epicondyle when the elbow is flexed at 90°.

Hegu：on the dorsum of the hand, between the 1st and 2nd metacarpal bones, and near the midpoint of the 2nd metacarpal bone.

Zusanli：3 cun below Dubi, one finger breadth from the anterior crest of the tibia.

Indication Lingering fever after several days' febrile diseases due to cold.

Method Quchi, Hegu are needled first with reducing techniques. Manipulate the needles for 1-2 minutes, retain them for 20 minutes. Then Zusanli is needled and reinforcing techniques are applied, retain the needle for 30 minutes.

四关
Siguan

组成 本穴组由合谷、太冲二穴组合而成。

位置 合谷：手背，第一、第二掌骨之间，约平第二掌骨中点处。

太冲：足背，第一、第二跖骨结合部之前凹陷中。

主治 疼痛症及兴奋性疾病，四肢寒颤，喑哑。

操作 刺法：针0.5～1寸，局部酸胀，针感或可向上传导。

灸法：灸3～5壮，艾条灸5～15分钟。

Composition This group of acupoints is composed of Hegu(LI4) and Taichong(LR3).

Location Hegu：on the dorsum of the hand, between the 1st and 2nd metacarpal bones, and near the midpoint

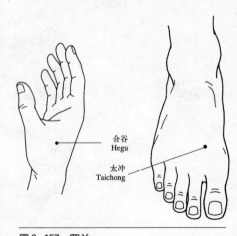

图 3-157 四关
Fig. 3-157 Siguan

of the 2nd metacarpal bone.

Taichong: on the instep of the foot, in the depression anterior to the commissure of the 1st and 2nd metatarsal bones.

Indication Pain and hyperexcitation, quivering of the four limbs due to cold, hoarseness.

Method Acupuncture: the needle is inserted 0.5–1 cun. The acu-esthesia of soreness and distension can be obtained in the part, it may radiate upwards too.

Moxibustion: 3–5 cones of moxibustion, or 5–15 minutes' moxibustion with moxa roll is applied.

谷庭
Guting

组成 本穴组由合谷、内庭二穴组合而成。

位置 合谷：手背，第一、第二掌骨之间，约平第二掌骨中点处。

内庭：足背第二、第三趾间缝纹端。

主治 面肿，肠鸣，鼻衄。

操作 合谷直刺0.5～1寸。内庭针0.5～0.8寸，得气为度。

Composition This group of acupoints is composed of Hegu(LI4) and Neiting(ST44).

Location Hegu: on the dorsum of the hand, between the 1st and 2nd metacarpal bones, and near the midpoint of the 2nd metacarpal bone.

Neiting: at the end of the margin of the web between the 2nd and 3rd toes.

Indication Swelling in the face, borborygmus, epistaxis.

Method Hegu is needled 0.5–1 cun perpendicularly.

Neiting is needled 0.5–0.8 cun till the acu-esthesia is obtained.

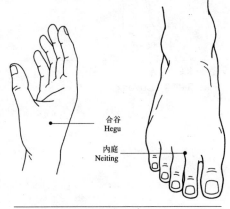

图3-158 谷庭
Fig. 3-158 Guting

祛痒
Quyang

组成 本穴组由血海、曲池、合谷、太冲、三阴交、风市

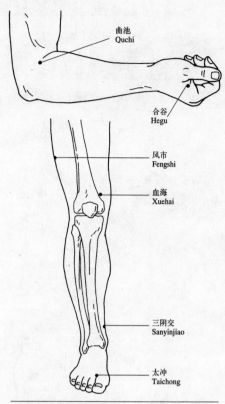

图3-159 祛痒
Fig. 3-159 Quyang

六穴组合而成。

位置 血海：髌骨内上缘上2寸。

三阴交：内踝高点上3寸，胫骨内侧面后缘。

曲池：屈肘，成直角，当肘横纹外端与肱骨外上髁连线的中点。

合谷：手背，第一、第二掌骨之间，约平第二掌骨中点处。

太冲：足背，第一、第二跖骨结合部之前凹陷中。

风市：大腿外侧正中，腘横纹水平线上7寸。

主治 皮肤瘙痒。

操作 刺法：曲池、血海针0.8～1.5寸。合谷、太冲针0.5～1寸，得气为度。

灸法：艾条灸10～20分钟。

Composition This group of acupoints is composed of Xuehai(SP10), Quchi(LI11), Hegu(LI4), Taichong(LR3), Sanyinjiao(SP6) and Fengshi(GB31).

Location Xuehai：2 cun above the superior medial corner of the patellla.

Sanyinjiao：3 cun above the tip of the medial malleolus, on the posterior border of the medial side of the tibia.

Quchi：at the midpoint of the line between the radial end of the cubital crease and the external humeral epicondyle when the elbow is flexed at 90°.

Hegu：on the dorsum of the hand, between the 1st and 2nd metacarpal bones, and near the midpoint of the 2nd metacarpal bone.

Taichong：on the instep of the foot, in the depression anterior to the commissure of the 1st and 2nd metatarsal bones.

Fengshi：on the midline of the lateral side of the thigh, 7 cun above the popliteal crease.

Indication Skin pruritus.

Method Acupuncture：Quchi and Xuehai are needled 0.8-1.5 cun.

Hegu and Taichong are needled 0.5-1 cun till the acu-esthesia is obtained.

Moxibustion：moxibustion with moxa roll for 10-20 minutes is applied.

肤痒
Fuyang

组成　本穴组由曲池、血海、三阴交三穴组合而成。

位置　曲池：屈肘，成直角，当肘横纹外端与肱骨外上髁连线的中点。

三阴交：内踝高点上3寸，胫骨内侧面后缘。

血海：髌骨内上缘上2寸。

主治　皮肤瘙痒。

操作　刺法：曲池、血海见"祛痒"。三阴交直刺0.8～1.5寸，得气为度。

灸法：艾条灸10～20分钟。

Composition　This group of acupoints is composed of Quchi(LI11), Xuehai(SP10) and Sanyinjiao(SP6).

Location　Quchi：at the midpoint of the line between the radial end of the cubital crease and the external humeral epicondyle when the elbow is flexed at 90°.

Sanyinjiao：3 cun above the tip of the medial malleolus, on the posterior border of the medial side of the tibia.

Xuehai：2 cun above the superior medial corner of the patellla.

Indication　Skin pruritus.

Methods　Acupuncture：Quchi and Xuehai：see Quyang.

Sanyinjiao is needled 0.5-1.5 cun perpendicularly till the acu-esthesia is obtained.

Moxibustion：moxibustion with moxa roll for 10-20 minutes is applied.

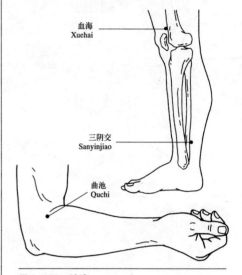

图 3-160　肤痒
Fig. 3-160　Fuyang

盗汗
Daohan

组成　本穴组由阴郄、后溪、照海三穴组合而成。

位置　阴郄：腕横纹上0.5寸，尺侧腕屈肌腱的桡侧。

后溪：握拳，第五指掌关节后尺侧，横纹头赤白肉际。

照海：内踝下缘凹陷中。

主治　盗汗。

操作　刺法：阴郄斜刺0.5～1寸。后溪直刺0.5～0.8寸。照海针0.3～0.5寸，得气为度。

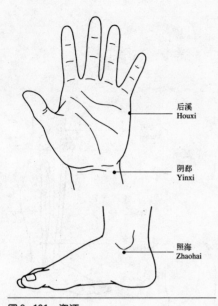

图3-161 盗汗
Fig. 3-161 Daohan

灸法：艾条灸10～20分钟。

按注 一说无照海穴。

Composition This group of acupoints is composed of Yinxi(HT6), Houxi(SI3) and Zhaohai(KI6).

Location Yinxi：0.5 cun above the palmar crease of the wrist, on the radial side of the tendon of the ulnar flexor muscle of the wrist.

Houxi：on the ulnar side of the proximal end of the 5th metacarpal bone, at the end of the palmar crease on the red and white skin when a fist is made.

Zhaohai：in the depression on the lower border of the medial malleolus.

Indication Night sweating.

Methods Acupuncture：Yinxi is needled 0.5－1 cun obliquely.

Houxi is needled 0.5－0.8 cun perpendicularly.

Zhaohai is needled 0.3－0.5 cun till the acu-esthesia is obatined.

Moxibustion：moxibustion with moxa roll for 10－20 minutes is applied.

Note In some books, Zhaohai is not included in Daohan.

● 多汗
Duohan

组成 本穴组由合谷、复溜二穴组合而成。

位置 合谷：手背，第一、第二掌骨之间，约平第二掌骨中点处。

复溜：太溪穴上2寸。

主治 多汗。

操作 合谷针0.5～1寸。复溜针0.8～1.5寸，得气为度。

Composition This group of acupoints is composed of Hegu(LI4) and Fuliu(KI7).

Location Hegu：on the dorsum of the hand, between the 1st and 2nd metacarpal bones, and near the midpoint of the 2nd metacarpal bone.

Fuliu：2 cun above Taixi.

Indication Excessive sweating.

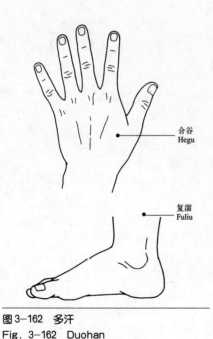

图3-162 多汗
Fig. 3-162 Duohan

Method Hegu is needled 0.5—1 cun. Fuliu is needled 0.8—1.5 cun till the acu-esthesia is obtained.

关照
Guanzhao

组成 本穴组由照海、外关二穴组合而成。

位置 照海：内踝下缘凹陷中。

外关：腕背横纹上2寸，桡骨与尺骨之间。

主治 胎衣不下。

操作 照海针0.3～0.5寸。外关针0.5～1.2寸，得气为度，留针30～60分钟，留针期间可多作运针手法。

Composition This group of acupoints is composed of Zhaohai(KI6) and Waiguan(TE5).

Location Zhaohai：in the depression on the lower border of the medial malleolus.

Waiguan：2 cun above the dorsal crease of the wrist, between the radius and ulna.

Indication Retained placenta.

Method Zhaohai is needled 0.3–0.5 cun. Waiguan is needled 0.5–1.2 cun till the acu-esthesia is obtained. Retain the needles for 30–60 minutes. Manipulating methods can be applied frequently during the retention of the needles.

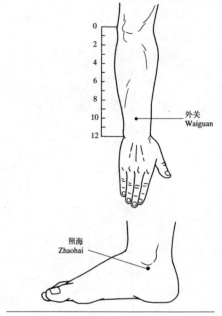

图 3-163 关照
Fig. 3-163 Guanzhao

溪跳
Xitiao

组成 本穴组由后溪、环跳二穴组合而成。

位置 后溪：握拳，第五指掌关节后尺侧，横纹头赤白肉际。

环跳：股骨大转子高点与骶管裂孔连线的外1/3与内2/3交界处。

主治 腿痛，坐骨神经痛。

操作 环跳见"悬跳"。后溪直刺0.5～0.8寸。得气为度。

Composition This group of acupoints is composed of Houxi(SI3) and Huantiao(GB30).

Location Houxi：on the ulnar side of the proximal

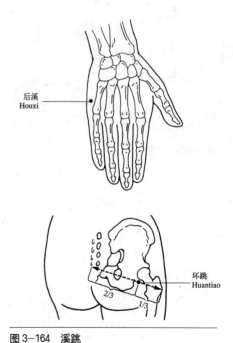

图 3-164 溪跳
Fig. 3-164 Xitiao

end of the 5th metacarpal bone, at the end of the palmar crease on the red and white skin when a fist is made.

Huantiao: at the junction of the lateral 1/3 and medial 2/3 of the line connecting the prominence of the great trochanter and the sacral hiatus.

Indication Pain in the leg and sciatica.

Method Huantiao: see Xuantiao. Houxi is needled 0.5—0.8 cun perpendicularly till the acu-esthesia is obtained.

解毒
Jiedu

组成 本穴组由曲池、合谷、足三里,行间四穴组合而成。

位置 曲池:屈肘,成直角,当肘横纹外端与肱骨外上髁连线的中点。

合谷:手背,第一、第二掌骨之间,约平第二掌骨中点处。

足三里:犊鼻穴下3寸,胫骨前嵴外一横指处。

行间:足背,第一、第二趾间缝纹端。

主治 疔疮,疖肿,痈疽遍布周身。

操作 先刺曲池、合谷,得气后用强刺激泻法;再刺足三里,得气后用强刺激泻法;最后刺行间,用泻法。均留针30分钟。留针期间行针2~3次,每次行针1—2分钟。

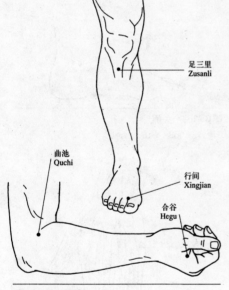

足三里
Zusanli

曲池
Quchi

行间
Xingjian

合谷
Hegu

图3—165 解毒
Fig. 3—165 Jiedu

Composition This group of acupoints is composed of Quchi(LI11), Hegu(LI4), Zusanli(ST36) and Xinjian(LR2).

Location Quchi: at the midpoint of the line between the radial end of the cubital crease and the external humeral epicondyle when the elbow is flexed at 90°.

Hegu: on the dorsum of the hand, between the 1st and 2nd metacarpal bones, and near the midpoint of the 2nd metacarpal bone.

Zusanli: 3 cun below Dubi, one finger breadth from the anterior crest of the tibia.

Xingjian: on the instep of the foot, on the end of the margin of the web between the 1st and 2nd toes.

Indication Furuncle, boil and carbuncle all over the body.

Method Quchi and Hegu is needled first with strong stimulating reducing techniques after the arrival of the acu–esthesia. Xingjian is needled finally and reducing techniques are applied. Retain the needles for 30 minutes, manipulate the needles 2–3 times during the retention, 1–2 minutes each manipulation.

● 手足髓孔
Shouzusuikong

组成　本穴组由手髓孔(阳谷)、足髓孔(昆仑)二穴组合而成。

位置　手髓孔：位于手腕背侧尺侧缘，尺骨小头与三角骨之间的凹陷处，即阳谷穴。

足髓孔：位于足外踝高点与跟腱之间凹陷中，即昆仑穴。

主治　中风后遗，四肢痿痹，头痛，眩晕。

操作　刺法：手髓孔针0.3~0.5寸，局部酸、胀感。足髓孔针0.5~1寸，局部酸、胀，并向足趾放散。

灸法：灸3~9壮，艾条灸5~15分钟。

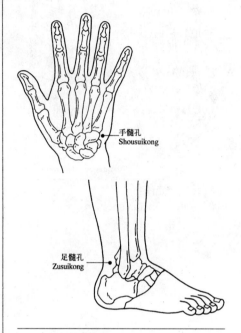

图3-166　手足髓孔
Fig. 3-166　Shouzusuikong

Composition　This group of acupoints is composed of Shousuikong (Yanggu) and Zusuikong (Kunlun).

Location　Shousuikong：on the ulnar side of the dorsum of the wrist, in the depression between the styloid process of the ulna and triangular bone, i.e. Yanggu (SI5).

Zusuikong：in the depression between the tip of the external malleolus and the Achilles's tendon, i.e. Kunlun (BL60).

Indication　Sequela of apoplexy, muscular atrophy and paralysis of the four limbs, headache and vertigo.

Method　Acupuncture：Shousuikong is needled 0.3–0.5 cun, the acu-esthesia of soreness and distension will be obtained in this part. Zusuikong is needled 0.5–1 cun, the acu-esthesia of soreness and distension will be obtained in this part and radiate to the toes.

Moxibustion：3–9 cones of moxibustion, or 5–15 minutes' moxibustion with moxa roll is applied.

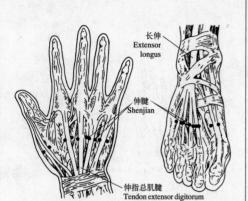

图3-167 手足伸腱
Fig. 3-167 Shouzushenjian

手足伸腱
Shouzushenjian

组成 本穴组由手、足伸肌腱两侧之左右十个点组合而成。

位置 手(足)患指(趾)的掌指(跖趾)关节后1寸伸肌腱的两侧各一穴。

主治 指头炎,腱鞘炎。

操作 刺法:直刺或斜刺0.2~0.3寸。

灸法:麦粒灸1~3壮,温灸3~5分钟。

按注 该穴可分为"手伸腱"与"足伸腱"。在"手伸腱",又可按大至小指(趾)序,分别称为"手伸腱1"、"手伸腱2"……"足伸腱"也依此类推。

Composition This group of acupoints is composed of ten points which are on both sides of the tendons of the extensor muscles of each hand or foot.

Location 1 cun posterior to the metacarpophalangeal (metatarsophalangeal) joints of the hands (feet), on both sides of the tendons of the extensor muscles.

Indication Dactylitis and tenosynovitis.

Method Acupuncture：the needle is inserted 0.2−0.3 cun perpendicularly or obliquely.

Moxibustion：1−3 cones of moxibustion, or 3−5 minutes' warm moxibustion is applied.

Note This group can be divided to Shoushenjian and Zushenjian. The points of Shoushenjian consist of Shoushenjian1, Shoushenjian2··· from the thumb to little finger. Zushenjian does the same way.

地神
Dishen

组成 本穴组由手足大指(趾)处的四个刺激点组成。

位置 手一穴位于拇指掌侧掌指关节横纹中点处。足一穴位于足大趾跖侧跖趾关节横纹中点处。

主治 自缢,腱鞘炎。

操作 刺法:直刺0.1~0.3寸,或点刺出血。

灸法:麦粒灸5~9壮。

Composition This group of acupoints is composed of

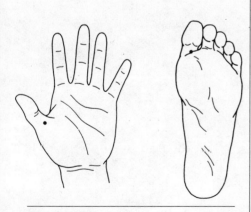

图3-168 地神
Fig. 3-168 Dishen

four points on the thumbs and great toes.

Location   The points on the hands are at the mid-points of the crease of the metacarpophalangeal joint on the palmar side of the thumbs. The points on the feet are at the midpoint of the crease of the metatarsophalangeal joint of the thenar side of the great toes.

Indication   Suicide by hanging oneself, tenosynovitis.

Methods   Acupuncture：the needle is inserted 0.1—0.3 cun, or the points can be pricked to bleed.

Moxibustion：5—9 wheat-sized moxa cones of moxibustion is applied.

🔴 手足大指(趾)爪甲穴
Shouzudazhi(zhi)zhuajiaxue

组成   本穴组由手足大指(趾)爪甲处的四个刺激点穴组合而成。

位置   位于手足大指(趾)爪甲根正中与皮肤交换处。

主治   卒中邪魅。

操作   艾炷灸7~14壮，炷置于半爪半肉之上。

Composition   This group of acupoints is composed of four points on the nail roots of the thumbs and great toes.

Location   On the junctions of the centre of the nail roots of the thumbs (great toes) of the hands (feet) and the skin.

Indication   Sudden diseases due to mental pathogenic factors.

Method   Moxibustion with 7—14 moxa cones is applied. The moxa cones are placed on the junctions of the nail and skin.

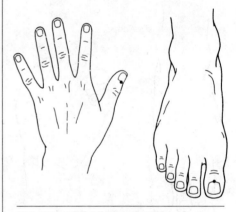

图 3-169   手足大指(趾)爪甲穴
Fig. 3-169   Shouzudazhi(zhi)zhuajiaxue

🔴 手足小指(趾)穴
Shouzuxiaozhi(zhi)xue

组成   本穴组由手足小指(趾)端的四个刺激点组合而成。

位置   位于手足小指(趾)尖端，距甲缘0.1寸处，双手、双足共4穴。

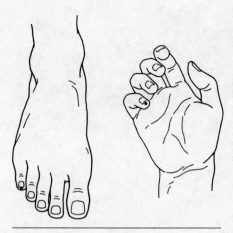

图 3-170 手足小指(趾)穴
Fig. 3-170 Shouzuxiaozhi(zhi)xue

主治 消渴，注食，疝气。
操作 艾炷灸7壮或随年壮。

Composition This group of acupoints is composed of four points on the tips of the little fingers and toes.

Location On the tips of the little fingers and toes, 0.1 cun from the border of the nail, 4 points each on the hands and feet.

Indication Diabetes, indigestion and hernia.

Method 7 cones of moxibustion is applied, the number of the cones can also be determined by the age of the patient.

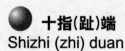 十指(趾)端
Shizhi (zhi) duan

组成 本穴组由手足十指(趾)尖端之十个点组合而成。
位置 位于手足十指(趾)尖端(同十宣穴与气端穴)。
主治 昏厥，休克急救。
操作 灸1~3壮。

Composition This group of acupoints is composed of ten points at the tips of the ten fingers and toes.

Location On the tips of the ten fingers and toes (including Shixuan and Qiduan).

Indications Syncope and shock.

Method 1-3 cones of moxibustion is applied.

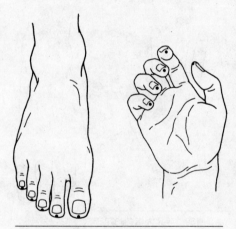

图 3-171 十指(趾)端
Fig. 3-171 Shizhi(zhi)duan

第四章　全身性组合穴

CHAPTER 4 COMPOSED ACUPOINTS ON THE WHOLE BODY

 固脱
Gutuo

组成　本穴组由气海、关元、神阙、百会、足三里五穴组合而成。

位置　气海：脐下1.5寸。

关元：脐下3寸。

神阙：脐的中间。

百会：后发际正中直上7寸。

足三里：犊鼻穴下3寸，胫骨前嵴外一横指处。

主治　虚脱。

操作　神阙用隔盐灸，余穴皆用大壮灸，不拘壮数。

Composition　This group of acupoints is composed of Qihai(GV6), Guanyuan(GV4), Shenque(GV8), Baihui(GV20) and Zusanli(ST36).

Location　Qihai：1.5 cun below the centre of the umbilicus.

Guanyuan：3 cun below the centre of the umbilicus.

Shenque：in the centre of the umbilicus.

Baihui：7 cun directly above the midpoint of the posterior hairline.

Zusanli：3 cun below Dubi, one finger breadth from the anterior crest of the tibia.

Indication　Prostration.

Method　Salt-cushioned moxibustion is applied to Shenque. Moxibustion with big moxa cones is applied to the other points without calculating the number of cones.

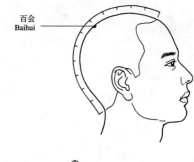
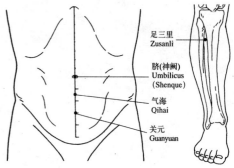

图4-1　固脱
Fig. 4-1　Gutuo

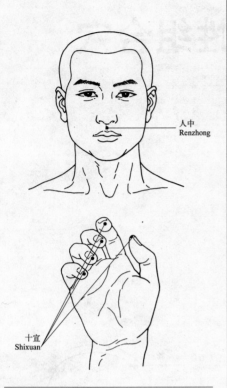

图 4-2 急救
Fig. 4-2 Jijiu

急救

Jijiu

组成　本穴组由人中、十宣二穴组合而成。

位置　人中：在人中沟的上 1/3 与中 1/3 交界处。

十宣：手十指尖端距指甲 0.1 寸。

主治　昏迷，急救。

操作　人中针尖向上斜刺 0.3～0.5 寸，痛胀感。十宣浅刺 0.1～0.2 寸，或用三棱针点刺到出血。

Composition　This group of acupoints is composed of Renzhong(GV26) and Shixuan(EX-UE11).

Location　Renzhong：at the junction of the upper third and middle third of the philtrum.

Shixuan：at the tips of the 10 fingers, about 0.1 cun from the free margin of the nails.

Indication　Coma and emergency diseases.

Method　Renzhong：the needle is obliquely inserted 0.3-0.5 cun upwards, the feeling is pain and distension. Shixuan：the needle is inserted 0.1-0.2 cun, or the points can be pricked to bleed.

回阳九针

Huiyangjiuzhen

组成　本穴组由哑门、中脘、环跳、合谷、劳宫、足三里、三阴交、太溪、涌泉九穴组合而成。

位置　哑门：后发际正中直上 0.5 寸。

中脘：脐上 4 寸。

环跳：股骨大转子高点与骶管裂孔连线的外 1/3 与内 2/3 交界处。

合谷：手背，第一、第二掌骨之间，约平第二掌骨中点处。

劳宫：第二、第三掌骨之间，握拳，中指尖下是穴。

足三里：犊鼻穴下 3 寸，胫骨前嵴外一横指处。

三阴交：内踝高点上 3 寸，胫骨内侧面后缘。

太溪：内踝高点与跟腱之间凹陷中。

涌泉：足底(去趾)前 1/3 处，足趾跖屈时呈凹陷处。

主治　休克。

操作　刺法：除环跳直刺 2～3 寸外，其余各穴分别针刺

0.5～1寸不等。

灸法：灸5～9壮。

Composition This group of acupoints is composed of Yamen(GV15), Zhongwan(CU12), Huantiao(GB30), Hegu (LI4), Laogong(PC8), Zusanli(ST36), Sanyinjiao(SP6), Taixi (KI3) and Yongquan(KI1).

Location Yamen：0.5 cun directly above the midpoint of the posterior hairline.

Zhongwan：4 cun above the centre of the umbilicus.

Huantiao：at the junction of the lateral 1/3 and medial 2/3 of the line connecting the prominence of the great trochanter and the sacral hiatus.

Hegu：on the dorsum of the hand, between the 1st and 2nd metacarpal bones, and near the midpoint of the 2nd metacarpal bone.

Laogong：between the 2nd and 3rd metacarpal bones, where the tip of the middle finger reaches when a fist is made.

Zusanli：3 cun below Dubi, one finger breadth from the anterior crest of the tibia.

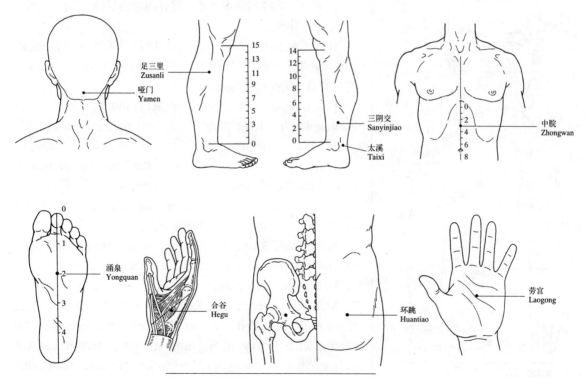

图4-3　回阳九针

Fig. 4-3 Huiyangjiuzhen

Sanyinjiao：3 cun above the tip of the medial malleolus, on the posterior border of the medial side of the tibia.

Taixi：in the midpoint between the tip of the medial malleolus and Achilles's tendon.

Yongquan：at the junction of the anterior one-third and one-third of the sole (the toes are not included), i.e. in the depression when the toes are extended downwards.

Indication Shock.

Method Acupuncture：Huantiao is needled 2−3 cun perpendicularly, the puncturing depth of the other points varies from 0.5 cun to 1 cun.

Moxibustion：5−9 cones of moxibustion is applied.

关中交
Guanzhongjiao

组成 本穴组由内关、人中、三阴交三穴组合而成。

位置 内关：腕横纹上2寸，掌长肌腱与桡侧腕屈肌腱之间。

人中：在人中沟的上1/3与中1/3交界处。

三阴交：内踝高点上3寸，胫骨内侧面后缘。

主治 中风。

操作 先刺内关0.5~1寸；继斜刺人中0.5寸，以重提插手法至流泪，或眼球湿润为度。三阴交以45°斜刺1~1.5寸，使下肢有3次抽动感为度。

Composition This group of acupoints is composed of Neiguan(PC6), Renzhong(GV26) and Sanyinjiao(SP6).

Location Neiguan：2 cun above the palmar crease of the wrist, between the tendons of the long palmar muscle and radial flexor muscle of the wrist.

Renzhong：at the junction of the upper one-third and middle one-third of the philtrum.

Sanyinjiao：3 cun above the tip of the medial malleolus, on the posterior border of the medial side of the tibia.

Indication Apoplexy.

Method Neiguan is needled 0.5−1 cun first. Then Renzhong is needled 0.5 cun obliquely, manipulating the needle with heavy lifting and inserting techniques till lachrymation or the eyes of the patient is moist. Sanyinjiao is needled 1−1.5 cun obliquely at the angle of 45° till the

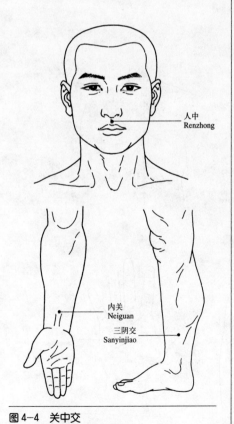

人中
Renzhong

内关
Neiguan

三阴交
Sanyinjiao

图4-4 关中交
Fig. 4-4 Guanzhongjiao

patient have the feeling of twitching in the lower limbs for three times.

🔵 中冲谷
Zhongchonggu

组成　本穴组由人中、中冲、合谷三穴组合而成。

位置　人中：在人中沟的上 1/3 与中 1/3 交界处。

中冲：中指尖端的中央。

合谷：手背，第一、第二掌骨之间，约平第二掌骨中点处。

主治　中风不醒人事，兼见牙关紧闭，口噤不开，两手握固，肢体强痉。

操作　中冲点刺放血；人中、合谷大幅度提插捻转，并久留针至神清。

Composition　This group of acupoints is composed of Renzhong(GV26), Zhongchong(PC9) and Hegu(LI4).

Location　Renzhong：at the junction of the upper one−third and middle one-third of the philtrum.

Zhongchong：at the tip of the middle finger.

Hegu：on the dorsum of the hand, between the 1st and 2nd metacarpal bones, and near the midpoint of the 2nd metacarpal bone.

Indication　Unconsciousness due to apoplexy, lockjaw and convulsion of the limbs.

Method　Zhongchong is pricked to bleed. Strong lifting, thrusting and rotating method is applied to Renzhong and Hegu, retain the needles till the recovery of the consciousness.

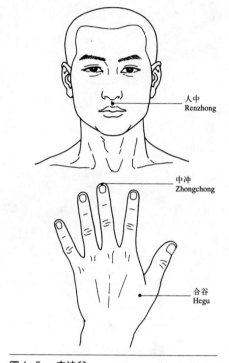

人中
Renzhong

中冲
Zhongchong

合谷
Hegu

图 4-5　中冲谷
Fig. 4-5　Zhongchonggu

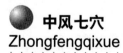 中风七穴
Zhongfengqixue

组成　本穴组由百会、风池、大椎、肩井、间使、曲池、足三里七穴组合而成。

位置　百会：后发际正中直上 7 寸。

风池：胸锁乳突肌与斜方肌之间凹陷中，平风府穴处。

大椎：第七颈椎棘突下。

肩井：大椎穴(督脉)与肩峰连线的中点。

间使：腕横纹上3寸，掌长肌腱与桡侧腕屈肌腱之间。

曲池：屈肘，成直角，当肘横纹外端与肱骨外上髁连线的中点。

足三里：犊鼻穴下3寸，胫骨前嵴外一横指处。

主治　中风半身不遂，语言障碍。

操作　各穴灸7壮。

Composition　This group of acupoints is composed of Baihui(GV20), Fengchi(GB20), Dazhui(GV14), Jianjing (GB21), Jianshi(PC5), Quchi(LI11) and Zusanli(ST36).

Location　Baihui：7 cun directly above the midpoint of the posterior hairline.

Fengchi：in the depression between the sternocleido-mastoid and trapezius muscles, at the horizontal level of Fengfu.

Dazhui：at the point below the spinous process of the 7th cervical vertebra.

Jianjing：at the midpoint between Dazhui and the acromion.

Jianshi：3 cun above the palmar crease of the wrist, between the tendons of the long palmar muscle and radial flexor muscle of the wrist.

Quchi：at the midpoint of the line between the radial end of the cubital crease and the external humeral epi-condyle when the elbow is flexed at 90°.

Zusanli：3 cun below Dubi, one finger breadth from the anterior crest of the tibia.

Indication　Hemiplegia due to apoplexy, speech difficulty.

Method　7 cones of moxibustion is applied to each point.

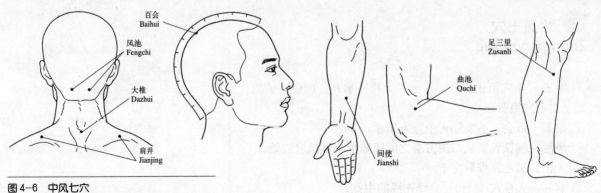

图4-6　中风七穴
Fig. 4-6　Zhongfengqixue

两点
Liangdian

组成　本穴组由翳风、合谷二穴组合而成。

位置　翳风：乳突前下方，平耳垂后缘的凹陷中。

合谷：手背，第一、第二掌骨之间，约平第二掌骨中点处。

主治　面瘫，面痉。

操作　针翳风穴时从骨边缘斜向对侧耳尖方向刺1～1.5寸，针感麻、胀、痛放散至耳与颞部；合谷穴针0.5～1.2寸，针感酸、麻、胀至指或肩部。

Composition　This group of acupoints is composed of Yifeng(TE17) and Hegu(LI4).

Location　Yifeng：anterior and inferior to the mastoid process, in the depression at the level of the posterior and lower border of the earlobe.

Hegu：on the dorsum of the hand, between the 1st and 2nd metacarpal bones, and near the midpoint of the 2nd metacarpal bone.

Indications　Facial paralysis, facial spasm.

Method　Yifeng：the needle is inserted 1−1.5 cun obliquely from the border of the bone to the opposite ear apex, the acu-esthesia of numbness, distension and pain should be induced to the ear and the temporal part of the head. Hegu：the needle is inserted 0.5−1.2 cun, the acu-esthesia of soreness, numbness, distension should be induced to the fingers or shoulder.

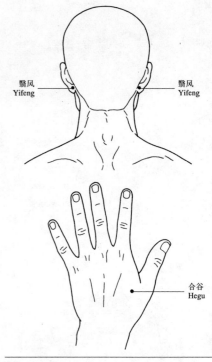

图4-7　两点
Fig. 4-7　Liangdian

两点加一圈
Liangdianjiayiquan

组成　本穴组由两点(翳风、合谷)加一圈(下关、颊车、地仓、四白)六穴组合而成。

位置　见"两点"和"一圈"。

主治　面瘫，面痉。

操作　针翳风穴时向对侧耳尖方向斜刺，合谷穴直刺，下关透颊车，下关透四白，地仓透颊车，地仓透四白。

Composition　This group of acupoints is composed of Liangdian (composed of Yifeng(TE17) and Hegu(LI4) and

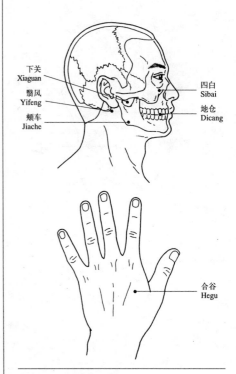

图4-8　两点加一圈
Fig. 4-8　Liangdianjiayiquan

Yiquan [composed of Xiaguan(ST7), Jiache(ST6), Dicang (ST4) and Sibai(ST2)].

Location　See Liangdian and Yiquan.

Indication　Facial paralysis, facial spasm.

Method　Yifeng：the needle is inserted obliquely towards the opposite ear apex；Hegu：the needle is inserted perpendicularly, and for other four points, the needles are penetrated from Xianguan to Jiache, Xiaguan to Sibai, Dicang to Jiache, Dicang to Sibai.

利舌
Lishe

组成　本穴组由廉泉、劳宫二穴组合而成。

位置　廉泉：舌骨体上缘的中点处。

劳宫：第二、第三掌骨之间，握拳，中指尖下是穴。

主治　舌强语塞。

操作　廉泉向下颌舌根方向直刺0.5～1寸，得气为度。

劳宫直刺0.3～0.8寸，得气为度。

Composition　This group of acupoints is composed of Lianquan(CV23) and Laogong(PC8).

Location　Lianquan：at the midpoint on the upper border of the hyoid bone.

Laogong：between the 2nd and 3rd metacarpal bones, where the tip of the middle finger reaches when a fist is made.

Indication　Stiff tongue and stuttering speech.

Method　Lianquan is needled 0.5－1 cun towards the tongue root perpendicularly till the acu-esthesia is obtained.

Laogong is needled 0.3－0.8 cun perpendicularly till the acu-esthesia is obtained.

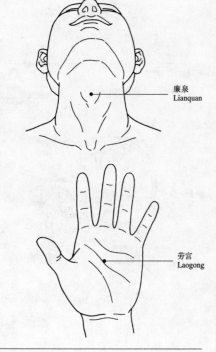

廉泉 Lianquan

劳宫 Laogong

图4-9 利舌
Fig. 4-9 Lishe

松舌
Songshe

组成　本穴组由哑门、廉泉、合谷三穴组合而成。

位置　哑门：后发际正中直上0.5寸。

廉泉：舌骨体上缘的中点处。

合谷：手背，第一、第二掌骨之间，约平第二掌骨中点处。

主治　舌强。

操作　廉泉见"利舌"。合谷见"启语"。哑门向下颌方向直刺0.5～1寸。均以得气为度。

Composition　This group of acupoints is composed of Yamen(GV15), Lianquan(CV23) and Hegu(LI4).

Location　Yamen：0.5 cun directly above the midpoint of the posterior hairline.

Lianquan：at the midpoint on the upper border of the hyoid bone.

Hegu：on the dorsum of the hand, between the 1st and 2nd metacarpal bones, and near the midpoint of the 2nd metacarpal bone.

Indication　Stiff tongue.

Method　Lianquan：see Lishe. Hegu：see Qiyu. Yamen is needled 0.5–1 cun towards the mandible perpendicularly till the acu-esthesia is obtained.

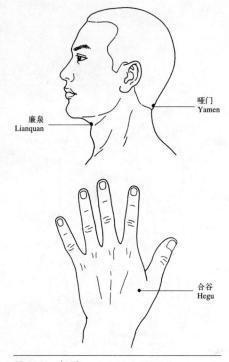

图4-10　松舌
Fig. 4-10　Songshe

廉冲
Lianchong

组成　本穴组由廉泉、中冲二穴组合而成。

位置　廉泉：舌骨体上缘的中点处。

中冲：中指尖端的中央。

主治　舌下肿痛。

操作　廉泉向下颌舌根方向直刺0.5～1寸，得气为度。中冲可用三棱针点刺出血。

Composition　This group of acupoints is composed of Lianquan(CV23) and Zhongchong(PC9).

Location　Lianquan：at the midpoint on the upper border of the hyoid bone.

Zhongchong：at the tip of the middle finger.

Indication　Sublingual swelling and pain.

Method　Lianquan is needled 0.5–1 cun towards the tongue root of the mandible perpendicularly till the acu-esthedis is obtained. Zhongchong can be pricked to bleed with a three-edged needle.

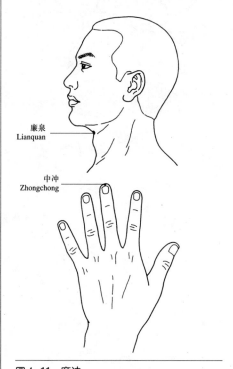

图4-11　廉冲
Fig. 4-11　Lianchong

启语

Qiyu

组成　本穴组由廉泉、合谷、哑门、内关、通里五穴组合而成。

位置　廉泉：舌骨体上缘的中点处。

合谷：手背，第一、第二掌骨之间，约平第二掌骨中点处。

哑门：后发际正中直上0.5寸。

内关：腕横纹上2寸，掌长肌腱与桡侧腕屈肌腱之间。

通里：腕横纹上1寸，尺侧腕屈肌腱的桡侧。

主治　失语。

操作　通里斜刺或沿皮刺0.5～0.8寸。其他各穴直刺0.5～1.2寸，得气为度。

按语　另一穴组无哑门、内关，其治亦同。

Composition　This group of acupoints is composed of Lianquan(CV23), Hegu(LI4), Yamen(GV15), Neiguan(PC6) and Tongli(HT5).

Location　Lianquan：at the midpoint on the upper border of the hyoid bone.

Hegu：on the dorsum of the hand, between the 1st and 2nd metacarpal bones, and near the midpoint of the 2nd metacarpal bone.

Yamen：0.5 cun directly above the midpoint of the posterior hairline.

Neiguan：2 cun above the palmar crease of the wrist, between the tendons of the long palmar muscle and radial flexor muscle of the wrist.

Tongli：1 cun above the palmar crease of the wrist, in the depression of the radial side of the tendon of the ulnar flexor muscle of the wrist.

Indication　Aphasia.

Method　Tongli is needled 0.5−0.8 cun obliquely or along the skin. The other points are needled 0.5−1.2 cun perpendicularly till the acu-esthesia is obtained.

Note　There's another group in which Yamen and Neiguan are not included, but the indication is the same as that of this one.

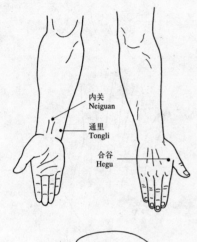

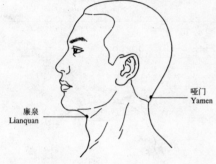

图 4-12　启语
Fig. 4-12　Qiyu

前额
Qiane

组成　本穴组由印堂、阳白、合谷、内庭四穴组合而成。

位置　印堂：两肩头连线的中点。

阳白：目正视，瞳孔直上，眉上1寸。

合谷：手背，第一、第二掌骨之间，约平第二掌骨中点处。

内庭：足背第二、第三趾间缝纹端。

主治　前额头痛，目痛。

操作　印堂、阳白针尖由上而下，沿皮刺之。合谷、内庭针0.5~1寸，得气为度。

Composition　This group of acupoints is composed of Yintang(EX-HN3), Yangbai(GB14), Hegu(LI4) and Neiting (ST44).

Location　Yintang：in the midpoint of the line connecting two ends of the eyebrows.

Yangbai：directly above the pupil, 1 cun above the eyebrow.

Hegu：on the dorsum of the hand, between the 1st and 2nd metacarpal bones, and near the midpoint of the 2nd metacarpal bone.

Neiting：at the end of the margin of the web between the 2nd and 3rd toes.

Indication　Pain in the forehead and ophthalmalgia.

Method　Yintang and Yangbai are needled downwards beneath the skin.

Hegu and Neiting are needled 0.5−1 cun till the acuesthesia is obtained.

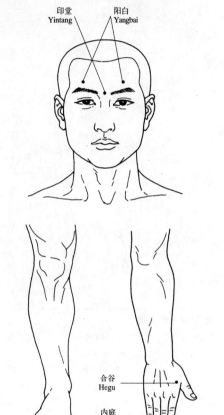

图 4-13　前额
Fig. 4-13　Qiane

 偏头痛
Piantoutong

组成　本穴组由太阳、率谷、中渚、足临泣四穴组合而成。

位置　太阳：眉梢与目外眦之间向后约1寸处凹陷中。

率谷：耳尖直上，入发际1.5寸。

中渚：握拳，第四、第五掌骨小头后缘之间凹陷中，液门穴后1寸。

足临泣：在第四、第五跖骨结合部前方，小趾伸肌腱外侧

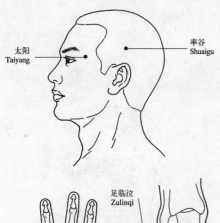

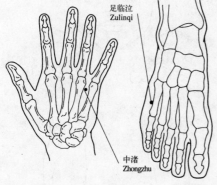

图 4-14 偏头痛
Fig. 4-14 Piantoutong

凹陷中。

主治 头颞痛，偏头痛。

操作 率谷可沿皮刺 0.3～0.5 寸。中渚、足临泣、太阳可直刺或斜刺 0.5～1 寸。

Composition This group of acupoints is composed of Taiyang(EX-HN5), Shuaigu(GB8), Zhongzhu(TE3) and Zulinqi(GB41).

Location Taiyang：in the depression 1 cun posterior to the juncture between the lateral end of the eyebrow and the outer canthus.

Shuaigu：directly above the ear apex, 1.5 cun above the hairline.

Zhongzhu：in the depression on the posterior border of the heads of the 4th and 5th metacarpal bones when a fist is made, 1 cun posterior to Yemen.

Zulinqi：anterior to the junction of the 4th and 5th metatarsal bones, in the depression lateral to the tendon of the extensor muscle of the little toe.

Indications Pain in the temporal part of the head and migraine.

Method Shuaigu is subcutaneously needled 0.3-0.5 cun. Zhongzhu, Zulinqi and Taiyang can be needled 0.5-1 cun perpendicularly or obliquely.

● **安巅**
Andian

组成 本穴组由百会、太冲二穴组合而成。

位置 百会：后发际正中直上 7 寸。

太冲：足背，第一、第二跖骨结合部之前凹陷中。

主治 巅顶头痛，头晕，高血压，抽搐，子宫下垂。

操作 刺法：百会向后沿皮刺 0.5～1 寸。太冲斜刺 0.5～1 寸。均以得气为度。

灸法：艾炷灸 5～9 壮，艾条灸 10～30 分钟(专用于治疗子宫下垂)。

Composition This group of acupoints is composed of Baihui(GV20) and Taichong(LR3).

Location Baihui：7 cun directly above the midpoint of the posterior hairline.

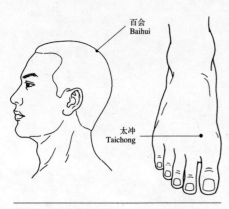

图 4-15 安巅
Fig. 4-15 Andian

Taichong: on the instep of the foot, in the depression anterior to the commissure of the 1st and 2nd metatarsal bones.

Indications Pain in the vertex, vertigo, hypertension, convulsion, prolapse of the uterus.

Methods Acupuncture: Baihui is needled 0.5−1 cun beneath the skin. Taichong is needled 0.5−1 cun obliquely till the acu-esthesia is obtained.

Moxibustion: moxibustion with 5−9 moxa cones, or moxibustion with moxa roll for 10−30 minutes (for prolapse of the uterus only) is applied.

后头痛
Houtoutong

组成 本穴组由风池、天柱、后溪、束骨四穴组合而成。

位置 风池：胸锁乳突肌与斜方肌之间凹陷中，平风府穴。

天柱：后发际正中直上 0.5 寸，旁开 1.3 寸，当斜方肌外缘凹陷中。

束骨：第五跖骨粗隆下，赤白肉际。

后溪：握拳，第五指掌关节后尺侧，横纹头赤白肉际。

主治 后头痛。

操作 风池、天柱直刺 0.5～1.2 寸，后溪针 0.5～0.8 寸，束骨针 0.3～0.5 寸。各以得气为度。

Composition This group of acupoints is composed of Fengchi(GB20), Tianzhu(BL10), Houxi(SI3) and Shugu(BL65).

Location Fengchi: in the depression between the sternocleidomastoid and trapezius muscles, at the norizontal level of Fengfu.

Tianzhu: 1.3 cun lateral to the point 0.5 directly cun above the midpoint of the posterior hairline, in the derpession lateral to the border of trapezius muscle.

Shugu: below the tuberosity of the 5th metatarsal bone, at the junction of the red and white skin.

Houxi: on the ulnar side of the proximal end of the 5th metacarpal bone, at the end of the palmar crease on the red and white skin when a fist is made.

Indication Pain in the posterior head.

Method Fengchi and Tianzhu are needled 0.5−1.2

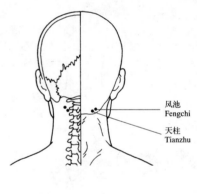

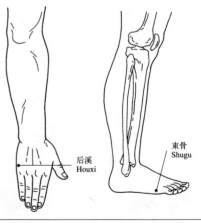

图 4-16 后头痛
Fig. 4-16 Houtoutong

cun perpendicularly till the acu-esthesia is obtained. Houxi is needled 0.5－0.8 cun. Shugu is needled 0.3－0.5 cun. Stop manipulating the needles after the acu-esthesia is obtained.

 寒头痛
Hantoutong

组成　本穴组由合谷、攒竹、太阳三穴组合而成。

位置　合谷：手背，第一、第二掌骨之间，约平第二掌骨中点处。

攒竹：眉头凹陷中。

太阳：眉梢与目外眦之间向后约1寸处凹陷中。

主治　伤寒头痛。

操作　先刺攒竹、太阳二穴，再刺合谷，均用泻法。若伤寒较重，头痛剧烈者，可用三棱针刺太阳出血。

Composition　This group of acupoints is composed of Hegu(LI4), Cuanzhu(BL2) and Taiyang(EX-HN5).

Location　Hegu：on the dorsum of the hand, between the 1st and 2nd metacarpal bones, and near the midpoint of the 2nd metacarpal bone.

Cuanzhu：in the depression of the medial end of the eyebrow.

Taiyang：in the depression 1 cun posterior to the juncture between the lateral end of the eyebrow and the outer canthus.

Indication　Headache of febrile diseases due to cold.

Method　Cuanzhu and Taiyang are needled first, then Hegu is needled. Reducing methods are applied to all the points. If the headache and the febrile diseases due to cold are severe, Taiyang may be pricked to bleed.

 强丰
Qiangfeng

组成　本穴组由强间、丰隆二穴组合而成。

位置　强间：脑户穴直上1.5寸。

丰隆：外踝高点上8寸，条口穴外1寸。

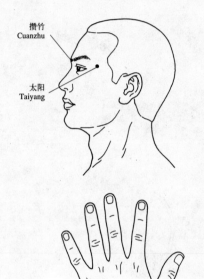

攒竹
Cuanzhu

太阳
Taiyang

合谷
Hegu

图4-17　寒头痛
Fig. 4-17　Hantoutong

主治　头痛如裹，缠绵难禁。

操作　先刺强间，重刺激用泻法，稍停片刻，再刺丰隆，亦用泻法，留针20分钟。

Composition　This group of acupoints is composed of Qiangjian(GV18) and Fenglong(ST40).

Location　Qiangjian：1.5 cun directly above Naohu.

Fenglong：8 cun above the tip of the external malleolus, 1 cun lateral to Tiaokou.

Indication　Band-wrapped and lingering headache.

Method　Qiangjian is needled first with strong reducing techniques. Fenglong is needled after a while, reducing techniques is applied to it too. Retain the needles for 20 minutes.

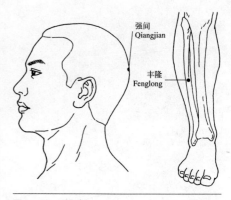

图4-18　强丰
Fig. 4-18　Qiangfeng

 头晕

Touyun

组成　本穴组由风池、印堂、内关三穴组合而成。

位置　风池：胸锁乳突肌与斜方肌之间凹陷中，平风府穴处。

内关：腕横纹上2寸，掌长肌腱与桡侧腕屈肌腱之间。

印堂：两眉头连线的中点。

主治　头晕。

操作　印堂针尖由上向下沿皮刺0.3～0.5寸。风池斜刺0.8～1.2寸，或平刺透风府穴。内关直刺0.5～1寸。各以得气为度。

Composition　This group of acupoints is composed of Fengchi(GB20), Yintang(EX-HN3) and Neiguan(PC6).

Location　Fengchi：in the depression between the sternocleidomastoid and trapezius muscles, at the horizontal level of Fengfu.

Neiguan：2 cun above the palmar crease of the wrist, between the tendons of the long palmar muscle and radial flexor muscle of the wrist.

Yintang：at the midpoint of the two inner ends of the eyebrows.

Indication　Dizziness.

Method　Yintang is subcutaneously needled 0.3－0.5 cun downwards. Fengchi is needled 0.8－1.2 cun obliquely,

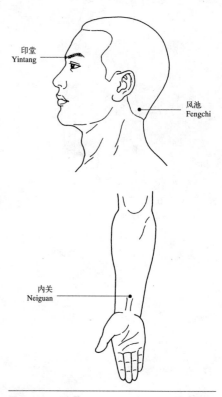

图4-19　头晕
Fig. 4-19　Touyun

or it can be penetrated horizontally to Fengfu. Neiguan is needled 0.5—1 cun perpendicularly. Stop manipulating the needles after the arrival of the acu-esthesia.

止晕
Zhiyun

组成　本穴组由百会、太阳、太冲、风池四穴组合而成。

位置　百会：后发际正中直上7寸。

太阳：眉梢与目外眦之间向后约1寸处凹陷中。

太冲：足背，第一、第二跖骨结合部之前凹陷中。

风池：胸锁乳突肌与斜方肌之间凹陷中，平风府穴处。

主治　头晕。

操作　百会、太阳沿皮刺0.5～1寸。太冲、风池刺0.5～1.2寸，得气为度。

Composition　This group of acupoints is composed of Baihui(GV20), Taiyang(EX-HN5), Taichong(LR3) and Fengchi(GB20).

Location　Baihui：7 cun directly above the midpoint of the posterior hairline.

Taiyang：in the depression 1 cun posterior to the juncture between the lateral end of the eyebrow and the outer canthus.

Taichong：on the instep of the foot, in the depression anterior to the commissure of the 1st and 2nd metatarsal bones.

Fengchi：in the depression between the sternocleido-mastoid and trapezius muscles, at the horizontal level of Fengfu.

Indication　Dizziness.

Method　Baihui and Taiyang are needled 0.5—1 cun beneath the skin. Taichong and Fengchi are needled 0.5—1.2 cun till the acu-esthesia is obtained.

百风溪
Baifengxi

组成　本穴组由百会、风池、太溪三穴组合而成。

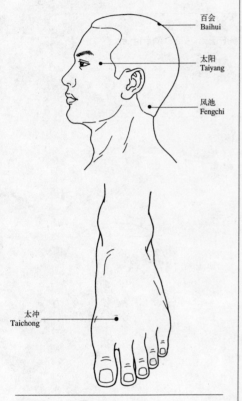

百会 Baihui
太阳 Taiyang
风池 Fengchi
太冲 Taichong

图4-20　止晕
Fig. 4-20　Zhiyun

位置　百会：后发际正中直上7寸。

风池：胸锁乳突肌与斜方肌之间凹陷中，平风府穴处。

太溪：内踝高点与跟腱之间凹陷中。

主治　头晕。

操作　百会沿皮刺0.5～1寸。太溪、风池，直刺0.5～1寸，得气为度。

Composition　This group of acupoints is composed of Baihui(GV20), Fengchi(GB20) and Taixi(KI3).

Location　Baihui：7 cun directly above the midpoint of the posterior hairline.

Fengchi：in the depression between the sternocleidomastoid and trapezius muscles, at the horizontal level of Fengfu.

Taixi：in the midpoint between the tip of the medial malleolus and Achilles's tendon.

Indication　Dizziness.

Method　Baihui is needled 0.5−1 cun beneath the skin.

Taixi and Fengchi are needled 0.5−1 cun till the acuesthesia is obtained.

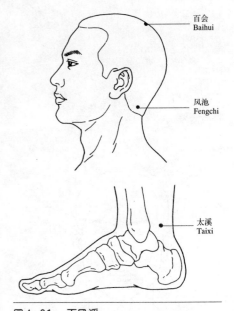

图4-21　百风溪
Fig. 4-21　Baifengxi

风谷
Fenggu

组成　本穴组由风池、合谷二穴组合而成。

位置　风池：胸锁乳突肌与斜方肌之间凹陷中，平风府穴处。

合谷：手背，第一、第二掌骨之间，约平第二掌骨中点处。

主治　头晕，目眩。

操作　直刺0.5～1寸，得气为度。

Composition　This group of acupoints is composed of Fengchi(GB20) and Hegu(LI4).

Location　Fengchi：in the depression between the sternocleidomastoid and trapezius muscles, at the horizontal level of Fengfu.

Hegu：on the dorsum of the hand, between the 1st and 2nd metacarpal bones, and near the midpoint of the 2nd metacarpal bone.

Indication　Dizziness and blurred vision.

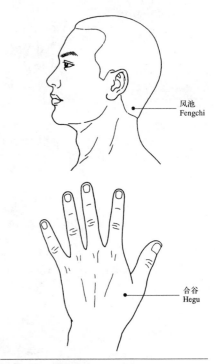

图4-22　风谷
Fig. 4-22　Fenggu

Method The needle is inserted 0.5−1 cun perpendicularly till the acu-esthesia is obtained.

● 眼明
Yanming

组成 本穴组由睛明、光明、合谷三穴组合而成。

位置 睛明：目内眦旁0.1寸。

光明：外踝高点上5寸，腓骨前缘。

合谷：手背，第一、第二掌骨之间，约平第二掌骨中点处。

主治 眼疾。

操作 光明针0.5~1寸，得气为度。睛明、合谷针法见"目清"。

Composition This group of acupoints is composed of Jingming(BL1), Guangming(GB37) and Hegu(LI4).

Location Jingming：0.1 cun lateral to the inner canthus.

Guangming：5 cun above the tip of the external malleolus, on the anterior border of the fibula.

Hegu：on the dorsum of the hand, between the 1st and 2nd metacarpal bones, and near the midpoint of the 2nd metacarpal bone.

Indication Eye diseases.

Method Guangming is needled 0.5−1 cun till the acu-esthesia is obtained. The acupuncture methods of Jingming and Hegu are the same as those of Muqing.

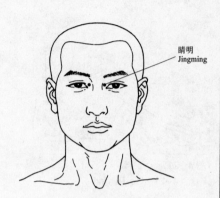

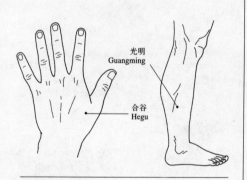

图4-23 眼明

Fig. 4-23 Yanming

● 目痛
Mutong

组成 本穴组由印堂、攒竹、丝竹空、太阳、行间五穴组合而成。

位置 印堂：两眉头连线的中点。

攒竹：眉头凹陷中。

丝竹空：眉梢处的凹陷中。

太阳：眉梢与目外眦之间向后约1寸处凹陷中。

行间：足背，第一、第二趾间缝纹端。

主治 目赤肿痛。

操作 各穴一般均用斜刺或沿皮刺0.5~1寸。行间可斜刺0.5~0.8寸，得气为度。

Composition This group of acupoints is composed of Yintang(EX-HN3), Cuanzhu(BL2), Sizhukong(TE23), Taiyang(EX-HN5) and Xingjian(LR2).

Location Yintang：at the midpoint of the line connecting the two medial ends of the eyebrows.

Cuanzhu：in the depression of the medial end of the eyebrow.

Sizhukong：in the depression of the lateral end of the eyebrow.

Taiyang：in the depression 1 cun posterior to the juncture between the lateral end of the eyebrow and the outer canthus.

Xingjian：on the instep of the foot, on the end of the margin of the web between the 1st and 2nd toes.

Indication Redness, swelling and pain of the eye.

Method Usually, the needle is inserted 0.5−1 cun obliquely or beneath the skin in each point.

Xingjian can be needled 0.5−0.8 cun obliquely till the acu−esthesia is obtained.

目清
Muqing

组成 本穴组由睛明、承泣、风池、合谷四穴组合而成。

位置 睛明：目内眦旁0.1寸。

承泣：目正视，瞳孔直下，当眶下缘与眼球之间。

风池：胸锁乳突肌与斜方肌之间凹陷中，平风府穴处。

合谷：手背，第一、第二掌骨之间，约平第二掌骨中点处。

主治 目赤，目痛，流泪。

操作 睛明、承泣缓缓进针，深0.5~0.8寸，不提插捻转。风池向同侧眼部针之，深0.5~1.2寸。合谷针0.5~1寸。各以得气为度。

Composition This group of acupoints is composed of Jingming(BL1), Chengqi(ST1), Fengchi(GB20) and Hegu(LI4).

Location Jingming：0.1 cun lateral to the inner canthus.

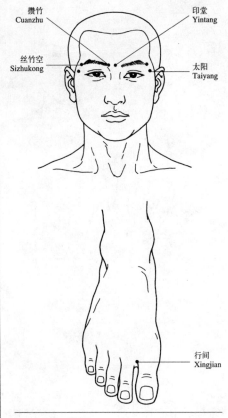

图4-24 目痛
Fig. 4-24 Mutong

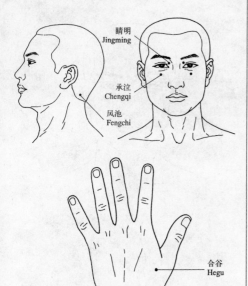

图 4-25　目清
Fig. 4-25　Muqing

Chengqi：directly below the pupil, between the eyeball and the infraorbital ridge.

Fengchi：in the depression between the sternocleidomastoid and trapezius muscles, at the horizontal level of Fengfu.

Hegu：on the dorsum of the hand, between the 1st and 2nd metacarpal bones, and near the midpoint of the 2nd metacarpal bone.

Indication　Redness and pain of the eye, lacrimation.

Method　Jingming and Chengqi are punctured slowly, the depth is 0.5−0.8 cun. Insert the needles to the depth without lifting, inserting or rotating the needles.

Fengchi is needled towards the eye on the same side, the depth is 0.5−1.2 cun.

Hegu is needled 0.5−1 cun. Stop manipulating the needles till the acu-esthesia is obtained.

● 肝泽
Ganze

组成　本穴组由肝俞、少泽二穴组合而成。

位置　肝俞：第九胸椎棘突下，旁开1.5寸。

少泽：小指尺侧指甲角旁约0.1寸。

主治　胬肉攀睛。

操作　肝俞向脊柱方向斜刺0.5~0.8寸，得气为度。少泽点刺出血。

Composition　This group of acupoints is composed of Ganshu(BL18) and Shaoze(SI1).

Location　Ganshu：1.5 cun lateral to the point below the spinous process of the 9th thoracic vertebra.

Shaoze：0.1 cun lateral to the ulnar corner of the fingernail of the little finger.

Indication　Pterygium.

Method　Ganshu is needled 0.5−0.8 cun towards the spine till the acu-esthesia is obtained. Shaoze is pricked to bleed.

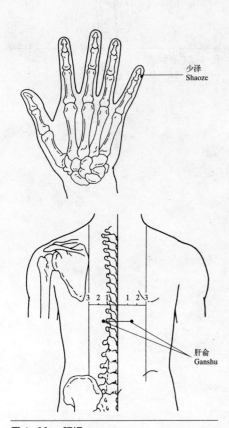

图 4-26　肝泽
Fig. 4-26　Ganze

鼻宁
Bining

组成　本穴组由印堂、迎香、合谷三穴组合而成。

位置　印堂：两眉头连线的中点。

合谷：手背，第一、第二掌骨之间，约平第二掌骨中点处。

迎香：鼻翼外缘中点，旁开0.5寸，当鼻唇沟中。

主治　鼻塞流涕，鼻渊等鼻病。

操作　印堂沿皮刺，迎香斜刺或沿皮刺，各深0.3～0.5寸。合谷直刺0.5～1寸，得气为度。

Composition　This group of acupoints is composed of Yintang(EX-HN3), Yingxiang(LI20) and Hegu(LI4).

Location　Yintang：at the midpoint of the line connecting the two medial ends of the eyebrows.

Yingxiang：at the midpoint of the lateral border of the ala nasi, in the nasolabial groove.

Hegu：on the dorsum of the hand, between the 1st and 2nd metacarpal bones, and near the midpoint of the 2nd metacarpal bone.

Indications　Nasal obstrucion and running nose, rhinorrhea, and other nose diseases.

Method　Yintang is needled beneath the skin. Yingxiang is needled obliquely or beneath the skin, the depth is 0.3−0.5 cun respectively. Hegu is needled 0.5−1 cun perpendicularly till the acu-esthesia is obtained.

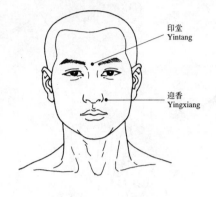
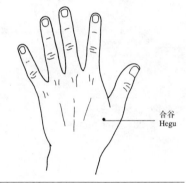

印堂 Yintang

迎香 Yingxiang

合谷 Hegu

图4-27　鼻宁
Fig. 4-27　Bining

天香谷
Tianxianggu

组成　本穴组由通天、迎香、合谷三穴组合而成。

位置　通天：承光穴后1.5寸。

迎香：鼻翼外缘中点，旁开0.5寸，当鼻唇沟中。

合谷：手背，第一、第二掌骨之间，约平第二掌骨中点处。

主治　鼻塞。

操作　通天向承光方向透刺1～1.5寸。迎香沿鼻唇沟刺0.5～1寸。合谷直刺0.5～1寸。各以得气为度，留针30分钟，留针期间可行捻转手法。

Composition　This group of acupoints is composed of

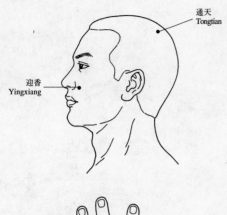

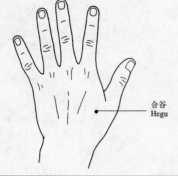

图4-28 天香谷
Fig. 4-28 Tianxianggu

Tongtian(BL7), Yingxiang(LI20) and Hegu(LI4).

Location Tongtian：1.5 cun posterior to Chengguang.

Yingxiang：at the midpoint of the lateral border of the ala nasi, in the nasolabial groove.

Hegu：on the dorsum of the hand, between the 1st and 2nd metacarpal bones, and near the midpoint of the 2nd metacarpal bone.

Indication Nasal obstruction.

Method Tongtian is penetrated 1−1.5 cun towards Chengguang.

Yingxiang is needled 0.5−1 cun along the nasolabial groove.

Hegu is needled 0.5−1 cun perpendicularly. Stop manipulating the needles after the arrival of the acuesthesia. Retain the needles for 30 minutes. Rotating techniques may be applied during the retention of the needles.

 鼻衄

Binü

组成 本穴组由合谷、上星、百劳、风府四穴组合而成。

位置 合谷：手背，第一、第二掌骨之间，约平第二掌骨中点处。

上星：前发际正中直上1寸。

百劳：在第七颈椎棘突下的大椎穴直上2寸，再旁开1寸处。

风府：后发际正中直上1寸。

主治 鼻衄。

操作 先仰卧位沿皮刺上星0.3~1厘米，得气后留针20分钟，或点刺出血。合谷针1.6~2.5厘米，使针感向肘、肩部放散，留针20分钟。然后取坐位，头微前倾，直刺百劳1.6~2.5厘米，留针20分钟；针风府使针尖向下颌方向缓慢刺入1.6~2.5厘米，针尖不可向上，以免刺入枕骨大孔而误伤延髓。如鼻衄不止则灸上星穴10壮，或悬灸10分钟。

Composition This group of acupoints is composed of Hegu(LI4), Shangxing(GV23), Bailao and Fengfu(GV16).

Location Hegu：on the dorsum of the hand, between the 1st and 2nd metacarpal bones, and near the midpoint of the 2nd metacarpal bone.

Shangxing：1 cun directly above the midpoint of the anterior hairline.

Bailao：1 cun lateral to the point 2 cun directly above Dazhui which is below the spinous process of the 7th cervical vertebra.

Indication   Epistaxis.

Method   Supine lying postion is selected first. Shangxing is needled 0.3－1 cm beneath the skin, retain the needle after the arrival of the acu-esthesia, or it can be pricked to bleed. Hegu is needled 1.6－2.5 cm, and the acu-esthesia should be induced to the elbow and shoulder, retain the needle for 20 minutes. Then sitting postion is selected, the head is bent forward slightly. Bailao is needled 1.6－2.5 cm perpendicularly, retain the needle for 20 minutes. Fengfu is needled 1.6－2.5 cun slowly with the tip of the needle towards the mandible, the tip of the needle shouldn't point upwards so as not to insert into the great occipital foramen and injury the medulla. If the epistaxis can't be relieved, 10 cones of moxibustion or suspended moxibusion for 10 minutes can be applied to Shangxing.

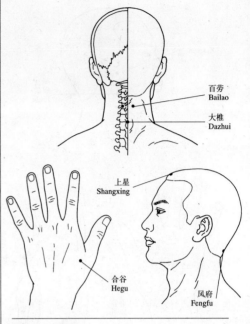

图4-29 鼻衄
Fig. 4-29 Binü

牙痛
Yatong

组成 本穴组由颊车、下关、合谷、内庭四穴组合而成。

位置 颊车：下颌角前上方一横指凹陷中，咀嚼时咬肌隆起最高点处。

下关：颧弓下缘，下颌骨髁状突之前方，切迹之间凹陷中。合口有孔，张口即闭。

合谷：手背，第一、第二掌骨之间，约平第二掌骨中点处。

内庭：足背第二、第三趾间缝纹端。

主治 牙痛。

操作 下关、颊车、合谷见"咀嚼"。内庭斜刺0.3～0.5寸，得气为度。

Composition   This group of acupoints is composed of Jiache(ST6), Xiaguan(ST7), Hegu and Neiting(ST44).

Location   Jiache：in the depression one finger breadth above the mandibular angle, where the masseter muscle is prominent when chewing.

Xiaguan: in the depression between the lower border of the zygomatic arch and the notch of condyloid process of the mandible. The depression can be felt when the mouth is shut, and will disappear when the mouth is open.

Hegu: on the dorsum of the hand, between the 1st and 2nd metacarpal bones, and near the midpoint of the 2nd metacarpal bone.

Neiting: at the end of the margin of the web between the 2nd and 3rd toes.

Indication   Toothache.

Method   Xiaguan, Jiache and Hegu: see Jujue. Neiting is inserted 0.3—0.5 cun obliquely till the acu-esthesia is obtained.

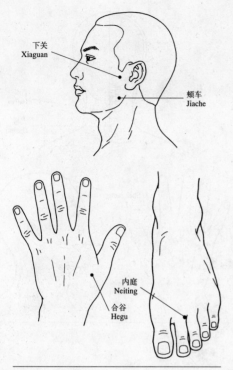

图 4—30   牙痛

Fig. 4—30   Yatong

 开关

Kaiguan

组成   本穴组由颊车、下关、合谷、人中、承浆五穴组合而成。

位置   颊车：下颌角前上方一横指凹陷中，咀嚼时咬肌隆起最高点处。

下关：颧弓下缘，下颌骨髁状突之前方，切迹之间凹陷中。合口有孔，张口即闭。

合谷：手背，第一、第二掌骨之间，约平第二掌骨中点处。

人中：在人中沟的上1/3与中1/3交界处。

承浆：颏唇沟的中点。

主治   牙关紧闭。

操作   下关、颊车、合谷见"咀嚼"。人中向鼻方向斜刺0.3寸。承浆向上或向下斜刺0.3~0.5寸，得气为度。

Composition   This group of acupoints is composed of Jiache(ST6), Xiaguan(ST7), Hegu(LI4), Renzhong(GV26) and Chengjiang(CV24).

Location   Jiache: in the depression one finger breadth above the mandibular angle, where the masseter muscle is prominent when chewing.

Xiaguan: in the depression between the lower border of the zygomatic arch and the notch of condyloid process of the mandible. The depression can be felt when the mouth is shut, and will disappear when the mouth is open.

Hegu：on the dorsum of the hand, between the 1st and 2nd metacarpal bones, and near the midpoint of the 2nd metacarpal bone.

Renzhong：at the junction of the upper one-third and middle one-third of the philtrum.

Chengjiang：at the midpoint of the mentolabial sulcus.

Indication　Trismus.

Method　Xiaguan, Jiache and Hegu：see Jujue. Renzhong is needled 0.3 cun obliquely towards the nose. Chengjiang is needled 0.3-0.5 cun upwards or downwards obliquely till the acu-esthesia is obtained.

流涎
Liuxian

组成　本穴组由人中、颊车、合谷三穴组合而成。

位置　人中：在人中沟的上1/3与中1/3交界处。

颊车：下颌角前上方一横指凹陷中，咀嚼时咬肌隆起最高点处。

合谷：手背，第一、第二掌骨之间，约平第二掌骨中点处。

主治　流涎。

操作　人中向鼻斜刺0.3寸。颊车向地仓方向透刺1.5～2.5寸。合谷直刺0.5～1.2寸，得气为度。

Composition　This group of acupoints is composed of Renzhong(GV26), Jiache(ST6) and Hegu(LI4).

Location　Renzhong：at the junction of the upper one-third and middle one-third of the philtrum.

Jiache：in the depression one finger breadth above the mandibular angle, where the masseter muscle is prominent when chewing.

Hegu：on the dorsum of the hand, between the 1st and 2nd metacarpal bones, and near the midpoint of the 2nd metacarpal bone.

Indication　Salivation.

Method　Renzhong is needled 0.3 cun obliquely towards the nose.

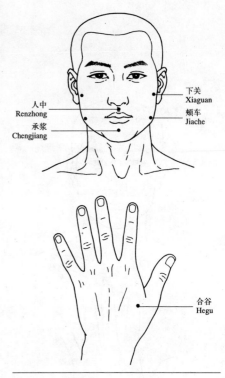

图4-31　开关
Fig. 4-31　Kaiguan

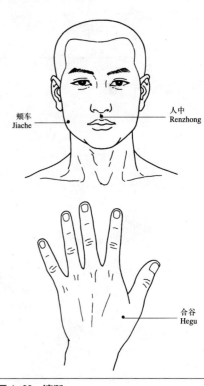

图4-32　流涎
Fig. 4-32　Liuxian

Jiache is penetrated 1.5−2.5 cun towards Dicang.

Hegu is needled 0.5−1.2 cun perpendicularly till the acu-esthesia is obtained.

陵中
Lingzhong

组成　本穴组由大陵、人中二穴组合而成。

位置　大陵：腕横纹中央，掌长肌腱与桡侧腕屈肌腱之间。

人中：在人中沟的上 1/3 与中 1/3 交界处。

主治　口臭。

操作　大陵斜刺 0.5～0.8 寸，人中见"流涎"穴人中之操作。

Composition　This group of acupoints is composed of Daling(PC7) and Renzhong(GV26).

Location　Daling：at the midpoint of the palmar crease of the wrist, between the tendons of the long palmar muscle and radial flexor muscle of the wrist.

Renzhong：at the junction of the upper one-third and middle one-third of the philtrum.

Indication　Foul breath.

Method　Daling is inserted 0.5−0.8 cun obliquely. Renzhong：see Liuxian.

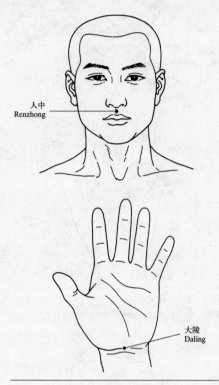

图 4−33　陵中
Fig. 4−33　Lingzhong

谷仓
Gucang

组成　本穴组由合谷、地仓二穴组合而成。

位置　合谷：手背，第一、第二掌骨之间，约平第二掌骨中点处。

地仓：口角旁 0.4 寸，巨髎穴直下取之。

主治　流涎。

操作　合谷直刺 0.5～1 寸，地仓沿皮向颊车方向透刺 1.5～2.5 寸，得气为度，留针 30 分钟。

Composition　This group of acupoints is composed of Hegu(LI4) and Dicang(ST4).

Location　Hegu：on the dorsum of the hand, between the 1st and 2nd metacarpal bones, and near the midpoint of the 2nd metacarpal bone.

Dicang: 0.4 cun lateral to the corner of the mouth, which is directly below Juliao.

Indication Salivation.

Method Hegu is needled 0.5—1 cun perpendicularly.

Dicang is penetrated 1.5—2.5 cun towards Jiache beneath the skin till the acu-esthesia is obtained. Retain the needles for 30 minutes.

口齿
Kouchi

组成 本穴组由颊车、地仓、下关、合谷四穴组合而成。

位置 地仓：口角旁 0.4 寸，巨髎穴直下取之。

颊车：下颌角前上方一横指凹陷中，咀嚼时咬肌隆起最高点处。

下关：颧弓下缘，下颌骨髁状突之前方，切迹之间凹陷中。合口有孔，张口即闭。

合谷：手背，第一、第二掌骨之间，约平第二掌骨中点处。

主治 面瘫，口角歪斜，流涎齿痛，咀嚼肌痉挛，张口不利。

操作 地仓向颊车方向沿皮透刺，针 1～3 寸。颊车也可向地仓方向沿皮透刺，针 1～3 寸。下关直刺或透刺均可，针 0.5～1 寸或 1～2 寸(透刺)。合谷巨刺，即左病右取，右病左取，针 0.5～1 寸，得气为度。

Composition This group of acupoints is composed of Jiache(ST6), Dicang(ST4), Xiaguan(ST7) and Hegu(LI4).

Location Dicang: 0.4 cun lateral to the corner of the mouth, which is directly below Juliao.

Jiache: in the depression one finger breadth above the mandibular angle, where the masseter muscle is prominent when chewing.

Xiaguan: in the depression between the lower border of the zygomatic arch and the notch of condyloid process of the mandible. The depression can be felt when the mouth is shut, and will disappear when the mouth is open.

Hegu: on the dorsum of the hand, between the 1st and 2nd metacarpal bones, and near the midpoint of the

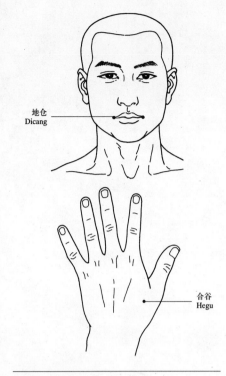

图 4-34 谷仓
Fig. 4-34 Gucang

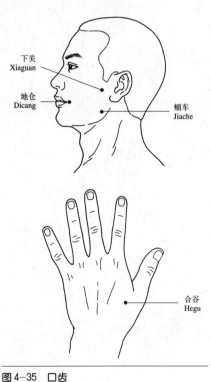

图 4-35 口齿
Fig. 4-35 Kouchi

2nd metacarpal bone.

Indications Facial paralysis, deviation of the mouth, salivation, toothache, convulsion of the masseter muscle, motor impairment of the mandibular joint.

Method Dicang is penetrated 1−3 cun towards Jiache beneath the skin. Jiache may be penetrated 1−3 cun towards Dicang beneath the skin too. Xiaguan can be needled perpendicularly or penetrated. The depth is 0.5−1 cun (needling perpendicularly) or 1−2 cun (penetration). Juci method is applied to Hegu, i. e. Hegu contralateral to the affected side is selected. The needle is inserted 0.5−1 cun till the acu-esthesia is obtained.

● 容谷
Ronggu

组成 本穴组由天容、合谷二穴组合而成。

位置 天容：下颌角后，胸锁乳突肌前缘。

合谷：手背，第一、第二掌骨之间，约平第二掌骨中点处。

主治 咽喉肿痛。

操作 直刺0.5～1寸，得气为度。

Composition This group of acupoints is composed of Tianrong(SI17) and Hegu(LI4).

Location Tianrong：posterior to the mandibular angle, in the front of the sternocleidomastoid muscle.

Hegu：on the dorsum of the hand, between the 1st and 2nd metacarpal bones, and near the midpoint of the 2nd metacarpal bone.

Indication Sore throat.

Method The needle is inserted 0.5−1 cun perpendicularly till the acu-esthesia is obtained.

● 开音
Kaiyin

组成 本穴组由扶突、合谷、间使三穴组合而成。

位置 扶突：喉结旁开3寸，当胸锁乳突肌的胸骨头与锁

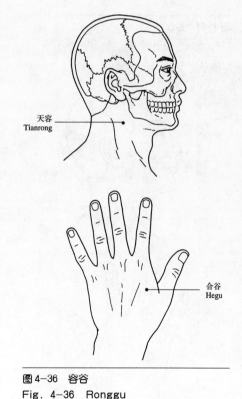

图4-36 容谷
Fig. 4-36 Ronggu

天容
Tianrong

合谷
Hegu

骨头之间。

合谷：手背，第一、第二掌骨之间，约平第二掌骨中点处。

间使：腕横纹上3寸，掌长肌腱与桡侧腕屈肌腱之间。

主治　失音。

操作　合谷、间使直刺0.5~1寸。扶突直刺针0.5~0.8寸。各以得气为度。

Composition　This group of acupoints is composed of Futu(ST32), Hegu(LI4) and Jianshi(PC5).

Location　Futu：3 cun lateral to the laryngeal protuberance, between the anterior and posterior heads of the sternocleidomastoid muscle.

Hegu：on the dorsum of the hand, between the 1st and 2nd metacarpal bones, and near the midpoint of the 2nd metacarpal bone.

Jianshi：3 cun above the palmar crease of the wrist, between the tendons of the long palmar muscle and radial flexor muscle of the wrist.

Indication　Hoarseness.

Method　Hegu and Jianshi are needled 0.5–1 cun perpendicularly till the acu-esthesia is obtained. Futu is needled 0.5–0.8 cun perpendicularly till the acu-esthesia is obtained.

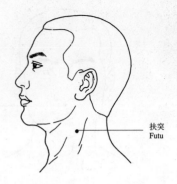

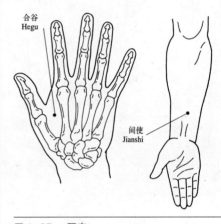

图4-37　开音
Fig. 4-37　Kaiyin

解痉急
Jiejingji

组成　本穴组由曲池、合谷、人中、复溜四穴组合而成。

位置　曲池：屈肘，成直角，当肘横纹外端与肱骨外上髁连线的中点。

合谷：手背，第一、第二掌骨之间，约平第二掌骨中点处。

人中：在人中沟的上1/3与中1/3交界处。

复溜：太溪穴上2寸。

主治　由伤寒或温病引起的壮热面赤，烦躁不宁，咬牙龂齿，睡中惊悸，手足躁扰，继则神志昏迷，双目直视，牙关紧闭，角弓反张，全身抽搐，呼吸急迫，脉弦数。

操作　先刺人中穴，用泻法，再针曲池、合谷穴用泻法，再针复溜穴，用平补平泻法，均留针20分钟或留针至抽搐停止。

Composition　This group of acupoints is composed of

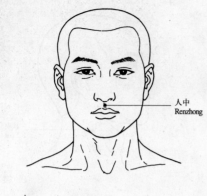

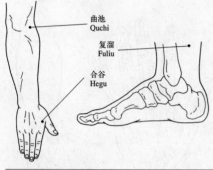

图 4-38 解痉急
Fig. 4-38 Jiejingji

Quchi(LI11), Hegu(LI4), Renzhong(GV26) and Fuliu(KI6).

Location Quchi：at the midpoint of the line between the radial end of the cubital crease and the external humeral epicondyle when the elbow is flexed at 90°.

Hegu：on the dorsum of the hand, between the 1st and 2nd metacarpal bones, and near the midpoint of the 2nd metacarpal bone.

Renzhong：at the junction of the upper one-third and middle one-third of the philtrum.

Fuliu：2 cun above Taixi.

Indication Symptoms of febrile diseases due to cold：high fever, redness of the face, irritability, clenched jaws, fear in the sleep, agitation of the four limbs, and loss of consciousness, upward staring of the eyes, trismus, opisthotonus, convulsion of the body, rapid breathing, string-taut and quick pulse.

Method Renzhong is needled first with reducing methods. Then reducing methods are applied to Quchi and Hegu. Mild rein forcing and reducing techniques are applied to Fuliu last. Retain the needles for 20 minutes or till the convulsion is relieved.

● 伤风
Shangfeng

组成 本穴组由风池、合谷、丝竹空三穴组合而成。

位置 风池：胸锁乳突肌与斜方肌之间凹陷中，平风府穴处。

合谷：手背，第一、第二掌骨之间，约平第二掌骨中点处。

丝竹空：眉梢处的凹陷中。

主治 发热恶风、头痛阵作，遇风则重。

操作 先刺风池、丝竹空，再刺合谷，均用泻法。若头痛甚者，可先刺丝竹空出血，再刺风池，后刺合谷，得气后均留针20分钟。

Composition This group of acupoints is composed of Fengchi(GB20), Hegu(LI4) and Sizhukong(TE23).

Location Fengchi：in the depression between the sternocleidomastoid and trapezius muscles, at the horizontal level of Fengfu.

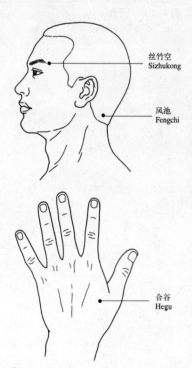

图 4-39 伤风
Fig. 4-39 Shangfeng

Hegu: on the dorsum of the hand, between the 1st and 2nd metacarpal bones, and near the midpoint of the 2nd metacarpal bone.

Sizhukong: in the depression of the lateral end of the eyebrow.

Indication Fever, aversion to wind, paroxysmal headache aggravated by wind.

Method First, Fengchi and Sizhukong, then Hegu is needled. Reducing methods are applied to the above points. For the patient with severe headache, Sizhukong may be pricked to bleed first, then Fengchi and Hegu are needled. Retain the needles for 20 minutes after the arrival of the acu-esthesia.

九针穴
Jiuzhenxue

组成　本穴组由少商、人中、与奇穴中商、老商和人中心五个刺激点组成。其中，少、中、老商穴即组合穴"三商"。
位置　少商：拇指桡侧指甲角旁约0.1寸。
人中：在人中沟的上1/3与中1/3交界处。
中商：在拇指背侧正中线、爪甲根后0.1寸处。
老商：在拇指外侧去爪甲0.1寸处。
人中心：中指中节之中点。
主治　流行性感冒。
操作　斜刺0.1~0.2寸，或点刺出血。

Composition This group of acupoints is composed of five points of Shaoshang (LU11), Renzhong(GV26) and the extraordinary points Zhongshang, Laoshang and Renzhongxin. Shaoshang, Zhongshang and Laoshang compose the group of Sanshang.

Location Shaoshang: on the the radial side of the thumb, 0.1 cun from the corner of the fingernail.

Renzhong: at the junction of the upper one-third and middle one-third of the philtrum.

Zhongshang: on the midline of the dorsum of the thumb, 0.1 cun posterior to the root of the fingernail.

Laoshang: on the lateral side of the thumb, 0.1 cun from the fingernail.

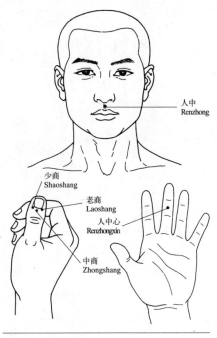

图4-40　九针穴
Fig. 4-40 Jiuzhenxue

Renzhongxin: at the midpoint of the 2nd phalange of the middle finger.

Indication   Influenza.

Method   The needle is inserted 0.1-0.2 cun obliquely, or the points can be pricked to bleed.

项僵
Xiangjiang

组成   本穴组由承浆、风府、后溪三穴组合而成。

位置   承浆：颏唇沟的中点。

风府：后发际正中直上1寸。

后溪：握拳，第五指掌关节后尺侧，横纹头赤白肉际。

主治   颈部感受风寒之邪，颈项僵硬疼痛，不能回首。

操作   先针承浆，只捻转不提插；再刺风府、后溪。均行刺1~2分钟，进针前可先行推拿手法以加强疗效。

Composition   This group of acupoints is composed of Chengjiang(CU24), Fengfu(GV16) and Houxi(SI3).

Location   Chengjiang: at the midpoint of the mentolabial sulcus.

Fengfu: 1 cun directly above the midpoint of the posterior hairline.

Houxi: on the ulnar side of the proximal end of the 5th metacarpal bone, at the end of the palmar crease on the red and white skin when a fist is made.

Indication   Stiffness, pain and motor impairment of the neck due to wind and cold.

Method   First Chengjiang is needled with rotating method and no lifting or inserting methods should be applied to it. Then Fengfu and Houxi are needled. Manipulate the needles for 1-2 minutes. Tuina techniques may be applied before the insertion so that the curative effect will be better.

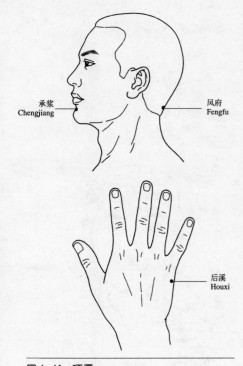

承浆
Chengjiang

风府
Fengfu

后溪
Houxi

图4-41 项僵
Fig. 4-41 Xiangjiang

项强
Xiangqiang

组成   本穴组由大椎、天柱、后溪、昆仑四穴组合而成。

位置　大椎：第七颈椎棘突下。

天柱：后发际正中直上0.5寸，旁开1.3寸，当斜方肌外缘凹陷中。

昆仑：外踝高点与跟腱之间凹陷中。

后溪：握拳，第五指掌关节后尺侧，横纹头赤白肉际。

主治　项强。

操作　刺法：天柱直刺针0.8～1.2寸。大椎、后溪、昆仑针0.5～1寸。各以得气为度。

灸法：艾条灸5～15分钟。

Composition　This group of acupoints is composed of Dazhui(GV14), Tianzhu(BL10), Houxi(SI3) and Kunlun (BL60).

Location　Dazhui：at the point below the spinous process of the 7th cervical vertebra.

Tianzhu：1.3 cun lateral to the the point 0.5 cun directly above the midpoint of the posterior hairline, in the depression lateral to the border of the trapezius muscle.

Kunlun：in the depression between the external malleolus and the heel tendon.

Houxi：on the ulnar side of the proximal end of the 5th metacarpal bone, at the end of the palmar crease on the red and white skin when a fist is made.

Indication　Neck rigidity.

Method　Acupuncture：Tianzhu is needled 0.8－1.2 cun perpendicularly. Dazhui, Houxi and Kunlun are needled 0.5－1 cun till the acu-esthesia is obtained.

Moxibustion：5－15 minutes' moxibustion with moxa roll is applied.

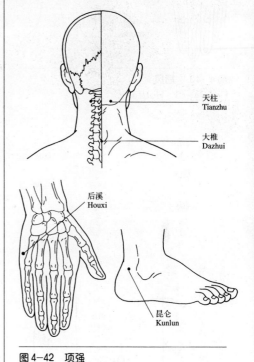

图4-42　项强
Fig. 4-42　Xiangqiang

 后风
Houfeng

组成　本穴组由后溪、风池二穴组合而成。

位置　后溪：握拳，第五指掌关节后尺侧，横纹头赤白肉际。

风池：胸锁乳突肌与斜方肌之间凹陷中，平风府穴处。

主治　落枕，颈项强急，颈椎病。

操作　先刺后溪，向合谷方向透刺，针1寸。后刺风池，针尖向鼻尖深1～1.5寸，得气为度。

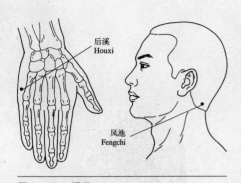

图4-43 后风
Fig. 4-43 Houfeng

Composition This group of acupoints is composed of Houxi(SI3) and Fengchi(GB20).

Location Houxi: on the ulnar side of the proximal end of the 5th metacarpal bone, at the end of the palmar crease on the red and white skin when a fist is made.

Fengchi: in the depression between the sternocleido-mastoid and trapezius muscles, at the horizontal level of Fengfu.

Indication Stiff neck, cervical spondylopathy.

Method First Houxi is penetrated 1 cun towards Hegu. Then Fengchi is needled with the tip of the needle towards the tip of the nose till the arrival of the acuesthesia.

● 退热
Tuire

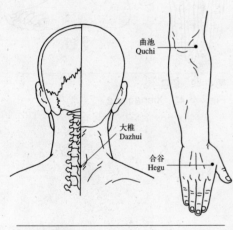

图4-44 退热
Fig. 4-44 Tuire

组成 本穴组由大椎、曲池、合谷三穴组合而成。

位置 大椎: 第七颈椎棘突下。

曲池: 屈肘, 成直角, 当肘横纹外端与肱骨外上髁连线的中点。

合谷: 手背, 第一、第二掌骨之间, 约平第二掌骨中点处。

主治 发热。

操作 大椎针0.5～1寸, 平补平泻法。曲池、合谷针0.5～1.2寸, 得气后行捻转或提插泻法。

Composition This group of acupoints is composed of Dazhui(GV14), Fengchi(GB20) and Hegu(LI4).

Location Dazhui: at the point below the spinous process of the 7th cervical vertebra.

Quchi: at the midpoint of the line between the radial end of the cubital crease and the external humeral epicondyle when the elbow is flexed at 90°.

Hegu: on the dorsum of the hand, between the 1st and 2nd metacarpal bones, and near the midpoint of the 2nd metacarpal bone.

Indication Fever.

Method Dazhui is needled 0.5−1 cun and even reinforcing-reducing techniques are applied to it. Quchi and Hegu are needled 0.5−1.2 cun. Reducing techniques by rotating or lifting and thrusting needles may be applied to them after the arrival of the acu-esthesia.

Shilao

组成　本穴组由间使、百劳二穴共三穴组合而成。

位置　间使：腕横纹上3寸，掌长肌腱与桡侧腕屈肌腱之间。

百劳：在第七颈椎棘突下的大椎穴直上2寸，再旁开1寸处。左右计二穴。

主治　疟疾。

操作　二穴于疟疾发作前2小时针之，直刺0.5～1.2寸，留针30分钟。

Composition　This group of acupoints is composed of Jianshi(PC5) and Bailao.

Location　Jianshi：3 cun above the palmar crease of the wrist, between the tendons of the long palmar muscle and radial flexor muscle of the wrist.

Bailao：1 cun lateral to the point 2 cun directly above Dazhui which is below the spinous process of the 7th cervical vertebra.

Indication　Malaria.

Method　The treatment is given 2 hours prior to the onset of malaria. The acupoints are needled 0.5−1.2 cun perpendicularly. Retain the needles for 30 minutes.

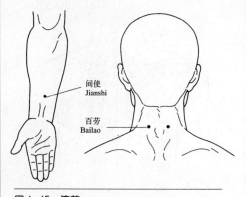

图4-45　使劳
Fig. 4-45　Shilao

Feixi

组成　本穴组由肺俞、膻中、天突、列缺、尺泽五穴组合而成。

位置　肺俞：第三胸椎棘突下，旁开1.5寸。

膻中：前正中线，平第四肋间隙。

天突：胸骨上窝正中。

列缺：桡骨茎突上方，腕横纹上1.5寸。

尺泽：肘横纹中，肱二头肌腱桡侧缘。

主治　肺系病证。

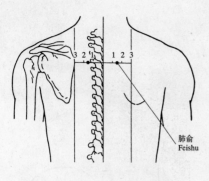

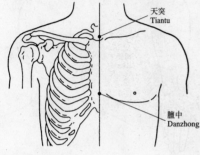

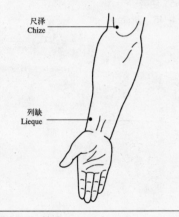

图4-46 肺系
Fig. 4-46 Feixi

操作　刺法：肺俞向脊柱方向斜刺0.5～0.8寸。天突、列缺沿皮刺0.3～0.5寸。膻中沿皮刺0.5～1寸。尺泽直刺0.8～1.2寸，得气为度。

灸法：肺俞、天突、膻中艾炷灸5～9壮，艾条灸10～20分钟。列缺、尺泽艾条灸10～20分钟。

Composition　This group of acupoints is composed of Feishu(BL13), Danzhong(CV17), Tiantu(CV22), Lieque (LU7) and Chize(LU5).

Location　Feishu：1.5 cun lateral to the point below the 3rd spinous process of the thoracic vertebra.

Danzhong：on the anterior midline, at the horizontal level of the 4th intercostal space.

Tiantu：in the centre of the suprasternal fossa.

Lieque：on the styloid process of the radius, 1.5 cun above the palmar crease of the wrist.

Chize：in the cubital crease, on the radial side of the tendon of the biceps muscle of the arm.

Indication　Diseases of the lung system.

Methods　Acupuncture：Feishu is needled 0.5-0.8 cun with the needle tip towards the spine.

Tiantu and Lieque are needled 0.3-0.5 cun beneath the skin.

Danzhong is needled 0.5-1 cun beneath the skin.

Chize is needled 0.8-1.2 cun perpendicularly till the acu-esthesia is obtained.

Moxibustion：5-9 cones of moxibustion, or 10-20 minutes' moxibustion with moxa roll is applied to Feishu, Tiantu and Danzhong. 10-20 minutes moxibustion with moxa roll is applied to Lieque and Chize.

● 镇咳
Zhenke

组成　本穴组由天突、列缺二穴组合而成。
位置　天突：胸骨上窝正中。
列缺：桡骨茎突上方，腕横纹上1.5寸。
主治　咳嗽。
操作　见"肺系"。
Composition　This group of acupoints is composed of

Tiantu(CU22) and Lieque(LU7).

Location　Tiantu：in the centre of the suprasternal fossa.

Lieque：on the styloid process of the radius, 1.5 cun above the crease of the wrist.

Indication　Cough.
Method　See Feixi.

止咳
Zhike

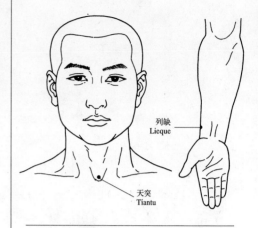

图 4-47　镇咳
Fig. 4-47　Zhenke

组成　本穴组由列缺、身柱、肺俞、太渊四穴组合而成。
位置　列缺：桡骨茎突上方，腕横纹上1.5寸。
身柱：第三胸椎棘突下。
肺俞：第三胸椎棘突下，旁开1.5寸。
太渊：掌后腕横纹桡侧端，桡动脉的桡侧凹陷中。
主治　咳嗽。
操作　刺法：列缺、太渊沿皮刺0.3～0.5寸。身柱由下向上刺0.5～0.8寸。肺俞向脊柱方向斜刺0.5～0.8寸，得气为度。
灸法：艾条温灸10～20分钟。

Composition　This group of acupoints is composed of Lieque(LU7), Shenzhu(GV12), Feishu(BL13) and Taiyuan (LU9).

Location　Lieque：on the styloid process of the radius, 1.5 cun above the palmar crease of the wrist.

Shenzhu：below the spinous process of the 3rd thoracic vertebra.

Feishu：1.5 cun lateral to the point below the 3rd spinous process of the thoracic vertebra.

Taiyuan：at the radial end of the palmar crease of the wrist, in the depression of the radial side of the radial artery.

Indication　Cough.

Methods　Acupuncture：Lieque and Taiyuan are needled 0.3—0.5 cun subcutaneously. Shenzhu is needled 0.5—0.8 cun upwards. Feishu is needled 0.5—0.8 cun towards the spine obliquely till the acu-esthesia is obtained.

Moxibustion：warm moxibustion with moxa roll for

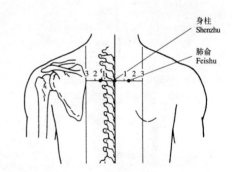

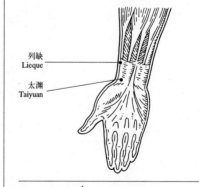

图 4-48　止咳
Fig. 4-48　Zhike

10—20 minutes is applied.

气管炎十九术
Qiguanyanshijiushu

组成　本穴组由廉泉、天突、人迎、水突、气舍、定喘、膻中、鸠尾、太渊、偏历、缺盆、大椎十九穴所组合而成。

位置　廉泉：舌骨体上缘的中点处。

天突：胸骨上窝正中。

人迎：喉结旁1.5寸，当颈总动脉之后，胸锁乳突肌前缘。

水突：人迎穴至气舍穴连线的中点，当胸锁乳突肌前缘。

气舍：人迎直下，锁骨上缘，在胸锁乳突肌的胸骨头与锁骨头之间。

膻中：前正中线，平第四肋间隙。

鸠尾：剑突下，脐上7寸。

缺盆：锁骨上窝正中处。

太渊：掌后腕横纹桡侧端，桡动脉的桡侧凹陷中。

偏历：在阳溪穴与曲池穴连线上，阳溪穴上3寸处。

大椎：第七颈椎棘突下。

定喘：大椎穴旁开0.5寸。

主治　急、慢性咳嗽，喘息。

操作　廉泉、天突、人迎、水突、气舍、膻中、鸠尾、缺盆，各针0.2~0.3寸，针感局部酸、麻。定喘、大椎穴针0.3~0.5寸，针感局部酸、胀。太渊、偏历针0.3~0.5寸，针感麻、酸至腕或指。

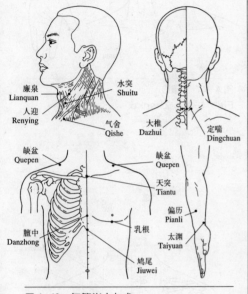

图4-49　气管炎十九术
Fig. 4-49　Qiguanyanshijiushu

Composition　This group of acupoints is composed of Lianquan(CV23), Tiantu(CV22), Renying(ST9), Shuitu(ST10), Qishe(ST11), Dingchuan(EX-B1), Danzhong(CV17), Jiuwei(CV15), Taiyuan(LU9), Pianli(LI6), Quepen(ST14) and Dazhui.

Location　Lianquan：at the midpoint at the upper border of the hyoid bone.

Tiantu：in the centre of the suprasternal fossa.

Renying：1.5 cun lateral to the laryngeal protuberance, which is posterior to the common carotid artery and anterior to the border of the sternocleidomastoid muscle.

Shuitu：at the midpoint of the line connecting Renying and Qishe, which is anterior to the border the sternocleidomastoid muscle.

Qishe: directly below Renying, in the depression between the sternal and clavicular heads of the sternocleidomastoid muscle.

Dingchuan: 0.5 cun lateral to Dazhui.

Danzhong: on the anterior midline, at the horizontal level of the 4th intercostal space.

Jiuwei: below the xiphoid process, 7 cun above the centre of the umbilicus.

Taiyuan: at the radial end of the palmar crease of the wrist, in the depression of the radial side of the radial artery.

Pianli: on the line connecting Yangxi and Quchi, 3 cun above Yangxi.

Qupen: in the centre of the clavicle fossa.

Dazhui: at the point below the spinous process of the 7th cervical vertebra.

Indication Acute and chronic cough and asthma.

Method Lianquan, Tiantu, Renying, Shuitu, Qishe, Danzhong, Jiuwei and Quepen are needled 0.2−0.3 cun, and the acu-esthesia of soreness and numbness in this part will be obtained. Dingchuan and Dazhui are needled 0.3−0.5 cun, the acu-esthesia of soreness and distension will be obatined in this part. Taiyuan and Pianli are needled 0.3−0.5 cun, the acu-esthesia of numbness and soreness will be induced to the wrist or fingers.

 补肺肾
Bufeishen

组成　本穴组由肺俞、孔最、肾俞、太溪四穴组合而成。
位置　肺俞：第三胸椎棘突下，旁开1.5寸。
肾俞：第二腰椎棘突下，旁开1.5寸。
孔最：尺泽与太渊连线上，腕横纹上7寸处。
太溪：内踝高点与跟腱之间凹陷中。
主治　老年哮喘，久喘，老年慢性气管炎。
操作　刺法：肺、肾俞向脊柱方向斜刺0.5～0.8寸，针感向四周扩散。孔最直刺1寸，太溪直刺0.5寸，得气后通以电针20分钟，每日1次。
灸法：肺俞、肾俞艾炷灸5～9壮，四穴艾条温灸5～15

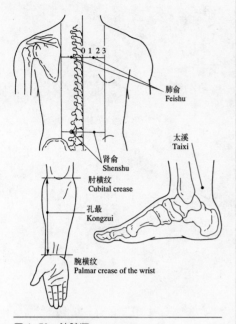

图 4-50 补肺肾
Fig. 4-50 Bufeishen

分钟。

Composition This group of acupoints is composed of Feishu(BL13), Kongzui(LU6), Shenshu(BL23) and Taixi (KI3).

Location Feishu：1.5 cun lateral to the point below the 3rd spinous process of the thoracic vertebra.

Shenshu：1.5 cun lateral to the point below the spinous process of the 2nd lumbar vertebra.

Kongzui：on the line connecting Chize and Taiyuan, 7 cun above the palmar crease of the wrist.

Taixi：in the midpoint between the tip of the medial malleolus and Achilles's tendon.

Indications Asthma, chronic bronchitis of the senile people.

Methods Acupuncture：Feishu and Shenshu are needled 0.5-0.8 cun obliquely with the needle tip towards the spine, and the acu-esthesia will radiate outwards. Kongzui is needled 1 cun perpendicularly, Taixi 0.5 cun perpendicularly. Electroacupuncture for 20 minutes is applied after the arrival of the acu-esthesia. Treat once every day.

Moxibustion：5-9 cones of moxibustion is applied to Feishu and Shenshu. Warm moxibustion with moxa roll for 5-15 minutes can be applied to all the four points.

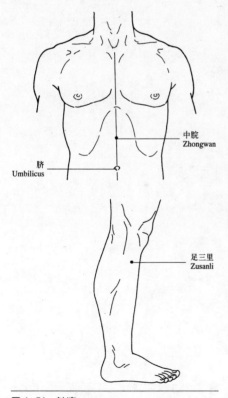

图 4-51 针痰
Fig. 4-51 Zhentan

🔵 针痰
Zhentan
・ ・ ・ ・ ・ ・

组成 本穴组由中脘、足三里穴组合而成。

位置 中脘：脐上4寸。

足三里：犊鼻穴下3寸，胫骨前嵴外一横指处。

主治 痰疾。

操作 针0.5~1.2寸，得气为度，留针30分钟。留针期间，可行提插捻转手法。

Composition This group of acupoints is composed of Zhongwan(CV12) and Zusanli(ST36).

Location Zhongwan：4 cun above the centre of the umbilicus.

Zusanli：3 cun below Dubi, one finger breadth from

the anterior crest of the tibia.

Indication　Diseases due to phlegm.

Method　The needle is inserted 0.5—1.2 cun till the acu-esthesia is obtained. Retain the needles for 30 minutes. Lifting, inserting and rotating techniques can be applied during the retention of the needles.

咯痰
Katan

组成　本穴组由肺俞、中脘、丰隆三穴组合而成。

位置　肺俞：第三胸椎棘突下，旁开1.5寸。

中脘：脐上4寸。

丰隆：外踝高点上8寸，条口穴外1寸。

主治　痰多。

操作　刺法：肺俞向脊柱方向斜刺0.5～0.8寸。中脘、丰隆针0.8～1.5寸，得气为度。

灸法：艾炷灸5～9壮，艾条灸10～20分钟。

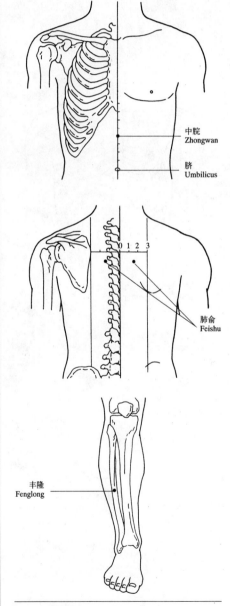

中脘
Zhongwan

脐
Umbilicus

肺俞
Feishu

丰隆
Fenglong

Composition　This group of acupoints is composed of Feishu(BL13), Zhongwan(CV12) and Fenglong(ST40).

Location　Feishu：1.5 cun lateral to the point below the 3rd spinous process of the thoracic vertebra.

Zhongwan：4 cun above the centre of the umbilicus.

Fenglong：8 cun above the tip of the external malleolus, 1 cun lateral to Tiaokou.

Indication　Copious phlegm.

Methods　Acupuncture：Feishu is needled 0.5—0.8 cun obliquely towards the spine. Zhongwan and Fenglong are needled 0.8—1.5 cun till the acu-esthesia is obtained.

Moxibustion：5—9 cones of moxibustion, or 10—20 minutes' moxibustion with moxa roll is applied.

化痰
Huatan

组成　本穴组由中脘、丰隆、足三里三穴组合而成。

位置　中脘：脐上4寸。

丰隆：外踝高点上8寸，条口穴外1寸。

图4-52　咯痰
Fig. 4-52　Katan

足三里：犊鼻穴下3寸，胫骨前嵴外一横指处。

主治　痰多。

操作　刺法：直刺0.8～1.5寸。

灸法：艾炷灸5～9壮，艾条灸10～20分钟。

Composition   This group of acupoints is composed of Zhongwan(CV12), Fenglong(ST40) and Zusanli(ST36).

Location   Zhongwan：4 cun above the centre of the umbilicus.

Fenglong：8 cun above the tip of the external malleolus, 1 cun lateral to Tiaokou.

Zusanli：3 cun below Dubi, one finger breadth from the anterior crest of the tibia.

Indication   Copious phlegm.

Methods   Acupuncture：the needle is inserted 0.8–1.5 cun perpendicularly.

Moxibustion：5–9 cones of moxibustion with moxa cone, or 10–20 minutes' moxibustion with moxa roll is applied.

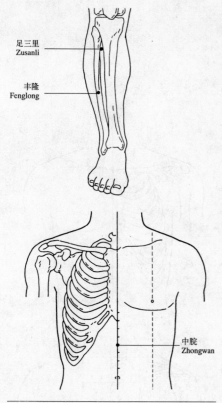

图4-53　化痰

Fig. 4-53　Huatan

● 尸劳
Shilao

组成　本穴组由涌泉、关元、丰隆三穴组合而成。

位置　涌泉：足底(去趾)前1/3处，足趾跖屈时呈凹陷处。

关元：脐下3寸。

丰隆：外踝高点上8寸，条口穴外1寸。

主治　肺痨结核。

操作　刺法：涌泉针0.5～0.8寸，痛酸感。关元、丰隆直刺1～1.5寸，得气为度。

灸法：关元、丰隆艾炷灸5～9壮，艾条灸10～30分钟。涌泉艾条灸10～30分钟。

Composition   This group of acupoints is composed of Yongquan(KI1), Guanyuan(CV4) and Fenglong(ST40).

Location   Yongquan：at the junction of the anterior one-third and middle one-third of the sole (the toes are not included), i.e. in the depression when the toes are extended downwards.

Guanyuan：3 cun below the centre of the umbilicus.

Fenglong：8 cun above the tip of the external malleolus,

1 cun lateral to Tiaokou.

Indication Pulmonary tuberculosis.

Method Acupuncture：Yongquan is needled 0.5−0.8 cun, the acu-esthesia is pain or soreness.

Guanyuan and Fenglong are needled 1−1.5 cun perpendicularly till the acu-esthesia is obtained.

Moxibustion：5−9 cones of moxibustion with moxa cone, or 10−30 minutes' moxibustion with moxa roll is applied to Guanyuan and Fenglong. 10−30 minutes' moxibustion with moxa roll is applied to Yongquan.

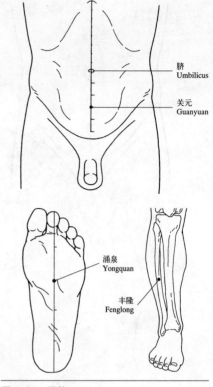

图 4-54 尸劳
Fig. 4-54 Shilao

五劳
Wulao

组成 本穴组由足三里、膏肓二穴组合而成。

位置 足三里：犊鼻穴下3寸，胫骨前嵴外一横指处。

膏肓：第四胸椎棘突下，旁开3寸。

主治 五劳羸瘦。

操作 艾炷灸5~9壮，艾条温灸10~30分钟。

Composition This group of acupoints is composed of Zusanli(ST36) and Gaohuang(BL43).

Location Zusanli：3 cun below Dubi, one finger breadth from the anterior crest of the tibia.

Gaohuang：3 cun lateral to the point below the spinous process of the 4th thoracic vertebra.

Indication Emaciation and consumptive diseases.

Method 5−9 cones of moxibustion, or 10−30 minutes' warm moxibustion with moxa roll is applied.

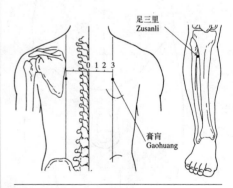

图 4-55 五劳
Fig. 4-55 Wulao

补虚
Buxu

组成 本穴组由关元、足三里二穴组合而成。

位置 足三里：犊鼻穴下3寸，胫骨前嵴外一横指处。

关元：脐下3寸。

主治 虚弱证。

操作 刺法：针1~1.5寸，行捻转或提插补法。

灸法：艾炷灸5~9壮，艾条灸10~30分钟。

Composition　This group of acupoints is composed of Guanyuan(CV4) and Zusanli(ST36).

Location　Zusanli：3 cun below Dubi, one finger breadth from the anterior crest of the tibia.

Guanyuan：3 cun below the centre of the umbilicus.

Indication　General weakness.

Method　Acupuncture：the needle is inserted 1−1.5 cun, reinforcing techniques by rotating, lifting and inserting the needles are applied.

Moxibustion：5−9 cones of moxibustion, or 10−30 minutes' moxibustion with moxa roll is applied.

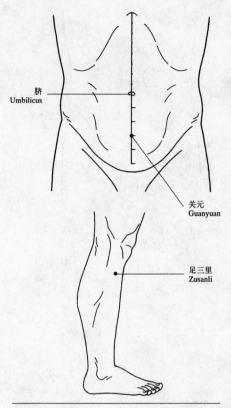

脐
Umbilicus

关元
Guanyuan

足三里
Zusanli

图 4-56 补虚
Fig. 4-56 Buxu

针虚
Zhenxu

组成　本穴组由气海、关元、委中，三穴组合而成。

位置　气海：脐下1.5寸。

委中：腘横纹中央。

关元：脐下3寸。

主治　虚证。

操作　气海针1～2寸，艾炷灸5～9壮。

委中麦粒灸5～9壮，艾炷温灸10～20分钟。

Composition　This group of acupoints is composed of Qihai(CV6), Guanyuan(CV4) and Weizhong(BL40).

Location　Qihai：1.5 cun below the centre of the umbilicus.

Weizhong：at the midpoint of the popliteal crease.

Guanyuan：3 cun below the centre of the umbilicus.

Indication　General asthenia.

Method　Qihai and Guanyuan are needled 1−2 cun. Moxibustion with 5−9 moxa cones can be applied to them.

Weizhong：5−9 cones of moxibustion, or 10−20 minutes' warm moxibustion with moxa roll is applied.

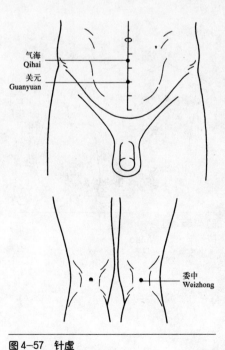

气海
Qihai

关元
Guanyuan

委中
Weizhong

图 4-57 针虚
Fig. 4-57 Zhenxu

肺俞原
Feishuyuan

组成　本穴组由肺俞、太渊二穴组合而成。

位置　肺俞：第三胸椎棘突下，旁开1.5寸。

太渊：掌后腕横纹桡侧端，桡动脉的桡侧凹陷中。

主治　肺系病证。

操作　刺法：斜刺0.5～0.8寸，局部酸胀感。

灸法：肺俞艾炷灸5～9壮，艾条温灸10～20分钟。太渊一般不灸。

Composition　This group of acupoints is composed of Feishu(BL13) and Taiyuan(LU9).

Location　Feishu：1.5 cun lateral to the point below the 3rd spinous process of the thoracic vertebra.

Taiyuan：at the radial end of the palmar crease of the wrist, in the depression of the radial side of the radial artery.

Indication　Diseases of the lung system.

Method　Acupuncture：the needle is inserted 0.5－0.8 cun obliquely. The acu-eshesia of soreness and distension will be obtained in this part.

Moxibustion：5－9 cones of moxibustion is applied to Feishu, moxibustion with moxa roll for 10－20 minutes can also be applied. Usually, moxibustion is not applied to Taiyuan.

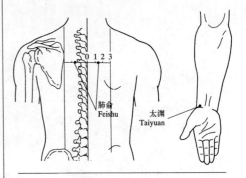

图4-58　肺俞原
Fig. 4-58　Feishuyuan

心俞原
Xinshuyuan

组成　本穴组由心俞、神门二穴组合而成。

位置　心俞：第五胸椎棘突下，旁开1.5寸。

神门：腕横纹尺侧端，尺侧腕屈肌腱的桡侧凹陷中。

主治　心脑神志病。

操作　刺法：针0.5～0.8寸。

灸法：心俞艾炷灸5～9壮，艾条温灸10～20分钟。神门一般不灸。

Composition　This group of acupoints is composed of Xinshu(BL15) and Shenmen(HT7).

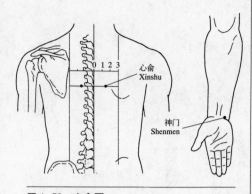

图 4-59 心俞原
Fig. 4-59 Xinshuyuan

Location Xinshu：1.5 cun lateral to the point below the spinous process of the 5th thoracic vertebra.

Shenmen：on the ulnar end of the palmar crease of the wrist, in the depression of the radial side of the tendon of the ulnar flexor muscle of the wrist.

Indication Diseases of the heart, brain and mind.

Method Acupuncture：the needle is inserted 0.5-0.8 cun.

Moxibustion：Xinshu：5-9 cones of moxibustion, 10-20 minutes' warm moxibustion with moxa roll is applied. Usually, moxibustion is not applied to Shenmen.

心包俞原
Xinbaoshuyuan

组成 本穴组由厥阴俞、大陵二穴组合而成。

位置 厥阴俞：第四胸椎棘突下，旁开1.5寸。

大陵：腕横纹中央，掌长肌腱与桡侧腕屈肌腱之间。

主治 心血管病证。

操作 刺法：斜刺0.5~0.8寸。

灸法：厥阴俞艾炷灸5~9壮，艾条温灸10~20分钟。大陵穴一般不灸。

Composition This group of acupoints is composed of Jueyinshu(BL14) and Daling(PC7).

Location Jueyinshu：1.5 cun lateral to the point below the spinous process of the 4th thoracic vertebra.

Daling：at the midpoint of the palmar crease of the wrist, between the tendons of the long palmar muscle and radial flexor muscle of the wrist.

Indication Diseases of heart and vessels.

Method Acupuncture：the needle is inserted 0.5-0.8 cun obliquely.

Moxibustion：Jueyinshu：5-9 cones of moxibustion, 10-20 minutes' warm moxibustion with moxa roll is applied. Usually, moxibustion is not applied to Daling.

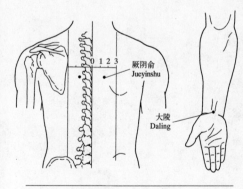

图 4-60 心包俞原
Fig. 4-60 Xinbaoshuyuan

● 脾俞原
Pishuyuan

组成 本穴组由脾俞、太白二穴组合而成。

位置 脾俞：第十一胸椎棘突下，旁开1.5寸。

太白：第一跖骨小头后缘，赤白肉际。

主治 脾脏及消化系病证。

操作 刺法：斜刺0.5～0.8寸。

灸法：脾俞艾炷灸5～9壮，艾条温灸10～20分钟。太白一般不灸。

Composition This group of acupoints is composed of Pishu(BL20) and Taibai(SP3).

Location Pishu：1.5 cun lateral to the point below the spinous process of the 11th thoracic vertebra.

Taibai：posterior to the head of the 1st metatarsal bone, on the junction of the red and white skin.

Indication Diseases of the spleen and digestive system.

Method Acupuncture：the needle is inserted 0.5-0.8 cun obliquely.

Moxibustion：Pishu：5-9 cones of moxibustion with moxa cone, 10-20 minutes' warm moxibustion with moxa roll is applied. Usually, moxibustion is not applied to Taibai.

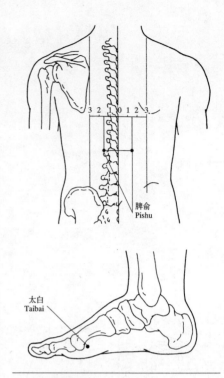

图4-61 脾俞原
Fig. 4-61 Pishuyuan

● 肾俞原
Shenshuyuan

组成 本穴组由肾俞、太溪二穴组合而成。

位置 肾俞：第二腰椎棘突下，旁开1.5寸。

太溪：内踝高点与跟腱之间凹陷中。

主治 肾脏及泌尿生殖系病证。

操作 刺法：针1.0～1.5寸。

灸法：肾俞艾炷灸5～9壮，艾条温灸10～20分钟。太溪穴一般少灸。

Composition This group of acupoints is composed of Shenshu(BL23) and Taixi(KI3).

Location Shenshu：1.5 cun lateral to the point below the spinous process of the 2nd lumbar vertebra.

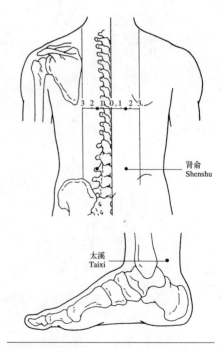

图4-62 肾俞原
Fig. 4-62 Shenshuyuan

Taixi: in the midpoint between the tip of the medial malleolus and Achilles's tendon.

Indication Diseases of the kidney and urogenital system.

Method Acupuncture: the needle is inserted 1–1.5 cun.

Moxibustion: Shenshu: 5–9 cones of moxibustion, 10–20 minutes' warm moxibustion with moxa roll is applied. Usually, less moxibustion of is applied to Taixi.

肝俞原
Ganshuyuan

组成 本穴组由肝俞、太冲二穴组合而成。

位置 肝俞：第九胸椎棘突下，旁开1.5寸。

太冲：足背，第一、第二跖骨结合部之前凹陷中。

主治 肝系病证，如肝炎，肝风，目疾，筋症等。

操作 刺法：针0.5~0.8寸。

灸法：肝俞艾炷灸5~9壮，艾条温灸10~20分钟。太冲一般不灸。

Composition This group of acupoints is composed of Guanshu (BL18) and Taichong (LR3).

Location Ganshu: 1.5 cun lateral to the point below the spinous process of the 9th thoracic vertebra.

Taichong: on the instep of the foot, in the depression anterior to the commissure of the 1st and 2nd metatarsal bones.

Indication Diseases of the liver system, such as hepatitis, Liver wind hyperactivity, Liver qi depression, liver yang hyperactivity, eye diseases and tendon diseases, etc..

Method Acupuncture: the needle is inserted 0.5–0.8 cun.

Moxibustion: Ganshu: 5–9 cones of moxibustion, 10–20 minutes' warm moxibustion with moxa roll is applied. Usually, moxibustion is not applied to Taichong.

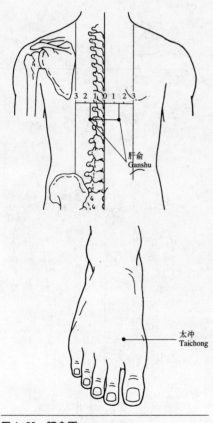

图4-63 肝俞原
Fig. 4-63 Ganshuyuan

膀胱俞原
Pangguangshuyuan

组成　本穴组由膀胱俞、京骨二穴组合而成。

位置　膀胱俞：第二骶椎棘突下，旁开1.5寸。

京骨：第五跖骨粗隆下，赤白肉际。

主治　膀胱、泌尿系病证。

操作　刺法：膀胱俞针1～2寸。京骨穴针0.3～0.5寸。

灸法：膀胱俞艾炷灸3～5壮，艾条温灸10～15分钟。京骨一般少灸或不灸。

Composition　This group of acupoints is composed of Pangguangshu (BL28) and Jinggu (BL64).

Location　Pangguangshu：1.5 cun lateral to the posterior midline below the 2nd sacral vertebra.

Jinggu：inferior to the tuberosity of the 5th metatarsal bone, at the junction of the red and white skin.

Indication　Diseases of the bladder and the urinary systems.

Method　Acupuncture：Pangguangshu is needled 1–2 cun, Jinggu 0.3–0.5 cun.

Moxibustion：Pangguangshu：moxibustion with 3–5 moxa cones, or warm moxibustion with moxa roll for 10–15 minutes is applied. Jinggu：usually, less or no moxubustion is applied.

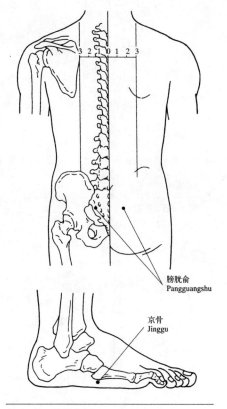

膀胱俞
Pangguangshu

京骨
Jinggu

图 4-64　膀胱俞原
Fig. 4-64　Pangguangshuyuan

胆俞原
Danshuyuan

组成　本穴组由胆俞、丘墟二穴组合而成。

位置　胆俞：第十胸椎棘突下，旁开1.5寸。

丘墟：外踝前下方，趾长伸肌腱外侧凹陷中。

主治　胆疾。

操作　刺法：斜刺0.5～0.8寸。

灸法：胆俞艾炷灸3～5壮，艾条温灸10～15分钟。丘墟一般少灸或温灸。

Composition　This group of acupoints is composed of Danshu (BL19) and Qiuxu (GB40).

Location　Danshu：1.5 cun lateral the point below the

spinous process of the 10th thoracic vertebra.

Qiuxu: anterior and inferior to the external malleolus, in the depression lateral to the tendon of the long extensor muscle of the toes.

Indication   Diseases of the gallbladder.

Method   Acupuncture: the needle is inserted 0.5—0.8 cun obliquely.

Moxibustion: Danshu: moxibustion with 3—5 moxa cones, or warm moxibustion with moxa roll for 10—15 minutes is applied. Qiuxu: usually, moxibustion of fewer cones or warm moxbustion is applied.

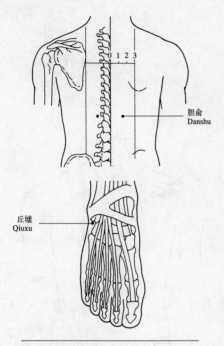

图 4-65　胆俞原
Fig. 4-65   Danshuyuan

大肠俞原
Dachangshuyuan

组成　本穴组由大肠俞、合谷二穴组合而成。

位置　大肠俞：第四腰椎棘突下，旁开1.5寸。

合谷：手背，第一、第二掌骨之间，约平第二掌骨中点处。

主治　肠及其他消化系病证。

操作　刺法：针0.8~1.5寸。大肠俞可深达2~3寸。

灸法：大肠俞艾炷灸3~5壮，艾条温灸10~15分钟。合谷一般少灸或不灸。

Composition   This group of acupoints is composed of Dachangshu (BL25) and Hegu (LI4).

Location   Dachangshu: 1.5 cun lateral to the spinous process of the 4th lumbar vertebra.

Hegu: on the dorsum of the hand, between the 1st and 2nd metacarpal bones, and near the midpoint of the 2nd metacarpal bone.

Indication   Diseases of the intestine and the digestive system.

Method   Acupuncture: the needle is inserted 0.8—1.5 cun. For Dachangshu, the depth may be 2—3 cun.

Moxibustion: Dachangshu: moxibustion with 3—5 moxa cones, or warm moxibustion with moxa roll for 10—15 minutes is applied. Hegu: usually, less moxibustion or no moxbustion is applied.

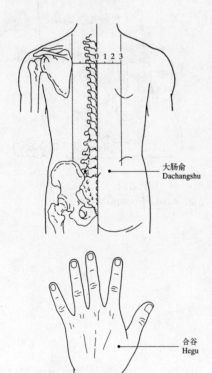

图 4-66　大肠俞原
Fig. 4-66   Dachangshuyuan

小肠俞原
Xiaochangshuyuan

组成　本穴组由小肠俞、腕骨组合而成。

位置　小肠俞：第一骶椎棘突下，旁开1.5寸。

腕骨：后溪穴直上，于第五掌骨基底与三角骨之间赤白肉际取之。

主治　小肠及其他消化系病证。

操作　刺法：针0.5～1寸。小肠俞可深至2寸。

灸法：小肠俞艾炷灸3～5壮，艾条温灸。腕骨一般不灸。

Composition　This group of acupoints is composed of Xiaochangshu (BL27) and Wangu (SI4).

Location　Xiaochangshu：1.5 cun lateral to the posterior midline, below the 1st sacral vertebra.

Wangu：directly above Houxi, on the junction of the red and white skin between the basal part of the 5th metacarpal bone and triangular bone.

Indication　Diseases of the small intestine and the digestive system.

Method　Acupuncture：the needle is inserted 0.5－1 cun. For Xiaochangshu, the depth may be 2 cun.

Moxibustion：Xiaochangshu：moxibustion with 3－5 moxa cones, or warm moxibustion is applied. Wangu：usually, moxibustion is not applied.

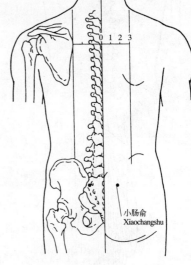
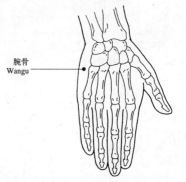

图4-67　小肠俞原
Fig. 4-67　Xiaochangshuyuan

胃俞原
Weishuyuan

组成　本穴组由胃俞、冲阳二穴组合而成。

位置　胃俞：第十二胸椎棘突下，旁开1.5寸。

冲阳：在解溪穴下方，踇长伸肌腱和趾长伸肌腱之间，当第二、第三跖骨与楔状骨间，足背动脉搏动处。

主治　胃及消化系病证。

操作　刺法：胃俞针0.5～1寸。冲阳横刺0.5～0.8寸。

灸法：胃俞艾炷灸5～9壮，艾条温灸10～20分钟。冲阳艾条温炎10～20分钟。

Composition　This group of acupoints is composed of Weishu (BL21) and Chongyang (ST42).

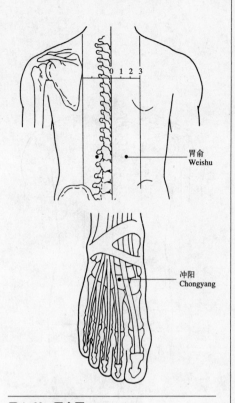

图 4-68 胃俞原
Fig. 4-68 Weishuyuan

Location Weishu：1.5 cun lateral to the point below the spinous process of the 12th thoracic vertebra.

Chongyang：inferior to Jiexi, between the tendons of the long extensor muscle of the great toe and the long extensor muscle of the toes, on the instep of the foot.

Indication Diseases of the stomach and digestive system.

Method Acupuncture：Weishu is needled 0.5−1 cun, Chongyang 0.5−0.8 cun transversely.

Moxibustion：Weishu：moxibustion with 3−5 moxa cones, or warm moxibustion with moxa roll for 10−20 minutes is applied. Chongyang：warm moxibustion with moxa roll for 10−20 minutes is applied.

三焦俞原
Sanjiaoshuyuan

组成 本穴组由三焦俞与阳池二穴组合而成。

位置 三焦俞：第一腰椎棘突下，旁开1.5寸。

阳池：腕背横纹中，指总伸肌腱尺侧缘凹陷中。

主治 三焦及水代谢病证。

操作 刺法：三焦俞针1～1.5寸。阳池针0.5～1寸。

灸法：三焦俞艾炷灸3～5壮，艾条温灸10～15分钟。阳池温灸10～15分钟。

Composition This group of acupoints is composed of Sanjiaoshu (BL22) and Yangchi (TE4).

Location Sanjiaoshu：1.5 cun lateral to the point below the spinous process of the 1st lumbar vertebra.

Yangchi：at the midpoint of the dorsal crease of the wrist, in the depression on the ulnar side of the tendon of the extensor muscle of the fingers.

Indication Diseases of Triple Energizer and water metabolism.

Method Acupuncture：Sanjiaoshu is needled 1−1.5 cun, Yangchi 0.5−1 cun.

Moxibustion：Sanjiaoshu：moxibustion with 3−5 moxa cones, or warm moxibustion with moxa roll for 10−15 minutes is applied. Yangchi：warm moxibustion with moxa roll for 10−15 minutes is applied.

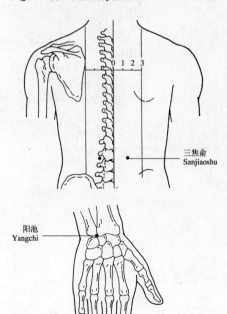

图 4-69 三焦俞原
Fig. 4-69 Sanjiaoshuyuan

骨髓会
Gusuihui

组成　本穴组由骨会大杼、髓会悬钟二穴组合而成。

位置　大杼：第一胸椎棘突下，旁开1.5寸。

悬钟：外踝高点上3寸，腓骨后缘。

主治　全身骨、髓病证。

操作　刺法：大杼斜刺0.5~0.8寸。悬钟0.5~1寸。

灸法：麦粒灸5~9壮，温灸10~20分钟。

Composition　This group of acupoints is composed of Dazhu (BL11), the Influential Point of Bone, and Xuanzhong (GB39), the Influential Point of Marrow.

Location　Dazhu：1.5 cun lateral to the spinous process of the 1st thoracic vertebra.

Xuanzhong：3 cun above the tip of the external malleolus, on the posterior border of the fibula.

Indication　Diseases of the bone and marrow of the whole body.

Method　Acupuncture：Dazhu is needled 0.5—0.8 cun obliquely, Xuanzhong 0.5—1 cun.

Moxibustion：5—9 wheat-sized moxa cones of moxibustion, or 10—20 minutes' warm moxibustion is applied.

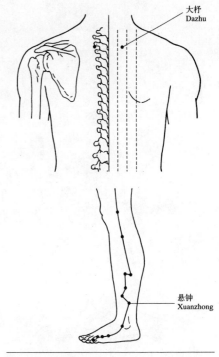

图4-70　骨髓会
Fig. 4-70　Gusuihui

筋骨会
Jinguhui

组成　本穴组由筋会阳陵泉、骨会大杼二穴组合而成。

位置　阳陵泉：腓骨小头前下方凹陷中。

大杼：第一胸椎棘突下，旁开1.5寸。

主治　全身筋病，骨病。

操作　刺法：阳陵泉针1~2寸。大杼斜刺0.5~0.8寸。

灸法：麦粒灸5~9壮，艾条温灸10~20分钟。

Composition　This group of acupoints is composed of Yanglingquan (GB34), the Influential Point of Tendon, and Dazhu (BL11), the Influential Point of Bone.

Location　Yanglingquan：in the depression anterior and inferior to the head of the fibula.

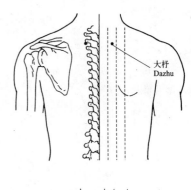

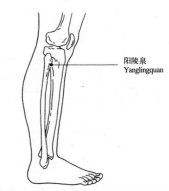

图4-71　筋骨会
Fig. 4-71　Jinguhui

Dazhu：1.5 cun lateral to the spinous process of the 1st thoracic vertebra.

Indications Diseases of the tendon and bone of the whole body.

Methods Acupuncture：Yanglingquan is needled 1—2 cun, Dazhu 0.5—0.8 cun obliquely.

Moxibustion：5—9 wheat-sized moxa cones of moxibustion, or 10—20 minutes' warm moxibustion is applied.

脉气会
Maiqihui

组成 本穴组由脉会太渊、气会膻中二穴组合而成。

位置 太渊：掌后腕横纹桡侧端，桡动脉的桡侧凹陷中。

膻中：前正中线，平第四肋间隙。

主治 全身气血病，血脉病。

操作 太渊：见"肺俞原"中太渊穴操作。

膻中：见"气血会"中膻中穴操作。

Composition This group of acupoints is composed of Taiyuan (LV9), the Influential Point of Vessels, and Danzhong (CV17), the Influential Point of Qi.

Location Taiyuan：at the radial end of the palmar crease of the wrist, in the depression of the radial side of the radial artery.

Danzhong：on the anterior midline, at the horizontal level of the 4th intercostal space.

Indication Diseases of qi, blood and vessels.

Method Taiyuan：see method for Taiyuan in Feishuyuan.

Danzhong：see method for Danzhong in Qixuehui.

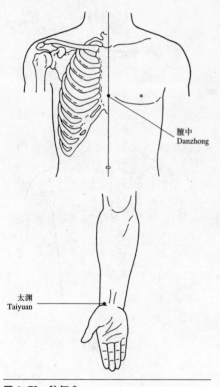

膻中
Danzhong

太渊
Taiyuan

图4-72 脉气会
Fig. 4-72 Maiqihui

筋气会
Jinqihui

组成 本穴组由筋会阳陵泉、气会膻中二穴组合而成。

位置 阳陵泉：腓骨小头前下方凹陷中。

膻中：前正中线，平第四肋间隙。

汉 英 对 照

主治 筋脉病与气病。

操作 阳陵泉：见"筋骨会"中阳陵泉操作。

膻中：见"脉气会"中膻中穴操作。

Composition This group of acupoints is composed of Yanglingquan (GB34), the Influential Point of Tendon, and Danzhong (CV17), the Influential Point of Qi.

Location Yanglingquan：in the depression anterior and inferior to the head of the fibula.

Danzhong：on the anterior midline, on the horizontal level of the 4th intercostal space.

Indication Diseases of the tendons, vessels and qi.

Method Yanglingquan：see method for Yanglingquan in Jinguhui.

Danzhong：see method for Danzhong in Maiqihui.

筋血会
Jinxuehui

组成 本穴组由筋会阳陵泉、血会膈俞二穴组合而成。

位置 阳陵泉：腓骨小头前下方凹陷中。

膈俞：第七胸椎棘突下，旁开1.5寸。

主治 筋病病证，肌肉病证。

操作 阳陵泉：见"筋骨会"中阳陵泉操作。

膈俞：见"气血会"中膈俞操作。

Composition This group of acupoints is composed of Yanglingquan (GB34), the Influential Point of Tendon, and Geshu (BL17), the Influential Point of Blood.

Location Yanglingquan：in the depression anterior and inferior to the head of the fibula.

Geshu：1.5 cun lateral to the point below the spinous process of the 7th thoracic vertebra.

Indication Blood syndromes of the tendon and muscle diseases.

Method Yanglingquan：see method for Yonglingquan in Jinguhui.

Geshu：see method for Geshu in Qixuehui.

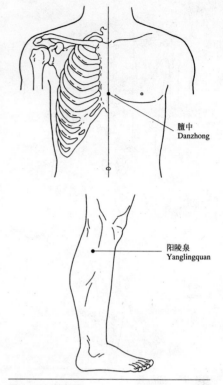

图 4-73 筋气会
Fig. 4-73 Jinqihui

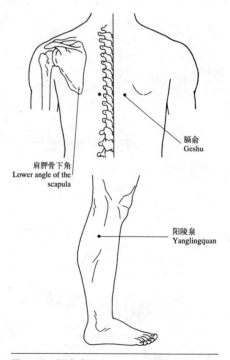

图 4-74 筋血会
Fig. 4-74 Jinxuehui

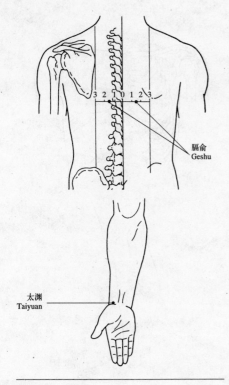

图4-75　血脉会
Fig. 4-75　Xuemaihui

● 血脉会
Xuemaihui

组成　本穴组由血会膈俞、脉会太渊二穴组合而成。

位置　膈俞：第七胸椎棘突下，旁开1.5寸。

太渊：掌后腕横纹桡侧端，桡动脉的桡侧凹陷中。

主治　血脉病证。

操作　见有关二穴操作法。

Composition　This group of acupoints is composed of Geshu (BL17), the Influential Point of Blood, and Taiyuan (LV9), the Influential Point of Vessels.

Location　Geshu：1.5 cun lateral to the point below the spinous process of the 7th thoracic vertebra.

Taiyuan：at the radial end of the palmar crease of the wrist, in the depression of the radial side of the radial artery.

Indication　Diseases of the blood and vessels.

Method　See methods related to the two points.

● 血髓会
Xuesuihui

组成　本穴组由血会膈俞、髓会悬钟二穴组合而成。

位置　膈俞：第七胸椎棘突下，旁开1.5寸。

悬钟：外踝高点上3寸，腓骨后缘。

主治　血液病、骨病等。

操作　膈俞：见"气血会"中膈俞穴操作。

悬钟：见"骨髓会"中悬钟穴操作。

Composition　This group of acupoints is composed of Geshu (BL17), the Influential Point of Blood, and Xuanzhong (GB39), the Influential Point of Marrow.

Location　Geshu：1.5 cun lateral to the point below the spinous process of the 7th thoracic vertebra.

Xuanzhong：3 cun above the tip of the external malleolus, on the posterior border of the fibula.

Indications　Diseases of the blood and bone.

Method　Geshu：see method for Geshu in Qixuehui.

Xuanzhong：see method for xuanzhong in Gusuihui.

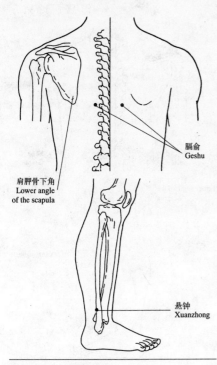

图4-76　血髓会
Fig. 4-76　Xuesuihui

● 交泰
Jiaotai

组成　本穴组由心俞、肾俞、神门、三阴交四穴组合而成。

位置　心俞：第五胸椎棘突下，旁开1.5寸。

肾俞：第二腰椎棘突下，旁开1.5寸。

神门：腕横纹尺侧端，尺侧腕屈肌腱的桡侧凹陷中。

三阴交：内踝高点上3寸，胫骨内侧面后缘。

主治　心肾不交之失眠，甚则彻夜不眠，梦遗滑精等。

操作　俯卧位取心俞米粒灸3壮。肾俞直刺0.5~1寸，提插捻转补法，得气后出针。仰卧位针三阴交1寸，得气后行提插捻转补法后即出针。神门直刺0.3~0.5寸，行提插捻转之泻法，得气后即出针。

按注　另组穴仅用心俞、肾俞。

Composition　This group of acupoints is composed of Xinshu (BL15), Shenshu (BL23), Shenmen (HT7) and Sanyinjiao (SP6).

Location　Xinshu：1.5 cun lateral to the point below the spinous process of the 5th thoracic vertebra.

Shenshu：1.5 cun lateral to the point below the spinous process of the 2nd lumbar vertebra.

Shenmen：on the ulnar end of the palmar crease of the wrist, in the depression of the radial side of the tendon of the ulnar flexor muscle of the wrist.

Sanyinjiao：3 cun above the tip of the medial malleolus, on the posterior border of the medial side of the tibia.

Indication　Insomnia due to disharmony between the heart and kidney, or even failing asleep during all night, nocturnal emission with dream, spermatorrhea without dream and seminal incontinence.

Method　Prone position is selected. 3 cones of moxibustion is applied to Xinshu. Shenshu is needled 0.5—1 cun perpendicularly, and reinforcing techniques by lifting, inserting and rotating the needles is applied. Withdraw the needle after the arrival of the acu-esthesia. Then supine position is selected, and Sanyinjiao is needled 1 cun. After the arrival of the acu-esthesia, apply the reinforcing techniques by lifting, inserting and rotating the needles, then withdraw the needle.

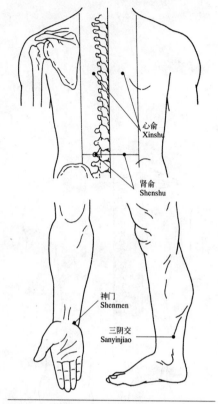

图4-77　交泰
Fig. 4-77　Jiaotai

Shenmen is needled 0.3—0.5 cun perpendicularly, and reducing techniques by lifting, inserting and rotating the needles is applied, withdraw the needle after the arrival of the acu-esthesia.

Note Another group is composed of Xinshu and Shenshu only.

● 消梦
Xiaomeng

组成 本穴组由心俞、神门、太冲三穴组合而成。

位置 心俞：第五胸椎棘突下，旁开1.5寸。

神门：腕横纹尺侧端，尺侧腕屈肌腱的桡侧凹陷中。

太冲：足背，第一、第二跖骨结合部之前凹陷中。

主治 多梦。

操作 刺法：心俞向脊柱方向斜刺0.5~0.8寸。神门斜刺0.5~0.8寸。太冲斜刺0.5~0.8寸。各以得气为度。

灸法：艾条灸10~20分钟。

Composition This group of acupoints is composed of Xinshu (BL15), Shenmen (HT7) and Taichong (LR3).

Location Xinshu：1.5 cun lateral to the point below the spinous process of the 5th thoracic vertebra.

Shenmen：on the ulnar end of the palmar crease of the wrist, in the depression of the radial side of the tendon of the ulnar flexor muscle of the wrist.

Taichong：on the instep of the foot, in the depression anterior to the commissure of the 1st and 2nd metatarsal bones.

Indications Excessive dreaming.

Methods Acupuncture：Xinshu is needled 0.5—0.8 cun obliquely towards the spine. Shenmen is needled 0.5—0.8 cun obliquely. Taichong is needled 0.5—0.8 cun obliquely. Stop manipulating the needles after the arrival of the acu-esthesia.

Moxibustion：moxibustion with moxa roll for 10—20 minutes is applied.

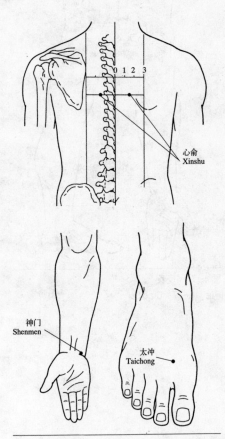

图 4-78 消梦
Fig. 4-78 Xiaomeng

心俞 Xinshu
神门 Shenmen
太冲 Taichong

椎池里
Zhuichili

组成　本穴组由大椎、曲池、足三里三穴组合而成。

位置　大椎：第七颈椎棘突下。

曲池：屈肘，成直角，当肘横纹外端与肱骨外上髁连线的中点。

足三里：犊鼻穴下3寸，胫骨前嵴外一横指处。

主治　嗜睡。

操作　曲池、足三里直刺1～1.5寸。大椎直刺0.5～1寸。各以得气为度。

Composition　This group of acupoints is composed of Dazhui (GV14), Quchi (LI11) and Zusanli (ST36).

Location　Dazhui：at the point below the spinous process of the 7th cervical vertebra.

Quchi：at the midpoint of the line between the radial end of the cubital crease and the external humeral epicondyle when the elbow is flexed at 90°

Zusanli：3 cun below Dubi, one finger breadth from the anterior crest of the tibia.

Indication　Somnolence.

Methods　Quchi and Zusanli are needled 1–1.5 cun perpendicularly. Dazhui is needled 0.5–1 cun perpendicularly. Stop manipulating the needles after the arrival of the acu-esthesia.

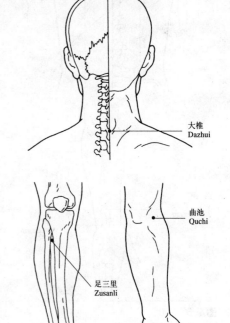

图4-79　椎池里
Fig. 4-79　Zhuichili

宽心
Kuanxin

组成　本穴组由心俞、内关、神门三穴组合而成。

位置　心俞：第五胸椎棘突下，旁开1.5寸。

内关：腕横纹上2寸，掌长肌腱与桡侧腕屈肌腱之间。

神门：腕横纹尺侧端，尺侧腕屈肌腱的桡侧凹陷中。

主治　心胆气虚善惊。

操作　坐位或俯卧位取心俞，得气后持续用补法，运针两分钟后出针，亦可悬灸5～10分钟。内关针1寸，神门针0.5寸，二穴均施提插捻转之平补平泻法，留针30分钟。

Composition　This group of acupoints is composed of

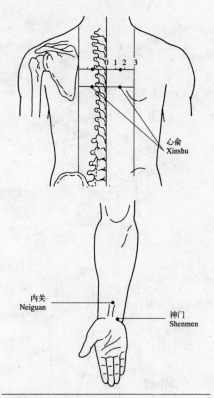

图 4-80 宽心
Fig. 4-80 Kuanxin

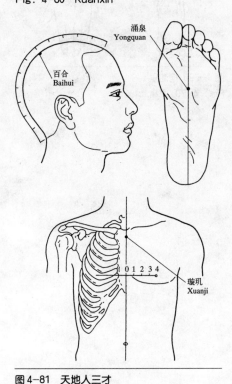

图 4-81 天地人三才
Fig. 4-81 Tiandirensancai

Xinshu (BL15), Neiguan (PC6) and Shenmen (HT7).

Location Xinshu：1.5 cun lateral to the point below the spinous process of the 5th thoracic vertebra.

Neiguan：2 cun above the palmar crease of the wrist, between the tendons of the long palmar muscle and radial flexor muscle of the wrist.

Shenmen：on the ulnar end of the palmar crease of the wrist, in the depression of the radial side of the tendon of the ulnar flexor muscle of the wrist.

Indication Fright and fear due to the deficiency of the heart and gallbladder.

Method Sitting or prone position is selected to locate Xinshu. After the arrival of the acu-esthesia, manipulate the needle for two minutes with reinforcing techniques, then withdraw the needle. Suspended moxibustion for 5-10 minutes can be also applied. Neiguan is needled 1 cun, Shenmen 0.5 cun. Even reinforcing-reducing techniques by lifting, inserting and rotating the needles can be applied to both points. Retain the needles for 30 minutes.

● 天地人三才
Tiandirensancai

组成 本穴组由百会(天)、涌泉(地)、璇玑(人)三穴组成。

位置 百会：后发际正中直上7寸。

涌泉：足底(去趾)前1/3处，足趾跖屈时呈凹陷处。

璇玑：前正中线，胸骨柄的中央。

主治 脏躁，带下，痛经，子宫下垂。

操作 刺法：针0.1～0.3寸，在刺时，或稍向前或后斜刺，局部有刺痛感。

灸法：灸3～5壮，艾条温灸5～15分钟。

Composition This group of acupoints is composed of Baihui (GV14) (Tian), Yongquan (KI1) (Di) and Xuanji (CV21) (Ren).

Location Baihui：7 cun directly above the midpoint of the posetrior hairline.

Yongquan：at the junction of the anterior one-third and middle one-third of the sole (the toes are not included), i.e. in the depression when the toes are extended downwards.

Xuanji: on the anterior midline, in the centre of the sternal handle.

Indication Hysteria, leukorrhea, dysmenorrhea, prolapse of the uterus.

Method Acupuncture: the needle is inserted 0.1–0.3 cun forwards or backwards slightly, and the acuesthesia will be obtained in this part.

Moxibustion: 3–5 cones of moxibustion, or 5–15 minutes' warm moxibustion with moxa roll is applied.

梅核气
Meiheqi

组成　本穴组由天突、内关、膻中、照海四穴组合而成。
位置　天突：胸骨上窝正中。
膻中：前正中线，平第四肋间隙。
内关：腕横纹上2寸，掌长肌腱与桡侧腕屈肌腱之间。
照海：内踝下缘凹陷中。
主治　梅核气。
操作　刺法：天突斜刺0.3~0.5寸。膻中沿皮刺0.5~1寸。照海直刺0.3~0.5寸。内关直刺0.5~1.2寸。各以得气为度。
灸法：艾条温灸10~20分钟。
按注　临床有以二穴组合者，即天突、内关或天突、膻中，或天突、照海，其效也佳。

Composition This group of acupoints is composed of Tiantu (CV22), Neiguan (PC6), Danzhong (CV17) and Zhaohai (KI6).

Location Tiantu: in the centre of the suprasternal fossa.

Danzhong: on the anterior midline, at the horizontal level of the 4th intercostal space.

Neiguan: 2 cun above the palmar crease of the wrist, between the tendons of the long palmar muscle and radial flexor muscle of the wrist.

Zhaohai: in the depression on the lower border of the medial malleolus.

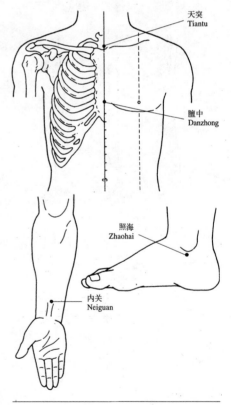

图 4-82　梅核气
Fig. 4-82　Meiheqi

Indication Globus hystericus.

Methods Acupuncture：Tiantu is needled 0.3−0.5 cun obliquely. Danzhong is needled 0.5−1 cun under the skin. Xuehai is needled 0.3−0.5 cun perpendicularly. Neiguan is needled 0.5−1.2 cun perpendicularly. Stop manipulating the needles after the arrival of the acu-esthesia.

Moxibustion：warm moxibustion with moxa roll for 10−20 minutes is applied.

Note In clinic, two points of the group can also work i.e. Tiantu and Neiguan, or Tiantu and Danzhong, or Tiantu and Zhaohai, the effect is good too.

 太极
Taiji

组成 本穴组由太白、中极二穴组合而成。
位置 太白：第一跖骨小头后缘，赤白肉际。
中极：脐下4寸。
主治 气冲。
操作 太白直刺0.5~0.8寸，局部酸胀痛感。中极直刺1~1.5寸，得气为度。

Composition This group of acupoints is composed of Taibai (SP3) and Zhongji (CV3).

Location Taibai：posterior to the head of the 1st metatarsal bone, on the junction of the white and red skin.

Zhongji：4 cun below the centre of the umbilicus.

Indication Up-rushing qi.

Method Taibai is needled 0.5−0.8 cun perpendicularly. The acu-esthesia of soreness, distension and pain can be obtained. Zhongji is needled 1−1.5 ucn perpendicuarly till the acu-esthesia is obtained.

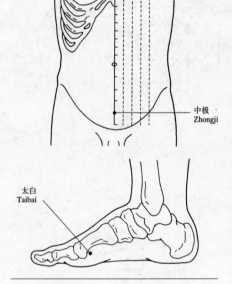

图4-83 太极
Fig. 4-83 Taiji

 使会
Shihui

组成 本穴组由间使、百会二穴组合而成。

位置　间使：腕横纹上3寸，掌长肌腱与桡侧腕屈肌腱之间。

百会：后发际正中直上7寸。

主治　痰火上扰发狂。

操作　百会逆经沿皮刺0.3~0.5寸，间使直刺0.5~0.7寸，得气后行泻法，二穴留针30分钟。

Composition　This group of acupoints is composed of Jianshi (PC5) and Baihui (GV20).

Location　Jianshi：3 cun above the palmar crease of the wrist, between the tendons of the long palmar muscle and radial flexor muscle of the wrist.

Baihui：7 cun directly above the midpoint of the posetrior hairline.

Indication　Mania due to upward disturbance of the phlegm fire.

Method　Baihui is needled backwards 0.3−0.5 cun beneath the skin, Jianshi 0.5−0.7 cun perpendicualry. Reducing techniques are applied after ther arrival of the acu-esthesia. Retain the needles for 30 minutes in the two points.

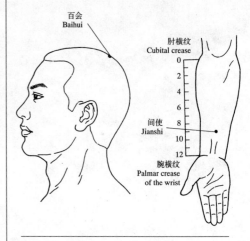

图 4−84　使会
Fig. 4−84　Shihui

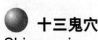
十三鬼穴
Shisanguixue

组成　本穴组由人中(鬼宫)、少商(鬼侯)、隐白(鬼垒)、大陵(鬼心)、申脉(鬼路)、风府(鬼枕)、颊车(鬼床)、承浆(鬼市)、劳宫(鬼窟)、上星(鬼堂)、男会阴女玉门(鬼藏)、曲池(鬼腿)、海泉(鬼封)十三穴组成。

位置　人中：在人中沟的上1/3与中1/3交界处。

承浆：颏唇沟的中点。

大陵：腕横纹中央，掌长肌腱与桡侧腕屈肌腱之间。

劳宫：第二、第三掌骨之间，握拳，中指尖下是穴。

少商：拇指桡侧指甲角旁约0.1寸。

隐白：踇趾内侧趾甲角旁约0.1寸。

上星：前发际正中直上1寸。

颊车：下颌角前上方一横指凹陷中，咀嚼时咬肌隆起最高点处。

曲池：屈肘，成直角，当肘横纹外端与肱骨外上髁连线的中点。

申脉：外踝下方凹陷中。

风府：后发际正中直上1寸。

海泉：舌下系带中点。

玉门：女性在外阴阴蒂头。

会阴：男性在阴囊根部与肛门的中间，女性在大阴唇后联合与肛门的中间。

主治　癫狂。

操作　一般针0.1～0.2寸，曲池、风府、颊车、大陵、会阴可针0.5～1寸。

按注　本穴组传统上只针不灸。另一组称鬼哭，只有少商、隐白二穴。

Composition　This group of acupoints is composed of Renzhong (GV26) (Guigong), Shaoshang (LU11) (Guihou), Yinbai (SP1) (Guilei), Daling (PC7) (Guixin), Shenmai (BL62) (Guilu), Fengfu (GV16) (Guizhen), Jiache (ST6) (Guichang), Chengjiang (CV24) (Guishi), Laogong (PC8) (Guiku), Shangxing (GV23) (Guitang), Huiyin (CV1)for male and Yumen for female (Guicang), Quchi (LI11) (Guitui) and Haiquan (Guifeng).

Location　Renzhong：at the junction of the upper one-third and middle one-third of the philtrum.

Chengjiang：at the midpoint of the mentolabial sulcus.

Daling：at the midpoint of the palmar crease of the wrist, between the tendons of the long palmar muscle and radial flexor muscle of the wrist.

Laogong：between the 2nd and 3rd metacarpal bones, where the tip of the middle finger reaches when a fist is made.

Shaoshang：on the the radial side of the thumb, 0.1 cun from the corner of the fingernail.

Yinbai：0.1 cun from the corner of the toenail of the medial side of the great toe.

Shangxing：1 cun directly above the midpoint of the anterior hairline.

Jiache：in the depression one finger breadth above the mandibular angle, where the masseter muscle is prominent when chewing.

Quchi：at the midpoint of the line between the radial end of the cubital crease and the external humeral epicondyle when the elbow is flexed at 90°.

Shenmai: in the depression on the lower border of the external malleolus.

Fengfu: 1 cun directly above the midpoint of the posterior hairline.

Haiquan: at the midpoint of the frenulum of the tongue.

Yumen: at the head of the clitoris in the pubes in female.

Huiyin: at the midpoint between the posterior border of the scrotum and anus in male, and between the posterior commissure of the large labia and anus in female.

Indication   Mania.

Method   Usually, the needle is inserted 0.1-0.2 cun. For Quchi, Fengfu, Jiache, Daling and Huiyin, the needle can be inserted 0.5-1 cun.

Note   This group is treated with only acupuncture, and no moxibustion is applied. There's another group called Guiku, which consists of Shaoshang (LU11) and Yinbai (SP1).

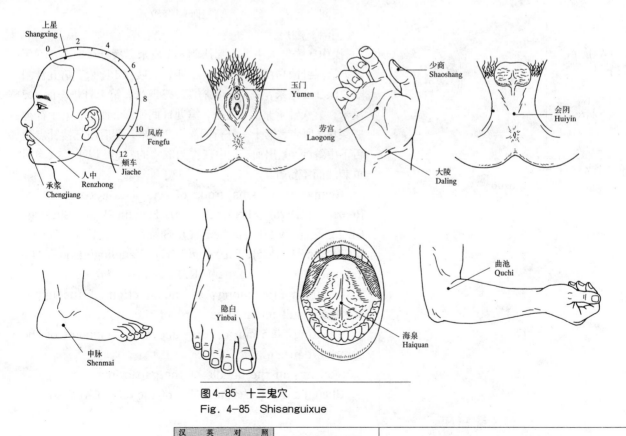

图 4-85　十三鬼穴
Fig. 4-85　Shisanguixue

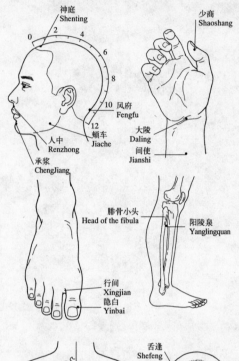

图4-86 十三穴
Fig. 4-86 Shisanxue

十三穴
Shisanxue

组成　本穴组由人中、神庭、风府、舌缝、承浆、颊车、少商、大陵、间使、乳中、阳陵泉、隐白、行间十三穴组合而成。

位置　人中：在人中沟的上1/3与中1/3交界处。

神庭：前发际正中直上0.5寸。

舌缝：舌下中缝处。

承浆：颏唇沟的中点。

风府：后发际正中直上1寸。

颊车：下颌角前上方一横指凹陷中，咀嚼时咬肌隆起最高点处。

少商：拇指桡侧指甲角旁约0.1寸。

大陵：腕横纹中央，掌长肌腱与桡侧腕屈肌腱之间。

间使：腕横纹上3寸，掌长肌腱与桡侧腕屈肌腱之间。

乳中：乳头中央。

阳陵泉：腓骨小头前下方凹陷中。

隐白：踇趾内侧趾甲角旁约0.1寸。

行间：足背，第一、第二趾间缝纹端。

主治　癫疾。

操作　先针人中，雀啄法刺入1厘米，次针少商深0.5厘米，第三针隐白深0.7厘米，第四针大陵深1厘米，第五针阳陵泉深3.3厘米，第六针风府深0.7厘米，第七针颊车深3.3厘米，第八针承浆深1厘米，第九针间使深2厘米，第十针神庭深0.7厘米，第十一针行间深1.2厘米，最后用三棱针点刺舌下中缝(舌缝)出血，乳中仅作为取穴的标志。以上二穴均用单刺法而不留针。

Composition　This group of acupoints is composed of Renzhong(GV26), Shenting(GV24), Fengfu(GV16), Shefeng, Chengjiang(CV24), Jiache(ST6), Shaoshang(LU11), Daling(PC7), Jianshi(PC5), Ruzhong(ST17), Yanglingquan(GV34), Yinbai(SP1) and Xingjian(LR2).

Location　Renzhong：at the junction of the upper one-third and middle one-third of the philtrum.

Shenting：0.5 cun directly above the midpoint of the anterior hairline.

Shefeng：in the middle of the gap below the tongue.

Chengjiang：at the midpoint of the mentolabial sulcus.

Fengfu: 1 cun directly above the midpoint of the posterior hairline.

Jiache: in the depression one finger breadth above the mandibular angle, where the masseter muscle is prominent when chewing.

Shaoshang: on the the radial side of the thumb, 0.1 cun from the corner of the fingernail.

Daling: at the midpoint of the palmar crease of the wrist, between the tendons of the long palmar muscle and radial flexor muscle of the wrist.

Jianshi: 3 cun above the palmar crease of the wrist, between the tendons of the long palmar muscle and radial flexor muscle of the wrist.

Ruzhong: in the centre of the nipple.

Yanglingquan: in the depression anterior and inferior to the head of the fibula.

Yinbai: 0.1 cun from the corner of the toenail of the medial side of the great toe.

Xingjian: on the instep of the foot, on the end of the margin of the web between the 1st and 2nd toes.

Indication Mania.

Method Renzhong is inserted 1 cm with sparrow-pecking method first. Shaoshang is needled 0.5 cm Secondly. Yinbai is needled 0.7 cm thirdly. Daling is needled 1 cm fourthly, Yanglingquan is needled 3.3 cm fifthly. Fengfu is needled 0.7 cm sixthly. Jiache is needled 3.3 cm seventhly. Chengjiang is needled 1 cm eighthly. Jianshi is needled 2 cm ninthly. Shenting is needled 0.7 cm tenthly. Xingjian is needled 1.2 cm eleventhly. Last, the middle cap below the tounge (Shefeng) is pricked to bleed. Ruzhong is used to locate the points only. The above two points are punctured with instantly-puncturing method, and needle are not retained in them.

柱神
Zhushen

组成 本穴组由身柱、本神二穴组合而成。
位置 身柱：第三胸椎棘突下。

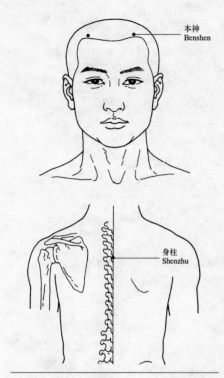

图 4-87 柱神
Fig. 4-87 Zhushen

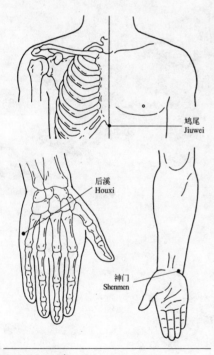

图 4-88 五痫
Fig. 4-88 Wuxian

tendon of the ulnar flexor muscle of the wrist.

Indication　Five kinds of epilepsy.

Method　Houxi is penetrated 0.5−1.2 cun towards Hegu. Jiuwei and Shenmen are needled 0.5−1.2 cun under the skin.

Note　An other group is composed of Jiuwei and Houxi only, the effect is good too.

镇痫
Zhenxian

组成　本穴组由鸠尾、涌泉二穴组合而成。

位置　鸠尾：剑突下，脐上7寸。

涌泉：足底(去趾)前1/3处，足趾跖屈时呈凹陷处。

主治　痫证。

操作　鸠尾针尖向下斜刺0.4～0.6寸，得气为度。涌泉直刺0.5～1寸，足底有痛胀感。

Composition　This group of acupoints is composed of Jiuwei (CV15) and Yongquan (KI1).

Location　Jiuwei：below the xiphoid process, 7 cun above the centre of the umbilicus.

Yongquan：at the junction of the anterior one-third and middle one-third of the sole (the toes are not included), i.e. in the depression when the toes are extended downwards.

Indication　Epilepsy.

Method　Jiuwei is needled 0.4−0.6 cun downwards obliquely till the acu-esthesia is obtained.

Yongquan is needled 0.5−1 cun perpendicularly, the acu-esthesia of pain and soreness will be obtained in the sole.

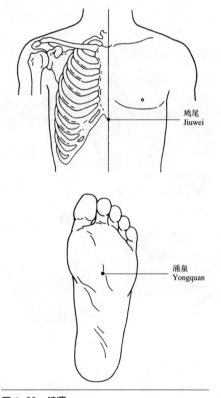

鸠尾
Jiuwei

涌泉
Yongquan

图 4−89　镇痫
Fig. 4−89　Zhenxian

心神
Xinshen

组成　本穴组由心俞、神门二穴组合而成。

位置　心俞：第五胸椎棘突下，旁开1.5寸。

神门：腕横纹尺侧端，尺侧腕屈肌腱的桡侧凹陷中。

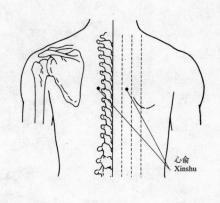

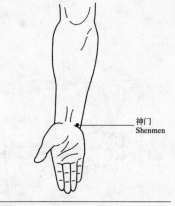

心俞
Xinshu

神门
Shenmen

图4-90 心神
Fig. 4-90 Xinshen

主治 呆滞如愚，精神恍惚，频频叹气，悲伤欲哭，胸闷急躁，虚烦不眠。

操作 斜向棘突针心俞0.5~0.8寸，得气后，用泻法持续运针2分钟，或用艾条悬灸5~10分钟。神门直刺0.3~0.5寸，或用艾条悬灸3~5分钟，留针30分钟。

Composition This group of acupoints is composed of Xinshu (BL15) and Shenmen (BL62).

Location Xinshu：1.5 cun lateral to the point below the spinous process of the 5th thoracic vertebra.

Shenmen：on the ulnar end of the palmar crease of the wrist, in the depression of the radial side of the tendon of the ulnar flexor muscle of the wrist.

Indication Dullness, trance, frequent sigh, sadness, irritability, insomnia due to deficiency.

Method Xinshu is needled 0.5−0.8 cun obliquely towards the spinous process. After the arrival of the acu−esthesia, manipulate the needle with reducing techniques for 2 minutes, or suspended moxibustion with moxa roll for 3−5 minutes can be applied to Xinshu. Shenmen is needled 0.3−0.5 cun perpendicularly, or suspended moxibustion with moxa roll for 3−5 minutes. The needle in Shenmen is retained for 30 minutes.

 安心

Anxin

组成 本穴组由心俞、厥阴俞、膻中、内关、神门五穴组合而成。

位置 心俞：第五胸椎棘突下，旁开1.5寸。

厥阴俞：第四胸椎棘突下，旁开1.5寸。

膻中：前正中线，平第四肋间隙。

内关：腕横纹上2寸，掌长肌腱与桡侧腕屈肌腱之间。

神门：腕横纹尺侧端，尺侧腕屈肌腱的桡侧凹陷中。

主治 心脏病。

操作 刺法：心俞、厥阴俞向脊柱方向斜刺0.5~0.8寸。膻中、神门沿皮刺0.5~1寸。内关、郄门直刺0.8~1.2寸。各以得气为度。

灸法：艾条温灸10~20分钟。

按注 临床另一穴组加郄门、间使，效同。

Composition   This group of acupoints is composed of Xinshu (BL15), Jueyinshu (BL14), Danzhong (CV17), Neiguan (PC6) and Shenmen (BL62).

Location   Xinshu: 1.5 cun lateral to the point below the spinous process of the 5th thoracic vertebra.

Jueyinshu: 1.5 cun lateral to the point below the spinous process of the 4th thoracic vertebra.

Danzhong: on the anterior midline, at the horizontal level of the 4th intercostal space.

Neiguan: 2 cun above the palmar crease of the wrist, between the tendons of the long palmar muscle and radial flexor muscle of the wrist.

Shenmen: on the ulnar end of the palmar crease of the wrist, in the depression of the radial side of the tendon of the ulnar flexor muscle of the wrist.

Indication   Heart diseases.

Method   Acupuncture: Xinshu and Jueyinshu are needled 0.5−0.8 cun obliquely towards the spine. Danzhong and Shenmen are needled 0.5−1 cun under the skin. Neiguan and Ximen are needled 0.8−1.2 cun till the acu-esthesia is obtained.

Moxibustion: warm moxibustion with moxa roll for 10−20 minutes is applied.

Note   There's another group is composed of the above points and Ximen, Jianshi, but the effect is similar.

三通谷
Santonggu

组成   本穴组由足通谷、腹通谷与胸通谷三穴组成。

位置   足通谷：第五跖趾关节前缘，赤白肉际处。

腹通谷：脐上5寸，前正中线旁开0.5寸。

胸通谷：在乳头直下2寸处。

主治   心痛，胸胁痛。

操作   刺法：足通谷直刺0.3～0.5寸。胸通谷斜刺0.5～0.8寸。

灸法：艾炷灸3～5壮，或温灸10～20分钟。

Composition   This group of acupoints is composed of Zutonggu (BL66), Futonggu (KI20) and Xiongtonggu.

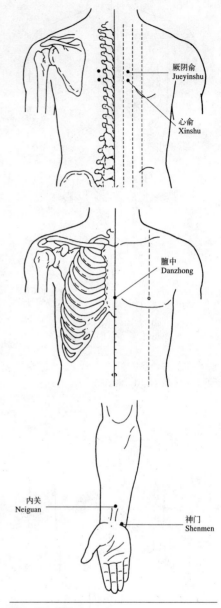

图4-91 安心
Fig. 4-91 Anxin

Location Zutonggu: anterior to the 5th metatar-sophalangeal joint, at the junction of the red and white skin.

Futonggu: 5 cun above the centre of the umbilicus, 0.5 cun lateral to the midline.

Xiongtonggu: 2 cun directly below the nipple.

Indication Headache, pain in the chest and hypochondriac region.

Method Acupuncture: Zutonggu is needled 0.3−0.5 cun perpendicularly, Xiongtonggu 0.5−0.8 cun obliquely.

Moxibustion: 3−5 cones of moxibustion, or 10−20 minutes' warm moxibustion is applied.

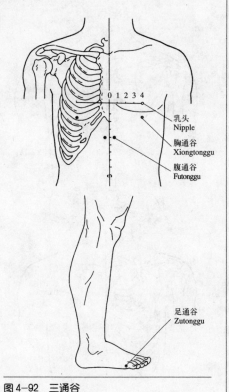

图4-92 三通谷
Fig. 4-92 Santonggu

● 陵脘 Lingwan

组成 本穴组由大陵、中脘二穴组合而成。

位置 大陵：腕横纹中央，掌长肌腱与桡侧腕屈肌腱之间。

中脘：脐上4寸。

主治 心胸疼痛。

操作 大陵直刺0.5~0.8寸。中脘直刺1~1.5寸。各以得气为度。

Composition This group of acupoints is composed of Daling (PC7) and Zhongwan (CV12).

Location Daling: at the midpoint of the palmar crease of the wrist, between the tendons of the long palmar muscle and radial flexor muscle of the wrist.

Zhongwan: 4 cun above the centre of the umbilicus.

Indication Pain in the heart and chest.

Method Daling is needled 0.5−0.8 cun perpendicularly. Zhongwan is needled 1−1.5 cun perpendicularly till the acu−esthesia is obtained.

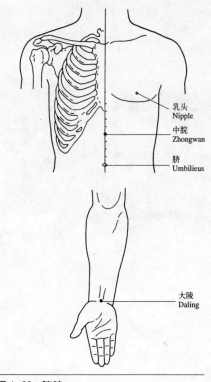

图4-93 陵脘
Fig. 4-93 Lingwan

● 膻关 Tanguan

组成 本穴组由膻中、内关二穴组合而成。

位置 膻中：前正中线，平第四肋间隙。

内关：腕横纹上2寸，掌长肌腱与桡侧腕屈肌腱之间。

主治　心胸疾病。

操作　直刺或斜刺0.5～1.0寸。

Composition　This group of acupoints is composed of Danzhong (CV17) and Neiguan (PC6).

Location　Danzhong：on the anterior midline, at the horizontal level of the 4th intercostal space.

Neiguan：2 cun above the palmar crease of the wrist, between the tendons of the long palmar muscle and radial flexor muscle of the wrist.

Indication　Diseases of the heart and chest.

Method　The needle is inserted 0.5－1 cun perpendicularly or obliquely.

膻门
Tanmen

组成　本穴组由膻中、郄门二穴组合而成。

位置　膻中：前正中线，平第四肋间隙。

郄门：腕横纹上5寸，掌长肌腱与桡侧腕屈肌腱之间。

主治　心胸疾病。

操作　直刺或斜刺0.5～1.2寸。

Composition　This group of acupoints is composed of Danzhong (CV17) and Ximen (PC4).

Location　Danzhong：on the anterior midline, at the horizontal level of the 4th intercostal space.

Ximen：5 cun above the palmar crease of the wrist, between the tendons of the long palmar muscle and radial flexor muscle of the wrist.

Indication　Diseases of the heart and chest.

Method　The needle is inserted 0.5－1.2 cun perpendicularly or obliquely.

脘渚
Wanzhu

组成　本穴组由中脘、中渚二穴组合而成。

位置　中脘：脐上4寸。

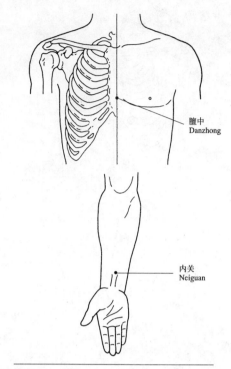

图4-94　膻关
Fig. 4-94　Tanguan

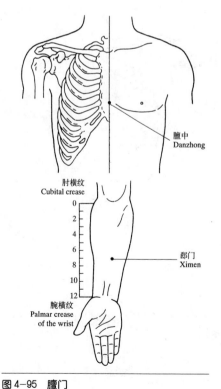

图4-95　膻门
Fig. 4-95　Tanmen

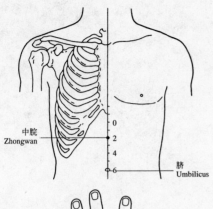

中脘
Zhongwan

脐
Umbilicus

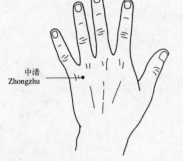

中渚
Zhongzhu

图4-96 脘渚
Fig. 4-96 Wanzhu

中渚：握拳，第四、第五掌骨小头后缘之间凹陷中，液门穴后1寸。

主治 脊间后心痛。

操作 中脘直刺1～1.5寸。中渚直刺0.5～0.8寸，得气为度。

Composition This group of acupoints is composed of Zhongwan (CV12) and Zhongzhu (TE3).

Location Zhongwan：4 cun above the centre of the umbilicus.

Zhongzhu：in the depression on the posterior border of the heads of the 4th and 5th metacarpal bones when a fist is made, 1 cun posterior to Yemen.

Indication Pain of the spine and heart.

Method Zhongwan is needled 1-1.5 cun perpendicularly.

Zhongzhu is needled 0.5-0.8 cun perpendicularly till the acu-esthesia is obtained.

宽胸
Kuanxiong

组成 本穴组由内关、郄门、膻中三穴组合而成。

位置 内关：腕横纹上2寸，掌长肌腱与桡侧腕屈肌腱之间。

郄门：腕横纹上5寸，掌长肌腱与桡侧腕屈肌腱之间。

膻中：前正中线，平第四肋间隙。

主治 胸闷，胸痛。

操作 见安心。

Composition This group of acupoints is composed of Neiguan (PC6), Ximen (PC4) and Danzhong (CV17).

Location Neiguan：2 cun above the palmar crease of the wrist, between the tendons of the long palmar muscle and radial flexor muscle of the wrist.

Ximen：5 cun above the palmar crease of the wrist, between the tendons of the long palmar muscle and radial flexor muscle of the wrist.

Danzhong：on the anterior midline, at the horizontal level of the 4th intercostal space.

Indication Stuffy chest, pain in the chest.

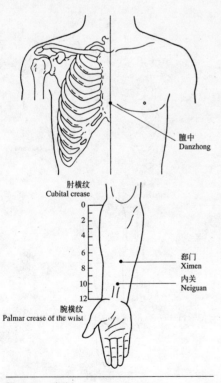

膻中
Danzhong

肘横纹
Cubital crease

郄门
Ximen

内关
Neiguan

腕横纹
Palmar crease of the wrist

图4-97 宽胸
Fig. 4-97 Kuanxiong

Method　See Anxin.

消闷
Xiaomen

　　组成　本穴组由中脘、内关二穴组合而成。
　　位置　中脘：脐上4寸。
　　内关：腕横纹上2寸，掌长肌腱与桡侧腕屈肌腱之间。
　　主治　胸闷，胃病。
　　操作　刺法：直刺0.5～1寸，得气为度。
　　灸法：艾炷灸3～5壮，艾条灸10～20分钟。

Composition　This group of acupoints is composed of Zhongwan (CV12) and Neiguan (PC6).

Location　Zhongwan：4 cun above the centre of the umbilicus.

Neiguan：2 cun above the palmar crease of the wrist, between the tendons of the long palmar muscle and radial flexor muscle of the wrist.

Indication　Stuffy chest, diseases of the stomach.

Method　Acupuncture：the needle is inserted 0.5-1 cun perpendicularly till the acu-esthesia is obtained.

Moxibustion：moxibustion with 3-5 moxa cones, or moxibustion with moxa roll for 10-20 minutes is applied.

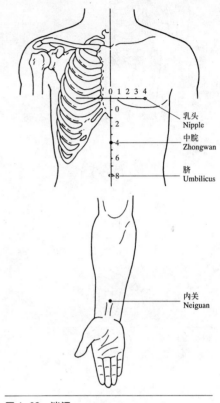
图4-98　消闷
Fig. 4-98　Xiaomen

平逆
Pingni

　　组成　本穴组由膻中、中脘、大陵三穴组合而成。
　　位置　膻中：前正中线，平第四肋间隙。
　　中脘：脐上4寸。
　　大陵：腕横纹中央，掌长肌腱与桡侧腕屈肌腱之间。
　　主治　咳逆频噫，上气咳逆阵作，胸胁胀痛，咳时引痛，噫气频频，脘腹满胀。
　　操作　膻中、大陵针0.6～0.9寸，用泻法。中脘针1.2～1.4寸，用补法，留针30分钟，灸用7～14壮。

Composition　This group of acupoints is composed of Danzhong (CV17), Zhongwan (CV12) and Daling (PC7).

　　Location　Danzhong：on the anterior midline, at

horizontal the level of the 4th intercostal space.

Zhongwan: 4 cun above the centre of the umbilicus.

Daling: at the midpoint of the palmar crease of the wrist, between the tendons of the long palmar muscle and radial flexor muscle of the wrist.

Indications Frequent cough and hiccup, distension and pain in the chest and hypochondriac region, pain when coughing, abdominal distension.

Method Danzhong and Daling are needled 0.6−0.9 cun with reducing techniques. Zhongwan is needled 1.2−1.4 cun with reinforcing techniques. Retain the needles for 30 minutes. 7−14 cones of moxibustion is applied.

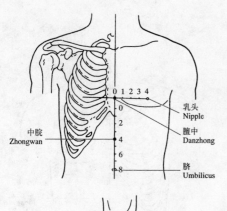

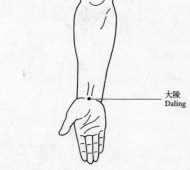

图4-99 平逆
Fig. 4-99 Pingni

膻里四关
Tanlisiguan

组成 本穴组由膻中、足三里、四关三穴组合而成。

位置 膻中：前正中线，平第四肋间隙。

足三里：犊鼻穴下3寸，胫骨前嵴外一横指处。

四关：即由合谷、太冲组合而成。

合谷：手背，第一、第二掌骨之间，约平第二掌骨中点处。

太冲：足背，第一、第二跖骨结合部之前凹陷中。

主治 呃逆。

操作 膻中沿皮刺。足三里直刺1~1.5寸。四关直刺0.5~1寸，得气为度，留针30分钟。

Composition This group of acupoints is composed of Danzhong (CV17), Zusanli (ST36) and Siguan.

Location Danzhong: on the anterior midline, at the horizontal level of the 4th intercostal space.

Zusanli: 3 cun below Dubi, one finger breadth from the anterior crest of the tibia.

Siguan: composed of Hegu and Taichong.

Hegu: on the dorsum of the hand, between the 1st and 2nd metacarpal bones, and near the midpoint of the 2nd metacarpal bone.

Taichong: on the instep of the foot, in the depression anterior to the commissure of the 1st and 2nd metatarsal bones.

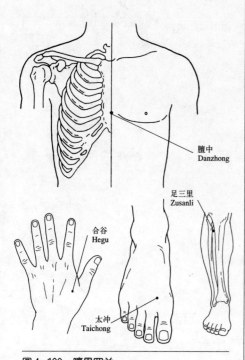

图 4-100 膻里四关
Fig. 4-100 Tanlisiguan

Indication　Hiccup.

Method　Danzhong is needled subcutaneously. Zusanli is needled 1–1.5 cun perpendicularly. Siguan 0.5–0.7 cun, till the acu-esthesia is obatined. Retain the needles for 30 minutes.

消嚏
Xiaoyi

组成　本穴组由天突、内关、膻中三穴组合而成。

位置　天突：胸骨上窝正中。

膻中：前正中线，平第四肋间隙。

内关：腕横纹上2寸，掌长肌腱与桡侧腕屈肌腱之间。

主治　嚏症。

操作　刺法：天突刺0.3～0.5寸。膻中沿皮刺0.5～1寸。内关针0.5～1寸。各以得气为度。

灸法：艾炷灸5～9壮，艾条灸10～30分钟。

Composition　This group of acupoints is composed of Tiantu (CV22), Neiguan (PC6) and Danzhong (CV17).

Location　Tiantu：in the centre of the suprasternal fossa.

Danzhong：on the anterior midline, at the horizontal level of the 4th intercostal space.

Neiguan：2 cun above the palmar crease of the wrist, between the tendons of the long palmar muscle and radial flexor muscle of the wrist.

Indication　Belching diseases.

Methods　Acupuncture：Tiantu is needled 0.3–0.5 cun. Danzhong is needled 0.5–1 cun under the skin. Neiguan is needled 0.5–1 cun. Stop manipulating the needles after the arrival of the acu-esthesia.

Moxibustion：5–9 cones of moxibustion, or 10–30 minutes' moxibustion with moxa roll is applied.

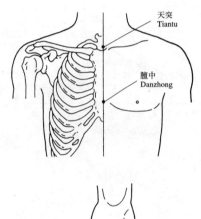
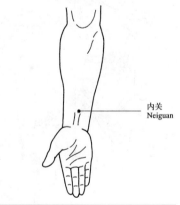

图4-101　消嚏
Fig. 4-101　Xiaoyi

翻胃穴
Fanweixue

组成　本穴组由上穴乳下与下穴内踝部前下方的一个刺激

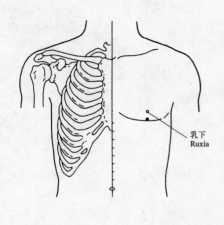

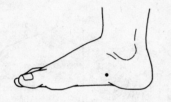

图 4-102 翻胃穴
Fig. 4-102 Fanweixue

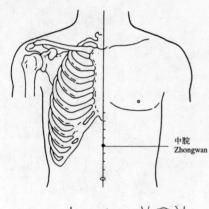

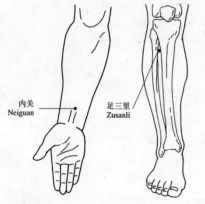

图 4-103 胃三针
Fig. 4-103 Weisanzhen

点组合而成。

位置 上穴：即"乳下"穴，位于乳头直下1寸处。

下穴：位于足内踝前下方3横指，在赤白肉际处。

主治 翻胃。

操作 艾炷灸5~9壮，或温灸10~30分钟。

Composition   This group of acupoints is composed of the upper point Ruxia and the lower point which is anterior and inferior to the medial malleolus.

Location   The upper point：Ruxia, 1 cun directly below the nipple.

The lower point：3 finger breadth anterior and inferior to the medial malleolus, at the junction of the red and white skin.

Indication   Nausea.

Method   5-9 cones of moxibustion, or 10-30 minutes' warm moxibustion is applied.

 胃三针
Weisanzhen

组成 本穴组由中脘、内关、足三里三穴组合而成。

位置 中脘：脐上4寸。

内关：腕横纹上2寸，掌长肌腱与桡侧腕屈肌腱之间。

足三里：犊鼻穴下3寸，胫骨前嵴外一横指处。

主治 各种胃病。

操作 中脘、内关直刺0.5~1寸。足三里直刺1~1.5寸。各以得气为度。

Composition   This group of acupoints is composed of Zhongwan(CV12), Neiguan(PC6) and Zusanli(ST36).

Location   Zhongwan：4 cun above the centre of the umbilicus.

Neiguan：2 cun above the palmar crease of the wrist, between the tendons of the long palmar muscle and radial flexor muscle of the wrist.

Zusanli：3 cun below Dubi, one finger breadth from the anterior crest of the tibia.

Indication   Diseases of the stomach.

Method   Zhongwan and Neiguan are needled 0.5-1 cun perpendicularly. Zusanli is needled 1-1.5 cun perpendicularly. Stop manipulating the needles after the arrival of the acu-esthesia.

胃宁
Weining

组成　本穴组由中脘、梁丘、足三里、胃俞四穴组合而成。

位置　中脘：脐上4寸。

梁丘：在髂前上棘与髌骨外缘连线上，髌骨外上缘上2寸。

足三里：犊鼻穴下3寸，胫骨前嵴外一横指处。

胃俞：第十二胸椎棘突下，旁开1.5寸。

主治　胃痛。

操作　刺法：中脘、梁丘、足三里直刺1~1.5寸。胃俞向脊柱方向斜刺0.5~0.8寸。

灸法：艾炷灸3~5壮，艾条灸10~20分钟。

Composition　This group of acupoints is composed of Zhongwan(CV12), Liangqiu(ST34), Zusanli(ST36) and Weishu(BL21).

Location　Zhongwan：4 cun above the centre of the umbilicus.

Liangqiu：on the line connecting the anteriosuperior iliac spine and the lateral corner of the patella, 2 cun above the superiolateral border of the patella.

Zusanli：3 cun below Dubi, one finger breadth from the anterior crest of the tibia.

Weishu：1.5 cun lateral to the point below the spinous process of the 12th thoracic vertebra.

Indications　Stomachache.

Methods　Acupuncture：Zhongwan, Liangqiu and Zusanli are needled 1−1.5 cun perpendicularly. Weishu is needled 0.5−0.8 cun obliquely with the needle tip towards the spine.

Moxibustion：moxibustion with 3−5 moxa cones, or moxibustion with moxa roll for 10−20 minutes is applied.

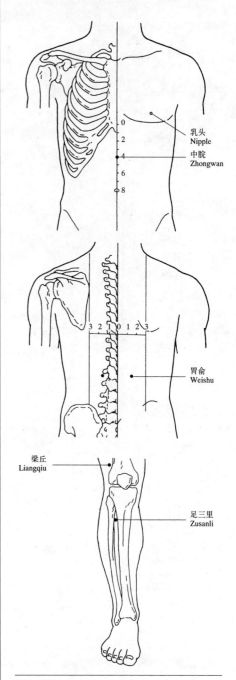

图 4-104　**胃宁**

Fig. 4-104　Weining

安胃

Anwei

组成 本穴组由胃俞、中脘、内关、足三里四穴组合而成。

位置 胃俞：第十二胸椎棘突下，旁开1.5寸。

中脘：脐上4寸。

内关：腕横纹上2寸，掌长肌腱与桡侧腕屈肌腱之间。

足三里：犊鼻穴下3寸，胫骨前嵴外一横指处。

主治 各种胃病。

操作 刺法：中脘、足三里、胃俞见"胃宁"。内关直刺0.5~1寸。各以得气为度。

灸法：艾炷灸3~5壮，艾条灸10~20分钟。

Composition This group of acupoints is composed of Weishu(BL21), Zhongwan(CV12), Neiguan(PC6) and Zusanli(ST36).

Location Weishu：1.5 cun lateral to the point below the spinous process of the 12th thoracic vertebra.

Zhongwan：4 cun above the centre of the umbilicus.

Neiguan：2 cun above the palmar crease of the wrist, between the tendons of the long palmar muscle and radial flexor muscle of the wrist.

Zusanli：3 cun below Dubi, one finger breadth from the anterior crest of the tibia.

Indications Diseases of the stomach.

Methods Acupuncture：Zhongwan, Zusanli and Weishu：see Weining. Neiguan is needled 0.5-1 cun. Stop manipulating the needles after the arrival of the acu-esthesia.

Moxibustion：Moxibustion with 3-5 moxa cones, or moxibustion with moxa roll for 10-20 minutes is applied.

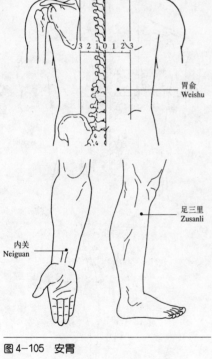

0
2
4
6
8

乳头
Nipple

中脘
Zhongwan

脐
Umbilicus

3 2 1 0 1 2 3

胃俞
Weishu

足三里
Zusanli

内关
Neiguan

图4-105 安胃
Fig. 4-105 Anwei

 提胃

Tiwei

组成 本穴组由中脘、足三里、胃上三穴组合而成。

位置 中脘：脐上4寸。

足三里：犊鼻穴下3寸，胫骨前嵴外一横指处。

胃上：在脐上2寸，任脉旁开4寸，当大横穴上2寸处。

主治　胃下垂。

操作　隔日针1次，每次留针20分钟左右，中间行针2~3次。胃上穴斜刺进针8~10厘米，采用中强刺激手法。

Composition　This group of acupoints is composed of Zhongwan(CV12), Zusanli(ST36) and Weishang.

Location　Weishang：2 cun above the centre of the umbilicus, 4 cun lateral to anterior midline, i.e. about 2 cun above Daheng.

Zhongwan：4 cun above the centre of the umbilicus.

Zusanli：3 cun below Dubi, one finger breadth from the anterior crest of the tibia.

Indication　Gastroptosis.

Method　Treat once every other day. Retain the needles for about 20 minutes each time. Manipulate the needles for 2−3 times during the retention. Weishang is needled 8−10 cm obliquely with the medium or strong stimulating intensity.

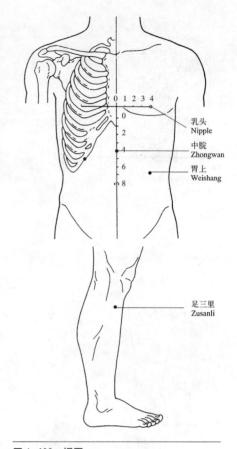

图4-106　提胃
Fig. 4-106　Tiwei

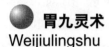

胃九灵术
Weijiulingshu

组成　本穴组由巨阙、中脘、下脘、梁门、强壮、保健六穴组成。

位置　巨阙：脐上6寸。

中脘：脐上4寸。

下脘：脐上2寸。

强壮：前臂伸侧桡侧线、肘横纹下3寸。

保健：小腿胫骨粗隆下3寸，胫骨前嵴外开3寸。

梁门：脐上4寸，前正中线旁开2寸。

主治　急、慢胃痛呕吐，泄泻，痢疾。

操作　刺法：巨阙、中脘、梁门、下脘穴针0.5~1寸，针感有局部沉、麻。强壮穴针0.5~0.8寸，针感麻、酸至腕。保健穴针0.5~1寸，针感麻、酸至外踝。

灸法：灸3~9壮，艾条灸10~20分钟。

按注　另一组穴加由胃九灵术的穴位加肓俞组成，治胃溃疡。

Composition　This group of acupoints is composed of Juque(CV14), Zhongwan(CV12), Xianwan(CV10), Liangmen(ST21), Qiangzhuang and Baojian.

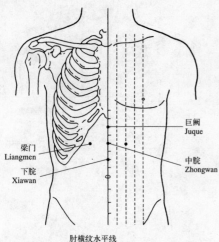

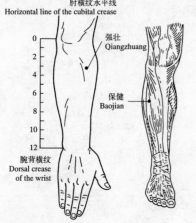

图 4-107　胃九灵术
Fig. 4-107　Weijiulingshu

Location　Juque：6 cun above the centre of the umbilicus.

Zhongwan：4 cun above the centre of the umbilicus.

Xiawan：2 cun above the centre of the umbilicus.

Qiangzhuang：on the radial side of the lateral aspect of the forearm, 3 cun below the cubital crease.

Baojian：3 cun below the medial condyle of the tibia, 2 cun lateral to the anterior crest of the tibia.

Liangmen：4 cun above the centre of the umbilicus, 2 cun lateral to the anterior midline.

Indication　Acute and chronic stomachache, vomiting, dirrhea, dysentery.

Method　Acupuncture：Juque, Zhongwan, Liangmen and Xiawan are needled 0.5−1 cun, the acu-esthesia of heaviness and numbness will be obtained in this part. Qiangzhuang is needled 0.5−0.8 cun, the acu-esthesia of numbness and soreness will be induced to the wrist. Baojian is needled 0.5−1 cun, the acu-esthesia of numbness and soreness will radiate to the external malleolus.

Moxibustion：3−9 cones of moxibustion, or moxibustion with moxa roll for 10−20 minutes is applied.

Note　Another group of acupoints is composed of points in Weijiulingshu and Huangshu. This group is used to treat gastric ulcer.

 治肝十七术
Zhiganshiqishu

组成　本穴组由胃九灵术(由任脉的巨阙、中脘、下脘、胃经的梁门和属于奇穴的强壮和保健穴组成)、肓俞、幽门、阴都、商曲和治肝十八穴组合而成。

位置　胃九灵术：见胃九灵术。

肓俞：脐旁 0.5 寸。

商曲：脐上 2 寸，前正中线旁开 0.5 寸。

阴都：脐上 4 寸，前正中线旁开 0.5 寸。

幽门：脐上 6 寸，前正中线旁开 0.5 寸。

治肝：胸部乳头直下肋弓缘下 2 分处，取右侧。

主治　急、慢性肝炎，肝硬化，脾肿大。

操作　刺法：巨阙、中脘、梁门、下脘穴针 0.5~1 寸，针感局部沉、麻。强壮穴针0.5～1寸，针感麻、酸至腕。保健穴针0.5～1寸，针感麻、酸至外踝。肓俞、幽门、商曲、阴都、治肝穴针0.5～1寸，针感局部沉麻。

灸法：灸3～9壮，艾条灸10～20分钟。

Composition This group of acupoints is composed of Weijiulingshu, Huangshu(KI16), Youmen(KI21), Yindu (KI19), Shangqu(KI17) and Zhiganxue.

Location Weijiulingshu：see Weijiulingshu.

Huangshu：0.5 cun lateral to the centre of the umbilicus.

Shangqu：2 cun above the centre of the umbilicus, 0.5 cun lateral to the anterior midline.

Yindu：4 cun above the centre of the umbilicus, 0.5 cun lateral to the anterior midline.

Youmen：6 cun above the centre of the umbilicus, 0.5 cun lateral to the anterior midline.

Zhiganxue：directly below the nipple on the chest, 0.2 cun below the costal arch, the point on the right side is selected.

Indication Acute and chronic hepatitis, hepatocirrhosis, splenomegaly.

Method Acupuncture：Juque, Zhongwan, Liangmen and Xiawan are needled 0.5−1 cun, the acu-esthesia of heaviness and numbness will be obtained in this part. Qiangzhuang is needled 0.5−0.8 cun, the acu-esthesia of numbness and soreness will radiate to the wrist. Baojian is needled 0.5−1 cun, the acu-esthesia of numbness and soreness will radiate to the external malleolus. Huangshu, Youmen, Shangqu, Yindu and Zhiganxue are needled 0.5−0.8 cun, the acu-esthesia of heaviness and distension will be obtained in the part.

Moxibustion：3−9 cones of moxibustion, or moxibustion with moxa roll for 10−20 minutes is applied.

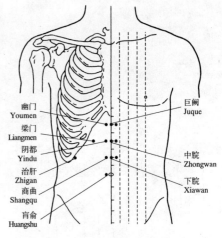
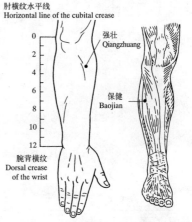

图4-108 治肝十七术
Fig. 4-108 Zhiganshiqishu

⬤ 泻黄
Xiehuang

组成 本穴组由公孙、至阳、脾俞、胃俞四穴组合而成。
位置 公孙：第一跖骨基底部的前下缘，赤白肉际。

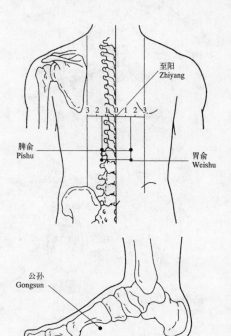

图4-109 泻黄
Fig. 4-109 Xiehuang

至阳：第七胸椎棘突下。

脾俞：第十一胸椎棘突下，旁开1.5寸。

胃俞：第十二胸椎棘突下，旁开1.5寸。

主治 黄疸。

操作 先刺脾俞、胃俞，向脊柱方向斜刺0.5~0.8寸，用补法。再刺公孙、至阳，深0.5~0.8寸用泻法，得气后出针。

Composition This group of acupoints is composed of Gongsun(SP3), Zhiyang(GV9), Pishu(BL20) and Weishu (BL21).

Location Gongsun：anterior and inferior to the base of the 1st metatarsal bone, on the junction of the red and white skin.

Zhiyang：below the spinous process of the 7th thoracic vertebra.

Pishu：1.5 cun lateral to the point below the spinous process of the 11th thoracic vertebra.

Weishu：1.5 cun lateral to the point below the spinous process of the 12th thoracic vertebra.

Indication Jaundice.

Method First Pishu and Weishu are needled 0.5−0.8 cun obliquely towards the spine with the reinforcing techniques. Then Gongsun and Zhiyang are needled 0.5−0.8 cun with reducing techniques. Withdraw the needles after the arrival of the acu-esthesia.

消疸
Xiaodan

组成 本穴组由至阳、太冲、阳陵泉、足三里四穴组合而成。

位置 至阳：第七胸椎棘突下。

太冲：足背，第一、第二跖骨结合部之前凹陷中。

阳陵泉：腓骨小头前下方凹陷中。

足三里：犊鼻穴下3寸，胫骨前嵴外一横指处。

主治 黄疸。

操作 刺法：至阳、太冲向上斜刺0.5~0.8寸。足三里、阳陵泉直刺1~1.5寸。各以得气为度。

灸法：艾炷灸3~5壮，艾条灸10~30分钟。

Composition This group of acupoints is composed of

Zhiyang(GV9), Taichong(LR3), Yanglingquan(GB34) and Zusanli(ST36).

Location　Zhiyang：below the spinous process of the 7th thoracic vertebra.

Taichong：on the instep of the foot, in the depression anterior to the commissure of the 1st and 2nd metatarsal bones.

Yanglingquan：in the depression anterior and inferior to the head of the fibula.

Zusanli：3 cun below Dubi, one finger breadth from the anterior crest of the tibia.

Indication　Jaundice.

Method　Acupuncture：Zhiyang and Taichong are needled 0.5−0.8 cun upwards obliquely. Zusanli and Yanglingquan are needled 1−1.5 cun perpendicularly. Stop manipulating the needles after the arrival of the acu-esthesia.

Moxibustion：moxibustion with 3−5 moxa cones, or moxibustion with moxa roll for 10−30 minutes is applied.

● 去黄十九术
Quhuangshijiushu

组成　本穴组由幽门、阴都、商曲、肓俞、巨阙、中脘、下脘、治肝、梁门、人中、阳陵泉、涌泉十九穴组合而成。

位置　幽门：脐上6寸，前正中线旁开0.5寸。

阴都：脐上4寸，前正中线旁开0.5寸。

商曲：脐上2寸，前正中线旁开0.5寸。

肓俞：脐旁0.5寸。

巨阙：脐上6寸。

中脘：脐上4寸。

下脘：脐上2寸。

治肝：乳头直下肋弓缘下0.2寸处(取右侧)。

梁门：脐上4寸，前正中线旁开2寸。

人中：在人中沟的上1/3与中1/3交界处。

阳陵泉：腓骨小头前下方凹陷中。

涌泉：足底(去趾)前1/3处，足趾跖屈时呈凹陷处。

主治　黄疸。

操作　幽门、阴都、商曲、肓俞、巨阙、中脘、下脘、治

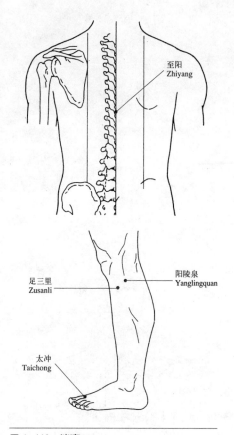

图4-110　消疸
Fig. 4-110　Xiaodan

肝、梁门穴针0.5～0.8寸，针感局部沉、胀。人中穴针0.1～0.2寸，针感痛。阳陵泉穴针1寸，针感麻、酸至外踝。涌泉穴针0.3～0.5寸，针感痛、麻至趾。

Composition This group of acupoints is composed of Youmen(KI21), Yindu(KI19), Shangqu(KI17), Huangshu (KI16), Juque(CV14), Zhongwan(CV12), Xiawan(CV10), Zhigan, Liangmen(ST34), Renzhong(GV26), Yanglingquan (GB34) and Yongquan(KI1).

Location Youmen：6 cun above the centre of the umbilicus, 0.5 cun lateral to the anterior midline.

Yindu：4 cun above the centre of the umbilicus, 0.5 cun lateral to the anterior midline.

Shangqu：2 cun above the centre of the umbilicus, 0.5 cun lateral to the anterior midline.

Huangshu：0.5 cun lateral to the centre of the umbilicus.

Juque：6 cun above the centre of the umbilicus.

Zhongwan：4 cun above the centre of the umbilicus.

Xiawan：2 cun above the centre of the umbilicus.

Zhigan：directly below the nipple, 0.2 cun below the costal arch, the point on the right side is selected.

Liangmen：4 cun above the centre of the umbilicus, 2 cun lateral to the anterior midline.

Renzhong：at the junction of the upper one-third and middle one-third of the philtrum.

Yanglingquan：in the depression anterior and inferior to the head of the fibula.

Yongquan：at the junction of the anterior one-third and middle one-third of the sole (the toes are not included), i.e. in the depression when the toes are extended downwards.

Indication Jaundice.

Method Youmen, Yindu, Shangqu, Huangshu, Juque, Zhongwan, Xiawan, Zhigan and Liangmen are needled 0.5—0.8 cun, the acu-esthesia of heaviness and distenstion will be obtained in the pat. Renzhong is needled 0.1—0.2 cun, the acu-esthesia is pain. Yanglingquan is needled 1 cun, the acu-esthesia of numbness and soreness will radiate to the external malleolus. Yongquan is needled 0.3—0.5 cun, the acu-esthesia of pain and numbness will radiate to the toes.

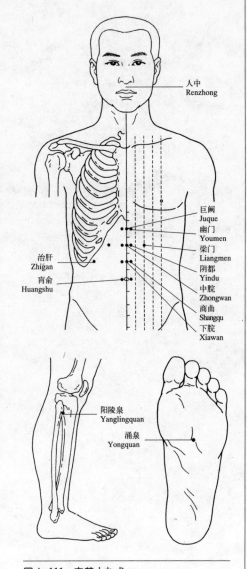

人中
Renzhong

巨阙
Juque
幽门
Youmen
梁门
Liangmen
阴都
Yindu
中脘
Zhongwan
商曲
Shangqu
下脘
Xiawan

治肝
Zhigan
肓俞
Huangshu

阳陵泉
Yanglingquan
涌泉
Yongquan

图4-111 去黄十九术
Fig. 4-111 Quhuangshijiushu

舒肝
Shugan

组成　本穴组由肝俞、太冲二穴组合而成。

位置　肝俞：第九胸椎棘突下，旁开1.5寸。

太冲：足背，第一、第二跖骨结合部之前凹陷中。

主治　肝病，胆囊病，高血压病，头痛眩晕等。

操作　刺法：肝俞向脊柱方向斜刺0.5～0.8寸。太冲向上斜刺0.5～1寸，得气为度。

灸法：肝俞艾炷灸5～9壮。太冲艾条灸5～15分钟。

Composition　This group of acupoints is composed of Ganshu(BL18) and Taichong(LR3).

Location　Ganshu：1.5 cun lateral to the point below the spinous process of the 9th thoracic vertebra.

Taichong：on the instep of the foot, in the depression anterior to the commissure of the 1st and 2nd metatarsal bones.

Indication　Diseases of the liver and gallbladder, hypertension, headache, vertigo.

Method　Acupuncture：Ganshu is needled 0.5—0.8 cun with the needle tip towards the spine obliquely.

Taichong is needled 0.5—1 cun obliquely upwards till the acu-esthesia is obtained.

Moxibustion：5—9 cones of moxibustion is applied to Ganshu. 5—15 minutes' moxibustion with moxa roll is applied to Taichong.

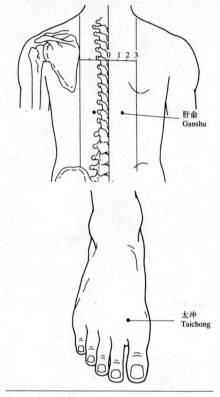

图4-112　舒肝
Fig. 4-112　Shugan

利胆
Lidan

组成　本穴组由胆俞、阳陵泉二穴组合而成。

位置　胆俞：第十胸椎棘突下，旁开1.5寸。

阳陵泉：腓骨小头前下方凹陷中。

主治　各种胆疾。

操作　刺法：胆俞向脊柱方向斜刺0.5～0.8寸。阳陵泉直刺1～1.5寸，得气为度。

灸法：艾炷灸5～9壮，艾条灸10～30分钟。

Composition　This group of acupoints is composed of

Danshu(BL19) and Yanglingquan(GB34).

Location Danshu：1.5 cun lateral the point below the spinous process of the 10th thoracic vertebra.

Yanglingquan：in the depression anterior and inferior to the head of the fibula.

Indication Gallbladder diseases.

Method Acupuncture：Danshu is needled 0.5−0.8 cun with the needle tip towards the spine. Yanglingquan is needled 1−1.5 cun perpendicularly till the acu-esthesia is obtained.

Moxibustion：moxibustion with 5−9 moxa cones, or moxibustion with moxa roll for 10−30 minutes is applied.

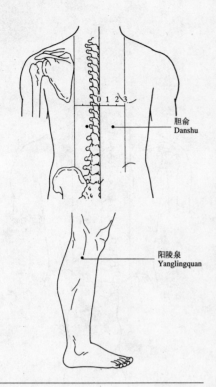

图4-113 利胆
Fig. 4-113 Lidan

● 胆三针
Dansanzhen

组成 本穴组由日月、期门、阳陵泉三穴组合而成。
位置 日月：乳头下方，第七肋间隙。
阳陵泉：腓骨小头前下方凹陷中。
期门：乳头直下，第六肋间隙。
主治 胆疾病。
操作 日月、期门平刺0.8～1寸。阳陵泉直刺1～1.5寸。各以得气为度。

Composition This group of acupoints is composed of Riyue(GB24), Qimen(LR14) and Yanglingquan(GB34).

Location Riyue：below the nipple, in the 7th intercostal space.

Yanglingquan：in the depression anterior and inferior to the head of the fibula.

Qimen：directly below the nipple, in the 6th intercostal space.

Indication Diseases of the gallbladder.

Method Riyue and Qimen are needled 0.8−1 cun horizontally.

Yanglingquan is needled 1−1.5 cun perpendicularly. Stop manipulating the needles after the arrival of the acu-esthesia.

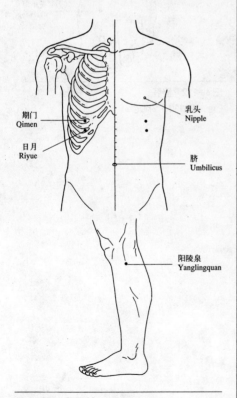

图4-114 胆三针
Fig. 4-114 Dansanzhen

胆痛
Dantong

组成　本穴组由日月、太冲、阳陵泉、胆囊四穴组成。

位置　日月：乳头下方，第七肋间隙。

阳陵泉：腓骨小头前下方凹陷中。

太冲：足背，第一、第二跖骨结合部之前凹陷中。

胆囊穴：腓骨小头前下方之阳陵泉穴下1～2寸处。

主治　胆绞痛。

操作　日月斜刺或平刺0.5～0.8寸。太冲直刺或斜刺0.5～0.8寸。阳陵泉、胆囊穴直刺1～2寸。各以得气为度。

Composition　This group of acupoints is composed of Riyue(GB24), Taichong(LR3), Yanglingquan(GB34) and Dannang(EX-LE6).

Location　Riyue：below the nipple, in the 7th intercostal space.

Yanglingquan：in the depression anterior and inferior to the head of the fibula.

Taichong　on the instep of the foot, in the depression anterior to the commissure of the 1st and 2nd metatarsal bones.

Dannangxue：1-2 cun below Yanglingquan which is in the depression anterior and inferior to the head of the fibula.

Indication　Colic gallbladder.

Method　Riyue is needled 0.5-0.8 cun obliquely or horizontally. Taichong is needled 0.5-0.8 cun perpendicularly or obliquely. Yanglingquan and Dannang are needled 1-2 cun perpendicularly. Stop manipulating the needles till the arrival of the acu-esthesia.

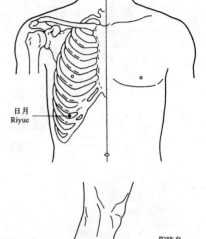

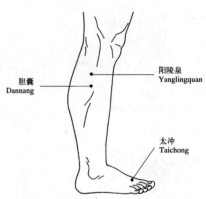

图4-115　胆痛
Fig. 4-115　Dantong

胆绞
Danjiao

组成　本穴组由胆俞、阳陵泉(或胆囊穴)二穴组合而成。

位置　胆俞：第十胸椎棘突下，旁开1.5寸。

阳陵泉：腓骨小头前下方凹陷中。

胆囊穴：见胆痛中奇穴胆囊穴。

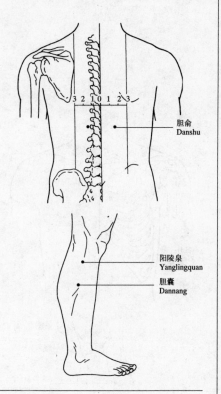

图4-116 胆绞
Fig. 4-116 Danjiao

主治　胆绞痛。

操作　胆俞针尖向脊椎方向斜刺0.5～0.8寸。阳陵泉或胆囊穴直刺1～2寸。各以得气为度。

Composition　This group of acupoints is composed of Danshu(BL19) and Yanglingquan(GB34) or Dannang(EX-LE6).

Location　Danshu：1.5 cun lateral to the point below the spinous process of the 10th thoracic vertebra.

Yanglingquan：in the depression anterior and inferior to the head of the fibula.

Dannang：see Dannang in Dantong.

Indication　Colic gallbladder.

Method　Danshu is needled 0.5-0.8 cun obliquely with the tip of the needle towards the spine. Yanglingquan or Dannang is needled 1-2 cun perpendicularly. Stop manipulating the needles after the arrival of the acu-esthesia.

● 膈孔
Gekong

组成　本穴组由膈俞、孔最二穴组合而成。

位置　膈俞：第七胸椎棘突下，旁开1.5寸。

孔最：尺泽穴与太渊穴连线上，腕横纹上7寸处。

主治　上焦血证，以肺系出血为主。

操作　斜刺0.5～0.8寸。

按注　本组穴属血会和郄穴组合。

Composition　This group of acupoints is composed of Geshu(BL17) and Kongzui(LV6).

Location　Geshu：1.5 cun lateral to the point below the spinous process of the 7th thoracic vertebra.

Kongzui：on the line connecting Chize and Taiyuan, 7 cun above the palmar crease of the wrist.

Indication：Blood syndromes of the upper jiao, the bleeding diseases of the lung system in particular.

Method　The needle is inserted 0.5-0.8 cun obliquely.

Note　This group is composed of the Influential Point of Blood and the Xi-Cleft Point.

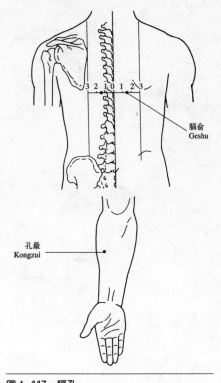

图4-117 膈孔
Fig. 4-117 Gekong

膈地
Gedi

组成　本穴组由膈俞、地机二穴组合而成。

位置　膈俞：第七胸椎棘突下，旁开1.5寸。

地机：阴陵泉穴下3寸。

主治　下焦血证(以治妇人出血为主)。

操作　斜刺0.5～0.8寸。

按注　本组穴也属血会和郄穴组合。

Composition This group of acupoints is composed of Geshu(BL17) an Diji(SP8).

Location Geshu：1.5 cun lateral to the point below the spinous process of the 7th thoracic vertebra.

Diji：3 cun below Yinlingquan.

Indication Blood syndromes of the lower jiao, especially the bleeding diseases of the female.

Method The needle is inserted 0.5—0.8 cun obliquely.

Note This group is composed of the Influential Point of Blood and the Xi-Cleft Point.

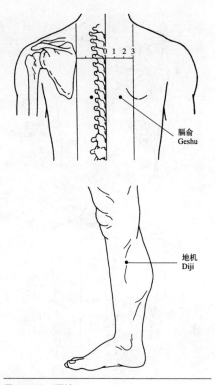

图4-118　膈地
Fig. 4-118 Gedi

归经
Guijing

组成　本穴组由隐白、脾俞、上脘、肝俞四穴组合而成。

位置　隐白：蹑趾内侧趾甲角旁约0.1寸。

上脘：脐上5寸。

脾俞：第十一胸椎棘突下，旁开1.5寸。

肝俞：第九胸椎棘突下，旁开1.5寸。

主治　脾阳不足之吐血、衄血。

操作　先取坐位或俯卧位，针脾俞、肝俞，针向脊柱斜刺0.4~0.6寸，使针感向下或沿肋骨向前放散。然后取仰卧位，针上脘1寸，使胀、麻感沿任脉向上、向下或向两侧放散，隐白针0.2～0.3寸，或灸2~3壮，或直接灸10分钟。

Composition This group of acupoints is composed of Yinbai(SP1), Pishu(BL20), Shangwan(CV13) and Ganshu (BL18).

Location Yinbai：0.1 cun from the corner of the toenail of the medial side of the great toe.

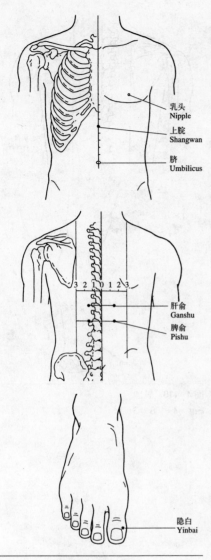

乳头
Nipple

上脘
Shangwan

脐
Umbilicus

3 2 1 0 1 2 3

肝俞
Ganshu

脾俞
Pishu

隐白
Yinbai

图4-119 归经
Fig. 4-119 Guijing

Shangwan: 5 cun above the centre of the umbilicus.

Pishu: 1.5 cun lateral to the point below the spinous process of the 11th thoracic vertebra.

Ganshu: 1.5 cun lateral to the point below the spinous process of the 9th thoracic vertebra.

Indication Haematemesis and epistaxis due to the deficiency of the spleen yang.

Method Sitting or prone position is selected first. Pishu and Ganshu are needled 0.4—0.6 cun towards the spine , and the acu-esthesia will spread downwards or forwards along the ribs. Then supine position is selected. Shangwan is needled 1 cun, and the acu-esthesia of distension and numbness will spread upwards, downwards along the anterlor midline, or to both lateral sides. Yinbai is needled 0.2—0.3 cun, or it can be treated with 10 minutes' direct moxibustion.

补中灸
Buzhongjiu

组成 本穴组由中脘、气海、足三里三穴组合而成。

位置 中脘：脐上4寸。

气海：脐下1.5寸。

足三里：犊鼻穴下3寸，胫骨前嵴外一横指处。

主治 脾胃气虚，纳呆，脘胀痞满，呃逆呕吐，大便溏泻，肠鸣，形体羸瘦，四肢无力，气短懒言；或兼低热不退，或身体沉重，下肢寒冷，或胃脘冷痛。

操作 每穴灸7～21壮。

Composition This group of acupoints is composed of Zhongwan(CV12), Qihai(CV6) and Zusanli(ST36).

Location Zhongwan: 4 cun above the centre of the umbilicus.

Qihai: 1.5 cun below the centre of the umbilicus.

Zusanli: 3 cun below Dubi, one finger breadth from the anterior crest of the tibia.

Indication Deficinecy of the spleen and stomach qi, anorexia, abdominal distension, hiccup, vomiting, loose stool, borborygmus, emaciation, weakness of the four limbs, shortness of breath, or with low fever, or with heavy feeling of the body, cold feeling of the lower limbs, or with stomachache due to cold.

Method：Moxibustion is applied to all the points, and 7-21 cones for each point.

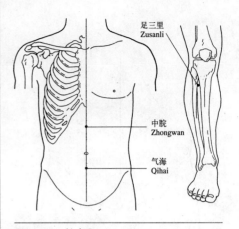

图 4-120 补中灸
Fig. 4-120 Buzhongjiu

● 寒水泻
Hanshuixie

组成　本穴组由气海、水分、足三里三穴组合而成。

位置　气海：脐下1.5寸。

水分：脐上1寸。

足三里：犊鼻穴下3寸，胫骨前嵴外一横指处。

主治　寒湿滞留胃肠，便泄清稀，水谷相杂，肠鸣腹痛，身寒喜暖。

操作　气海、水分用温灸20~30分钟。足三里用艾炷灸5~9壮，或温灸至局部红润为佳。

Composition　This group of acupoints is composed of Qihai(CV6), Shuifen(CV9) and Zusanli(ST36).

Location　Qihai：1.5 cun below the centre of the umbilicus.

Shuifen：1 cun above the centre of the umbilicus.

Zusanli：3 cun below Dubi, one finger breadth from the anterior crest of the tibia.

Indication　Cold and damp stagnation in the intestine and stomach, loose stool with undigested food, borborygmus, abdominal pain, cold feeling of the body which may be relieved by warmth.

Method　Warm moxibustion for 20-30 minutes is applied to Qihai and Shuifen. 5-9 cones of moxibustion, or warm moxibustion is applied to Zusanli till the skin becomes reddish in the part.

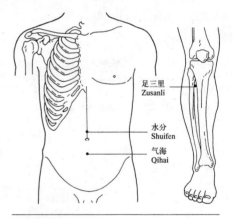

图 4-121 寒水泻
Fig. 4-121 Hanshuixie

● 肠三针
Changsanzhen

组成　本穴组由天枢、关元、上巨虚三穴组合而成。

位置　天枢：脐旁2寸。

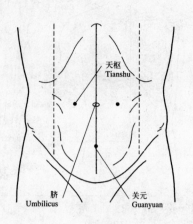

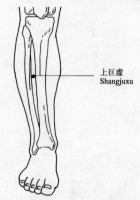

图4-122 肠三针
Fig. 4-122 Changsanzhen

关元：脐下3寸。
上巨虚：足三里穴下3寸。
主治　腹痛，肠炎，痢疾，便秘。
操作　天枢、关元直刺0.8～1.2寸。上巨虚直刺1～1.5寸。各以得气为度。

Composition　This group of acupoints is composed of Tianshu(ST25), Guanyuan(CV4) and Shangjuxu(ST37).

Location　Tianshu：2 cun lateral to the centre of the umbilicus.

Guanyuan：3 cun below the centre of the umbilicus.
Shangjuxu：3 cun below Zusanli.

Indication　Abdominal pain, enteritis, dysentery, constipation.

Method　Tianshu and Guanyuan are needled 0.8-1.2 cun perpendicularly.

Shangjuxu is needled 1-1.5 cun perpendicularly. Stop manipulating the needles till the arrival of the acuesthesia.

消胀
Xiaozhang

组成　本穴组由天枢、气海、内关、足三里四穴组合而成。
位置　天枢：脐旁2寸。
足三里：犊鼻穴下3寸，胫骨前嵴外一横指处。
气海：脐下1.5寸。
内关：腕横纹上2寸，掌长肌腱与桡侧腕屈肌腱之间。
主治　腹胀。
操作　内关针0.5～0.8寸。天枢、气海、足三里针1～1.5寸。各以得气为度，留针30分钟，中间每隔5～10分钟，运针1次。

Composition　This group of acupoints is composed of Tianshu(ST25), Qihai(CV6), Neiguan(PC6) and Zusanli(ST36).

Location　Tianshu：2 cun lateral to the centre of the umbilicus.

Zusanli：3 cun below Dubi, one finger breadth from the anterior crest of the tibia.

Qihai：1.5 cun below the centre of the umbilicus.

Neiguan：2 cun above the palmar crease of the wrist, between the tendons of the long palmar muscle and radial flexor muscle of the wrist.

Indication Abdominal distension.

Method Neiguan is needled 0.5−0.8 cun.

Tianshu, Qihai and Zusanli are needled 1−1.5 cun till the acu-esthesia is obtained. Retain the needles for 30 minutes. Manipulate the needles every 5−10 minutes during the retention of the needles.

消块
Xiaokuai

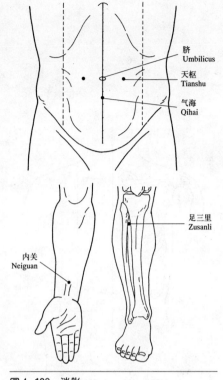

图 4-123 消胀
Fig. 4-123 Xiaozhang

组成 本穴组由大陵、中脘、三阴交三穴组合而成。

位置 大陵：腕横纹中央，掌长肌腱与桡侧腕屈肌腱之间。

中脘：脐上4寸。

三阴交：内踝高点上3寸，胫骨内侧面后缘。

主治 腹有积块，初起软而不坚，久则按之觉硬，痛处不移，面黯消瘦，体倦乏力，饮食减少，时有寒热。女子或见经闭不行。

操作 仰卧位针三阴交，然后取中脘、大陵，得气后诸穴均留针30分钟，三阴交亦可加灸。

Composition This group of acupoints is composed of Daling(PC7), Zhongwan(CV12) and Sanyinjiao(SP6).

Location Daling：at the midpoint of the palmar crease of the wrist, between the tendons of the long palmar muscle and radial flexor muscle of the wrist.

Zhongwan：4 cun above the centre of the umbilicus.

Sanyinjiao：3 cun above the tip of the medial malleolus, on the posterior border of the medial side of the tibia.

Indications Abdominal mass which is soft first, and turns hard then, darkish complexion, emaciation, weakness, anorexia, fever, possible amenorrhea in female.

Method Sanyinjiao is puntured when the supine position is selected. Then Zhongwan and Daling is needled. Retain the needleds for 30 minutes after the arrival of the acu-esthesia. Sanyinjiao may be treated with moxibustion too.

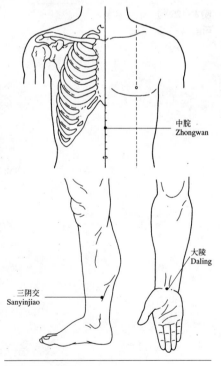

图 4-124 消块
Fig. 4-124 Xiaokuai

止痢
Zhili

组成 本穴组由下脘、天枢、照海三穴组合而成。

位置 下脘：脐上2寸。

天枢：脐旁2寸。

照海：内踝下缘凹陷中。

主治 急性痢疾，腹痛下痢赤白，里急后重，肛门灼热，小便短赤。

操作 先针下脘、天枢，直刺1~1.2寸，均用泻法；再针照海；直刺0.3~0.5寸。平补平泻，行针1~2次，留针30分钟。

Composition This group of acupoints is composed of Xiawan(CV10), Tianshu(ST25) and Zhaohai(KI6).

Location Xiawan：2 cun above the centre of the umbilicus.

Tianshu：2 cun lateral to the centre of the umbilicus.

Zhaohai：in the depression on the lower border of the medial malleolus.

Indication Acute dysentery, abdominal pain, frequent stools containeing blood and mucus, tenesmus, burning sensation in the anus, scanty and yellow urine.

Method Xiawan and Tianshu is needled 1−1.2 cun perpendicularly first with reducing techniques. Then Zhaohai is needled 0.3−0.5 cun with even reinforcing-reducing techniques. Manipulate the needles for 1−2 times, Retain the needles for 30 minutes.

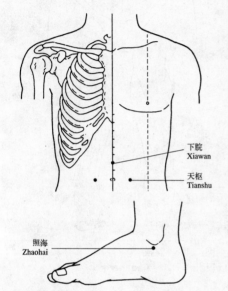

图4-125 止痢
Fig. 4-125 Zhili

小腹镇痛七灵术
Xiaofuzhentongqilingshu

组成 本穴组由石门、府舍、理中、行间、太冲五穴组合而成。

位置 石门：脐下2寸。

府舍：冲门穴外上方0.7寸，前正中线旁开4寸。

行间：足背，第一、第二趾间缝纹端。

理中：胫骨粗隆下3寸，胫骨前嵴外开1寸处。

太冲：在人中沟的上1/3与中1/3交界处。

主治 小腹痛，肠痛，痛经。

操作 石门、府舍针0.5~1寸,针感向下抽、胀;理中针1~1.5寸,针感麻酸至外踝;行间穴进针后向上斜刺0.5~1寸透向太冲穴,针感抽、胀至趾。

Composition This group of acupoints is composed of Shimen(CV5), Fushe(SP13), Lizhong and Xingjian(LR2) penetrating to Taichong(LR2).

Location Shimen: 2 cun below the centre of the umbilicus.

Fushe: 0.7 cun lateral and superior to Chongmen, 4 cun lateral to the anterior midline.

Xingjian: on the instep of the foot, on the end of the margin of the web between the 1st and 2nd toes.

Lizhong: 3 cun below the medial condyle of the tibia, 2 cun lateral to the anterior crest of the tibia.

Taichong: on the instep of the foot, in the depression anterior to the commissure of the 1st and 2nd metatarsal bones.

Indication Pain in the lower abdomen, appendicitis, dysmenorrhea.

Method Shimen and Fushe are needled 0.5−1 cun, the acu-esthesia of distension will spread downwards. Lizhong is needled 1−1.5 cun, the acu-esthesia of numbness and soreness will radiate to the external malleolus. Xingjian is penetrated 0.5−1 cun to Taichong upwards obliquely, the acu-esthesia of twitching and distenstion will radiate to the toes.

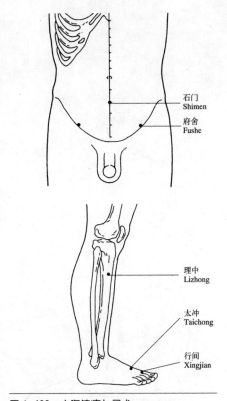

图4-126 小腹镇痛七灵术
Fig. 4-126 Xiaofuzhentongqilingshu

滑泻
Huaxie

组成 本穴组由百会、脾俞、肾俞三穴组合而成。
位置 百会:后发际正中直上7寸。
脾俞:第十一胸椎棘突下,旁开1.5寸。
肾俞:第二腰椎棘突下,旁开1.5寸。
主治 泄泻日久,水谷不化,大便滑脱不禁。
操作 先针脾俞,深0.5~0.8寸。肾俞针1~1.5寸,用补法,留针30分钟,同时加温灸10~15分钟。最后再将艾条点灸百会10分钟。

Composition This group of acupoints is composed of

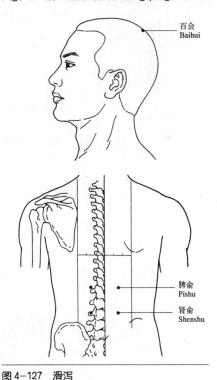

图4-127 滑泻
Fig. 4-127 Huaxie

Baihui(GV20), Pishu(BL20) and Shenshu(BL23).

Location Baihui：7 cun directly above the midpoint of the posetrior hairline.

Pishu：1.5 cun lateral to the point below the spinous process of the 11th thoracic vertebra.

Shenshu：1.5 cun lateral to the point below the spinous process of the 2nd lumbar vertebra.

Indication Prolonged diarrhea with undigested food, incontinent defecation.

Method Pishu is needled 0.5−0.8 cun first. Shenshu is needled 1−1.5 cun with reinforcing techniques. Retain the needles for 30 mnitues, and warm moxibustion for 10−15 minutes is applied at the same time. Point-moxibustion with moxa roll for 10 minutes is applied to Baihui last.

⬤ 枢沟
Shugou

组成 本穴组由天枢、支沟二穴组合而成。

位置 天枢：脐旁2寸。

支沟：腕背横纹上3寸，桡骨与尺骨之间。

主治 便秘。

操作 直刺1~1.5寸，得气后用泻法。

Composition This group of acupoints is composed of Tianshu(ST25) and Zhigou(TE6).

Location Tianshu：2 cun lateral to the centre of the umbilicus.

Zhigou：2 cun above the dorsal crease of the wrist, between the radius and ulna.

Indication Constipation.

Method The needle is inserted 1−1.5 cun. Reducing techniques are applied after the arrival of the acu-esthesia.

⬤ 肛痔
Gangzhi

组成 本穴组由二白、百会、志室、长强四穴组合而成。

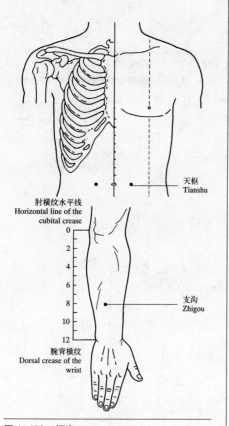

天枢
Tianshu

肘横纹水平线
Horizontal line of the cubital crease

0
2
4
6
8
10
12

支沟
Zhigou

腕背横纹
Dorsal crease of the wrist

图 4-128 枢沟
Fig. 4-128 Shugou

位置　二白：腕横纹上四寸，桡侧屈腕肌腱二侧。

长强：尾骨尖下0.5寸，约当尾骨尖端与肛门的中点。

百会：后发际正中直上7寸。

志室：第二腰椎棘突下，旁开3寸。

主治　脱肛及痔疮。

操作　俯卧位，艾条悬灸百会10~20分钟，针二白，然后针志室、长强。诸穴用补法，得气后留针30分钟，长强亦可用灸。

Composition　This group of acupoints is composed of Erbai(EX-UE2), Baihui(GV20), Zhishi(BL52) and Changqiang(GV1).

Location　Erbai：4 cun above the palmar crease of the wrist, on each side of the tendon of the radial flexor muscle of the wrist.

Changqiang：0.5 cun below the tip of the coccyx, at the midpoint of the line connecting the tip of the coccyx and anus.

Baihui：7 cun directly above the midpoint of the posetrior hairline.

Zhishi：3 cun lateral to the point below the spinous process of the 2nd lumbar vertebra.

Indication　Prolapse of the rectum and hemorrhoids.

Method　The prone position is selected. Baihui is treated with suspended moxibustion with moxa roll for 10−20 minutes. Erbai is needled, then Zhishi and Changqian. Reinforcing techniques are applied to all the points. Retain the needles for 30 minutes after the arrival of the acu-esthesia. Moxibustion can be applied to Changqiang too.

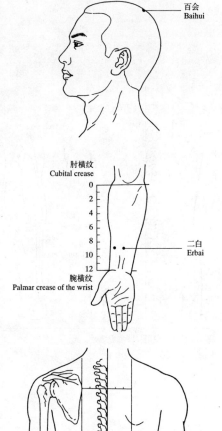

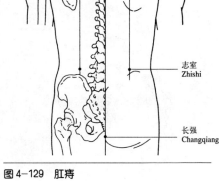

图4-129　肛痔
Fig. 4-129　Gangzhi

脱肛
Tuogang

组成　本穴组由长强、承山二穴组合而成。

位置　长强：尾骨尖下0.5寸，约当尾骨尖端与肛门的中点。

承山：腓肠肌两肌腹之间凹陷的顶端。

主治　脱肛。

操作　刺法：长强斜刺1~1.5寸，连续运针5~10分钟。

承山直刺1~1.5寸。各以得气为度。

灸法：艾条温灸10~30分钟。

Composition This group of acupoints is composed of Changqiang(GV1) and Chengshan(BL57).

Location Changqiang：0.5 cun below the tip of the coccyx, at the midpoint of the line connecting the tip of the coccyx and anus.

Chengshan：on the top of the depression below the belly of the gastrocnemius muscle.

Indication Prolapse of the rectum.

Method Acupuncture：Changqiang is needled 1−1.5 cun obliquely, manipulating the needle for 5−10 minutes continuously. Chengshan is needled 1−1.5 cun perpendicularly. Stop manipulating the needles after the arrival of the acu-esthesia.

Moxibustion：warm moxibustion with moxa roll for 10−30 minutes is applied.

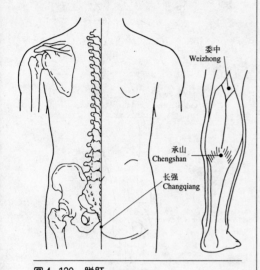

图4-130 脱肛
Fig. 4-130 Tuogang

会尾
Huiwei

组成 本穴组由百会、鸠尾二穴组合而成。

位置 百会：后发际正中直上7寸。

鸠尾：剑突下，脐上7寸。

主治 脱肛日久。

操作 先温灸百会1小时，后温灸鸠尾5~10分钟。

Composition This group of acupoints is composed of Baihui(GV20) and Jiuwei(CV15).

Location Baihui：7 cun directly above the midpoint of the posetrior hairline.

Jiuwei：below the xiphoid process, 7 cun above the centre of the umbilicus.

Indication Chronic prolapse of the rectum.

Method Baihui is treated with warm moxibustion for an hour first, then Jiuwei is treated with warm moxibustion for 5−10 minutes.

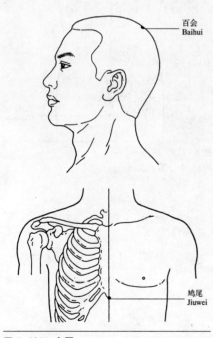

图4-131 会尾
Fig. 4-131 Huiwei

肛痒
Gangyang

组成　本穴组由百会、长强、次髎三穴组合而成。

位置　百会：后发际正中直上7寸。

长强：尾骨尖下0.5寸，约当尾骨尖端与肛门的中点。

次髎：第二骶后孔中，约当髂后上棘下与督脉连线的中点。

主治　肛门瘙痒。

操作　刺法：百会、长强沿皮刺0.5~1寸。次髎向第二骶后孔斜刺0.8~1.5寸，得气为度。

灸法：艾炷灸5~9壮，艾条温灸10~30分钟。

Composition　This group of acupoints is composed of Baihui(GV20), Changqiang(GV1) and Ciliao(BL32).

Location　Baihui：7 cun directly above the midpoint of the posetrior hairline.

Changqiang：0.5 cun below the tip of the coccyx, at the midpoint of the line connecting the tip of the coccyx and anus.

Ciliao：in the 2nd posterior sacral foramen, at the midpoint between the posterioinferior iliac spine and the posterior midline.

Indication　Itch in the anus.

Methods　Acupuncture：Baihui and Changqiang are needled 0.5−1 cun under the skin. Ciliao is needled 0.5−1.5 cun towards the 2nd posterior sacral foramen obliquely till the acu-esthesia is obtained.

Moxibustion：moxibustion with 5−9 moxa cones, or moxibustion with moxa roll for 10−30 minutes is applied.

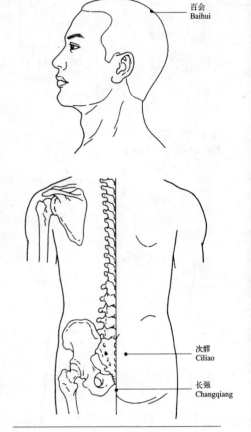

图4-132　肛痒
Fig. 4-132　Gangyang

肛痛
Gangtong

组成　本穴组由孔最、腰俞二穴组合而成。

位置　孔最：尺泽穴与太渊穴连线上，腕横纹上7寸处。

腰俞：当骶管裂孔处。

主治　肛门疼痛。

操作　刺法：腰俞由下向上沿皮刺0.5~0.8寸。孔最直刺0.5~1.2寸。得气为度。

灸法：艾条灸10~20分钟。

Composition This group of acupoints is composed of Kongzui(LV6) and Yaoshu(GV2).

Location Kongzui：on the line connecting Chize and Taiyuan, 7 cun above the palmar crease of the wrist.

Yaoshu：at the point of the sacral hiatus.

Indication Pain in the anus.

Method Acupuncture：Yaoshu is needled 0.5－0.8 cun upwards beneath the skin. Kongzui is needled 0.5－1.2 cun perpendicularly till the acu-esthesia is obtained.

Moxibustion：moxibustion with moxa roll for 10－20 minutes is applied.

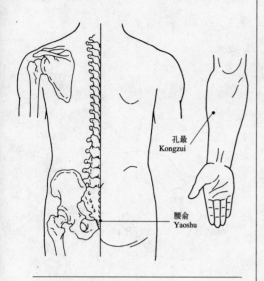

图4-133 肛痛
Fig. 4-133 Gangtong

针水
Zhenshui

组成 本穴组由水分、阴陵泉二穴组合而成。

位置 水分：脐上1寸。

阴陵泉：胫骨内侧髁下缘凹陷中。

主治 水疾。

操作 直刺0.5~1.2寸，得气为度，留针30分钟，可行提插捻转手法。

Composition This group of acupoints is composed of Shuifen(CV9) and Yinlingquan(SP9).

Location Shuifen：1 cun above the centre of the umbilicus.

Yinlingquan：in the depression below the medial condyle of the tibia.

Indication Diseases of water.

Method The needle is inserted 0.5－1.2 cun till the acu-esthesia is obtained. Retain the needle for 30 minutes. Lifing, inserting and rotating techniques may be applied.

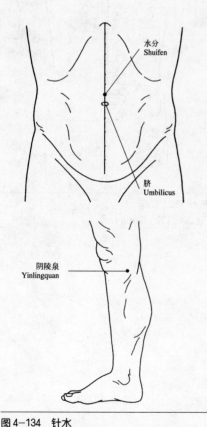

图4-134 针水
Fig. 4-134 Zhenshui

蛊胀
Guzhang

组成 本穴组由三阴交、水分、足三里三穴组合而成。

位置　三阴交：内踝高点上 3 寸，胫骨内侧面后缘。

水分：脐上 1 寸。

足三里：犊鼻穴下 3 寸，胫骨前嵴外一横指处。

主治　鼓胀。

操作　刺法：直刺 0.8～1.5 寸，得气为度。

灸法：艾炷灸 300 壮(累针灸 1 月量)，艾条灸 10～20 分钟。

Composition　This group of acupoints is composed of Sanyinjiao(SP6), Shuifen(CV9) and Zusanli(ST36).

Location　Sanyinjiao：3 cun above the tip of the medial malleolus, on the posterior border of the tibia.

Shuifen：1 cun above the centre of the umbilicus.

Zusanli：3 cun below Dubi, one finger breadth from the anterior crest of the tibia.

Indication　Ascites.

Method　Acupuncture：the needle is inserted 0.8–1.5 cun till the acu-esthesia is obtained.

Moxibustion　300 cones of moxibustion in one month, or moxibustion with moxa roll for 10–20 minutes is applied.

水气
Shuiqi

组成　本穴组由水沟、水分、神阙三穴组合而成。

位置　水沟：在人中沟的上 1/3 与中 1/3 交界处。

水分：脐上 1 寸。

神阙：脐的中间。

主治　水臌。

操作　先用艾条悬灸神阙 20～30 分钟，或隔姜灸 10～15 壮，艾炷如黄豆大；然后针刺水分，如腹大胀满，皮肤光亮，则用灸；针刺水沟得气后捻转 1 分钟后出针，亦可用艾条温灸。

Composition　This group of acupoints is composed of Renzhong(GV26), Shuifen(CV9) and Shenque(CV8).

Location　Renzhong：at the junction of the upper one-third and middle one-third of the philtrum.

Shuifen：1 cun above the centre of the umbilicus.

Shenque：in the centre of the umbilicus.

Indication　Ascites.

Method　First suspended moxibustion with moxa roll

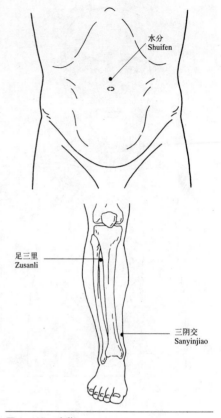

图 4-135　蛊胀

Fig. 4-135　Guzhang

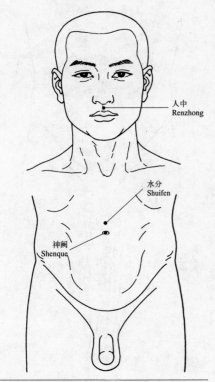

图4-136 水气
Fig. 4-136 Shuiqi

for 20-30 minutes is applied to Shenque, Shenque can also be treated with ginger-cushioned moxibustion, and the cone is about as big as the soybean. Then Shuifen is needled. For the patient of the abdominal distension with smooth and bright skin, moxibustion is applied. Renzhong is punctured and after the arrival of the acu-esthesia, the needle is rotated for 1 minute and then withdrew. Renzhong can also be treated with moxibustion with moxa roll or warm moxibustion.

● 水溜
Shuiliu

组成　本穴组由水分、复溜二穴组合而成。

位置　水分：脐上1寸。

复溜：太溪穴上2寸。

主治　腹水。

操作　刺法：直刺0.8~1.5寸，得气为度。

灸法：艾条灸10~20分钟。

Composition　This group of acupoints is composed of Shuifen(CV9) and Fuliu(KI7).

Location　Shuifen：1 cun above the centre of the umbilicus.

Fuliu：2 cun above Taixi.

Indication　Ascites.

Method　Acupuncture：the needle is inserted 0.8－1.5 cun till the acu-esthesia is obtained.

Moxibustion：moxibustion with moxa roll for 10－20 minutes is applied.

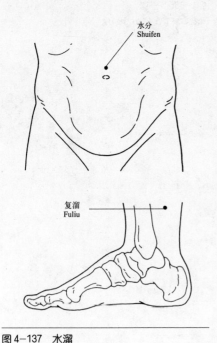

图4-137 水溜
Fig. 4-137 Shuiliu

● 浮肿
Fuzhong

组成　本穴组由肾俞、阴陵泉、复溜三穴组合而成。

位置　肾俞：第二腰椎棘突下，旁开1.5寸。

阴陵泉：胫骨内侧髁下缘凹陷中。

复溜：太溪穴上2寸。

主治　浮肿。

操作 刺法：直刺0.8~1.5寸，得气为度。

灸法：艾条灸10~20分钟。

Composition This group of acupoints is composed of Shenshu(BL23), Yinlingquan(SP9) and Fuliu(KI7).

Location Shenshu：1.5 cun lateral to the point below the spinous process of the 2nd lumbar vertebra.

Yinlingquan：in the depression below the medial condyle of the tibia.

Fuliu：2 cun above Taixi.

Indication Edema.

Method Acupuncture：the needle is inserted 0.8–1.5 cun till the acu-esthesia is obtained.

Moxibustion：moxibustion with moxa roll for 10–20 minutes is applied.

 ### 浮肿九灵术
Fuzhongjiulingshu

组成 本穴组由关元、中极、水分、水道、三阴交、行间六穴组合而成。

位置 关元：脐下3寸。

中极：脐下4寸。

水分：脐上1寸。

水道：脐下3寸，前正中线旁开2寸。

三阴交：内踝高点上3寸，胫骨内侧面后缘。

行间：足背，第一、第二趾间缝纹端。

主治 肾性水肿。

操作 刺法：关元、中极、水道穴针0.5~1.5寸，针感抽、胀至耻骨联合。水分穴针0.5~1寸，针感局部沉、胀。三阴交穴针0.5~1.2寸，针感麻、酸至内踝。行间穴进针后向上斜刺透向太冲穴，针感抽、胀至趾。

灸法：灸3~9壮，艾条温灸10~20分钟。

Composition This group of acupoints is composed of Guanyuan(CV4), Zhongji(CV3), Shuifen(CV9), Shuidao(ST28), Sanyinjiao(SP6) and Xingjian(LR2).

Location Guanyuan：2 cun below the centre of the umbilicus.

Zhongji：4 cun below the centre of the umbilicus.

Shuifen：1 cun above the centre of the umbilicus.

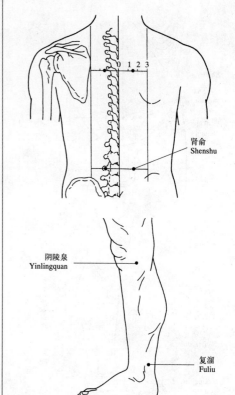

图4-138 浮肿
Fig. 4-138 Fuzhong

肾俞 Shenshu

阴陵泉 Yinlingquan

复溜 Fuliu

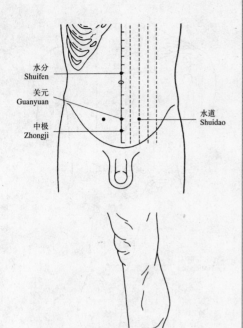

图 4-139 浮肿九灵术
Fig. 4-139 Fuzhongjiulingshu

Shuidao：3 cun below the centre of the umbilicus, 2 cun lateral to the anterior midline.

Sanyinjiao：3 cun above the tip of the medial malleolus, on the posterior border of the medial side of the tibia.

Xingjian：on the instep of the foot, on the end of the margin of the web between the 1st and 2nd toes.

Indication　Renal edema.

Method　Acupuncture：Guanyuan, Zhongji and Shuidao are needled 0.5-1.5 cun, the acu-esthesia of distension will spread to the symphysis pubis. Shuifen is needled 0.5-1 cun, and the acu-esthesia is the heaviness and distension in the part. Sanyinjiao is needled 0.5-1.2 cun, the acu-esthesia of numbness and soreness will spread to the medial malleolus. Xingjian is penetrated to Taichong upwards obliquely, the acu-esthesia of twitching and distension will radiate to the toes.

Moxibustion：3-9 cones of moxibustion, or warm moxibustion with moxa roll for 10-20 minutes is applied.

然交
Ranjiao

组成　本穴组由然谷、阴交二穴组合而成。

位置　然谷：足舟骨粗隆下缘凹陷中。

阴交：脐下1寸。

主治　肾病，肾虚。

操作　刺法：然谷直刺0.5～0.8寸，局部酸胀痛感。阴交直刺0.5～1.2寸，得气为度。

灸法：然谷麦粒灸3～5壮。阴交艾炷灸3～5壮。

Composition　This group of acupoints is composed of Rangu(KI2) and Yinjiao(CV7).

Location　Rangu：in the depression inferior to the tuberosity of the navicular bone.

Yinjiao：1 cun below the centre of the umbilicus.

Indications　Diseases of the kidney, deficiency of the kidney.

Methods　Acupuncture：Rangu is needled 0.5-0.8 cun perpendicularly, the acu-esthesia of soreness, distension and pain will be obtained in this part.

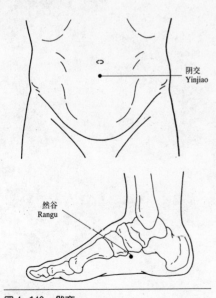

图 4-140 然交
Fig. 4-140 Ranjiao

Yinjiao is needled 0.5−1.2 cun perpendicularly till the acu-esthesia is obtained.

Moxibustion：3−5 cones wheat-sized moxa of moxibustion is applied to Rangu. 3−5 cones of moxibustion is applied to Yinjiao.

● 肾绞
Shenjiao

组成　本穴组由京门、水泉、肾俞、三阴交四穴组合而成。
位置　京门：第十二肋端。
水泉：太溪直下1寸。
肾俞：第二腰椎棘突下，旁开1.5寸。
三阴交：内踝高点上3寸，胫骨内侧面后缘。
主治　肾绞痛。
操作　京门斜刺0.5~0.8寸。水泉针0.5~0.8寸。肾俞、三阴交针1~1.5寸，得气为度。京门、肾俞针后可拔罐。
按注　临床也可只选取肾俞、三阴交二穴即可见效者。

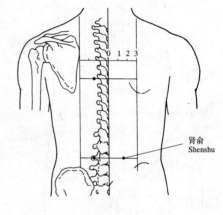

Composition　This group of acupoints is composed of Jingmen(GB25)，Shuiquan(KI5)，Shenshu(BL23) and Sanyinjiao(SP6).

Location　Jingmen：on the end of the 12th rib.

Shuiquan：1 cun directly below Taixi.

Shenshu：1.5 cun lateral to the point below the spinous process of the 2nd lumbar vertebra.

Sanyinjiao：3 cun above the tip of the medial malleolus, on the posterior border of the medial side of the tibia.

Indication　Renal colic.

Methods　Jingmen is needled 0.5−0.8 cun obliquely. Shuiquan is needled 0.5−0.8 cun. Shenshu and Sanyinjiao are needled 1−1.5 cun till the acu-esthesia is obtained. Cupping can be applied to Jingmen and Shenshu after acupuncture.

Note　In clinic use, Shenshu and Sanyinjiao may also take effect.

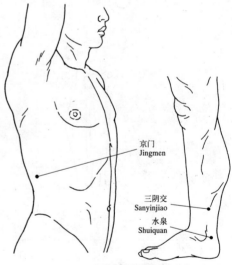

图4-141　肾绞
Fig. 4-141　Shenjiao

济阴阳
Jiyinyang

组成　本穴组由心俞、肾俞、关元、三阴交四穴组合而成。

位置　心俞：第五胸椎棘突下，旁开1.5寸。

肾俞：第二腰椎棘突下，旁开1.5寸。

关元：脐下3寸。

三阴交：内踝高点上3寸，胫骨内侧面后缘。

主治　心肾两虚之遗精。

操作　针心俞0.5~0.8寸，肾俞1~1.5寸，得气后持续运针2分钟。针关元、三阴交，得气为度，留针20~30分钟。

Composition　This group of acupoints is composed of Xinshu(BL15), Shenshu(BL23), Guanyuan(CV4) and Sanyinjiao(SP6).

Location　Xinshu：1.5 cun lateral to the point below the spinous process of the 5th thoracic vertebra.

Shenshu：1.5 cun lateral to the point below the spinous process of the 2nd lumbar vertebra.

Guanyuan：2 cun below the centre of the umbilicus.

Sanyinjiao：3 cun above the tip of the medial malleolus, on the posterior border of the medial side of the tibia.

Indication　Seminal emission due to the deficiency of the heart and kidney.

Method　Fisrt, Xinshu is needled 0.5-0.8 cun, Shenshu 1-1.5 cun. Manipulating the needles for 2 minutes continuously after the arrival of the acu-esthesia. Then Guanyuan and Sanyinjiao are needled till the acu-esthesia is obtained. Retain the needles for 20-30 minutes.

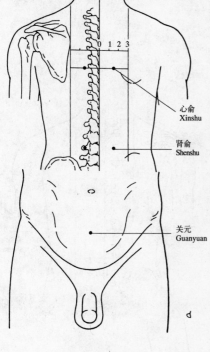

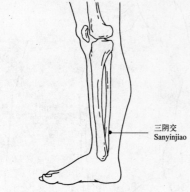

图4-142　济阴阳
Fig. 4-142　Jiyinyang

益肾
Yishen

组成　本穴组由肾俞、志室、太溪三穴组合而成。

位置　肾俞：第二腰椎棘突下，旁开1.5寸。

志室：第二腰椎棘突下，旁开3寸。

太溪：内踝高点与跟腱之间凹陷中。

主治　泌尿生殖系统各种病证，肾绞痛。

操作　刺法：肾俞见"肾绞"。志室斜刺0.5~0.8寸。太溪直刺0.5～1寸，得气为度。

灸法：艾条灸10～20分钟。

按注 临床用本穴组中的志室、太溪也可治疗肾绞痛，其效甚佳。

Composition This group of acupoints is composed of Shenshu(BL23), Zhishi(BL52) and Taixi(KI3).

Location Shenshu：1.5 cun lateral to the point below the spinous process of the 2nd lumbar vertebra.

Zhishi：3 cun lateral to the point below the spinous process of the 2nd lumbar vertebra.

Taixi：in the midpoint between the tip of the medial malleolus and Achilles's tendon.

Indications All kinds diseases of the urogenital system, renal colic.

Methods Acupuncture：Shenshu：see Shenjiao. Zhishi is needled 0.5–0.8 cun obliquely. Taixi is needled 0.5–1 cun perpendicularly till the acu-esthesia is obtained.

Moxibustion：moxibustion with moxa roll for 10–20 minutes is applied.

Note In clinic use, Zhishi and Taixi of this group is used to treat renal colic, the effect is quite good.

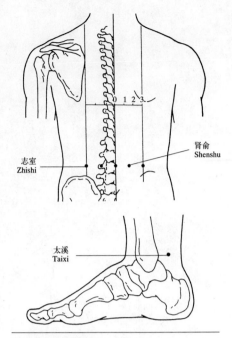

图4-143 益肾
Fig. 4-143 Yishen

利阴
Liyin

组成 本穴组由中极、关元、三阴交三穴组合而成。

位置 中极：脐下4寸。

关元：脐下3寸。

三阴交：内踝高点上3寸，胫骨内侧面后缘。

主治：泌尿生殖系统病证，如遗精，阳痿，早泄，尿失禁及妇科病等。

操作 刺法：三阴交直刺1～1.5寸，得气为度。中极、关元针感向外阴放散为佳。

灸法：艾炷灸5～9壮，艾条灸10～30分钟。

Composition This group of acupoints is composed of Zhongji(CV3), Guanyuan(CV4) and Sanyinjiao(SP6).

Location Zhongji：4 cun below the centre of the umbilicus.

Guanyuan：3 cun below the centre of the umbilicus.

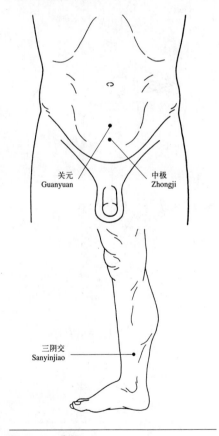

图4-144 利阴
Fig. 4-144 Liyin

Sanyinjiao: 3 cun above the tip of the medial malleolus, on the posterior border of the medial side of the tibia.

Indication Diseases of the urogenital system, such as seminal emission, impotence, premature ejaculation, incontinence of urine and female diseases.

Method Acupuncture: The needle is inserted 1—1.5 cun perpendicularly. Stop manipulating the needle in Sanyinjiao till the acu-esthesia is obtained.

The curative effect will be better if the acu-esthesia of Zhongji and Guanyuan transmits to the pubes.

Moxibustion: 5—9 cones of moxibustion, or 10—30 minutes moxibustion with moxa roll is applied.

● 涩溲
Sesou

组成 本穴组由中极、肾俞、阴陵泉三穴组合而成。

位置 中极：脐下4寸。

肾俞：第二腰椎棘突下，旁开1.5寸。

阴陵泉：胫骨内侧髁下缘凹陷中。

主治 肾气不足之小便频数，尿频而清长，或兼尿遗失禁，伴面色㿠白，头晕耳鸣，气短喘逆，腰膝无力，四肢不温。

操作 先针肾俞1～1.5寸，得气后持续运针1分钟，然后温针灸3～5壮；再针中极，得气后使针感放散至阴部，留针20～30分钟，温针3～5壮；针阴陵泉要使针感放射至足，留针20～30分钟。

Composition This group of acupoints is composed of Zhongji(CV3), Shenshu(BL23) and Yinlingquan(SP9).

Location Zhongji: 4 cun below the centre of the umbilicus.

Shenshu: 1.5 cun lateral to the point below the spinous process of the 2nd lumbar vertebra.

Yinlingquan: in the depression below the medial condyle of the tibia.

Indication Symptoms of deficiency of kidney qi: frequent urination, thin and excessive urine, or with incontinence of urination, whitish complexion, dizziness, tinnitus, shortness of breath, asthma, weakness in the lower back and knees, coldness in the four limbs.

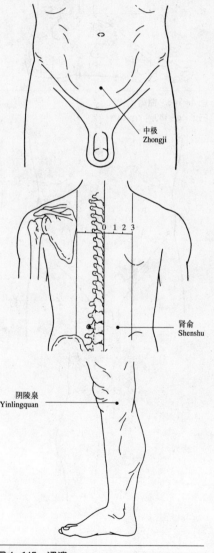

图4-145 涩溲
Fig. 4-145 Sesou

Method   Shenshu is needled 1−1.5 cun first. Manipulate the needle for 1 minute continuously after the arrival of the acu-esthesia. Then Zhongji is needled, and the acu-esthesia should radiate to the pubes. Retain the needles for 20−30 minutes, 3−5 cones of warm needle moxibustion is applied. The acu-esthesia of Yinlingquan should transmit to the foot, and retain the needles for 20−30 minutes.

尿频
Niaopin

组成   本穴组由中极、大赫、曲泉三穴组合而成。

位置   中极：脐下4寸。

大赫：脐下4寸，前正中线旁开0.5寸。

曲泉：屈膝，当膝内侧横纹头上方凹陷中。

主治   尿频。

操作   刺法：中极、大赫直刺1~1.5寸，感应放散至尿道口。曲泉直刺0.5~1寸。

灸法：艾条温灸10~20分钟。

Composition   This group of acupoints is composed of Zhongji(CV3), Dahe(KI12) and Ququan(LR8).

Location   Zhongji：4 cun below the centre of the umbilicus.

Dahe：4 cun below the centre of the umbilicus, 0.5 cun lateral to the anterior midline.

Ququan：when the knee is flexed, in the depression above the medial end of the popliteal crease.

Indication   Frequent urination.

Methods   Acupuncture：Zhongji and Dahe is needled 1−1.5 cun perpendicularly, the acu-esthesia shoud spread to the urethra. Ququan is needled 0.5−1 cun perpendicularly.

Moxibustion：warm moxibustion with moxa roll for 10−20 minutes is applied.

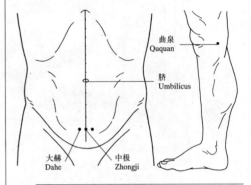

图4-146 尿频
Fig. 4-146 Niaopin

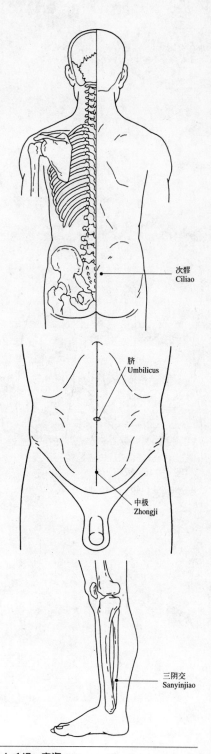

图4-147 安泡
Fig. 4-147 Anpao

● 安泡
Anpao

组成 本穴组由次髎、中极、三阴交三穴组合而成。

位置 次髎：第二骶后孔中，约当髂后上棘下与督脉的中点。

中极：脐下4寸。

三阴交：内踝高点上3寸，胫骨内侧面后缘。

主治 尿频尿闭，小便不利，遗精，阳痿早泄，月经不调，带多等。

操作 刺法：次髎向第二骶后孔斜刺1～1.5寸。中极尿频时直刺感应到尿道口，尿闭时斜刺1～1.5寸。三阴交直刺1～1.5寸，得气为度。

灸法：艾炷灸3～5壮，艾条灸10～20分钟。

Composition This group of acupoints is composed of Ciliao(BL32), Zhongji(CV3) and Sanyinjiao(SP6).

Location Ciliao：in the 2nd posterior sacral foramen, at the midpoint between the posterioinferior iliac spine and the posterior midline.

Zhongji：4 cun below the centre of the umbilicus.

Sanyinjiao：3 cun above the tip of the medial malleolus, on the posterior border of the medial side of the tibia.

Indication Frequent urination, anuria, seminal emission, impotence, premature ejaculation, irregular menstruation, excessive leukorrhea.

Method Acupuncture：Ciliao is needled 1－1.5 cun towards the 2nd posterior sacral foramen. Zhongji：for the frequent urination, the needle is inserted perpendicularly till the acu－esthesia spreads to the urethra；for the anuria, the needle is inserted 1－1.5 cun obliquely. Sanyinjiao is inserted 1－1.5 cun perpendicularly till the acu-esthesia is obtained.

Moxibustion：moxibustion with 3－5 moxa cones, or moxibustion with moxa roll for 10－20 minutes is applied.

气闭
Qibi

组成　本穴组由阴陵泉、气海、三阴交三穴组合而成。

位置　阴陵泉：胫骨内侧髁下缘凹陷中。

三阴交：内踝高点上3寸，胫骨内侧面后缘。

气海：脐下1.5寸。

主治　肾气不足之小便不通，尿意频频排出无力。

操作　先针气海1.2～1.5寸，使针感向阴部放散，如不效则加灸3～5壮；然后针阴陵泉、三阴交各1～1.2寸，行提插捻转之补法。诸穴均留针20～30分钟。

Composition　This group of acupoints is composed of Yinlingquan(SP9), Qihai(CV6) and Sanyinjiao(SP6).

Location　Yinlingquan：in the depression below the medial condyle of the tibia.

Sanyinjiao：3 cun above the tip of the medial malleolus, on the posterior border of the tibia.

Qihai：1.5 cun below the centre of the umbilicus.

Indication　Retention of urine, incapability of urination due to deficiency of kidney qi.

Method　First, Qihai is needled 1.2−1.5 cun, the acu-esthesia shoud spread to the pubes, 3−5 cones of moxibustion can be applied if acupuncture doesn't take effect. Then Yinlingquan and Sanyinjiao are needled 1−1.2 cun, reinforcing techniques by lifting, inserting and rotating the needles is applied. Reatin the needles for 20−30 minutes.

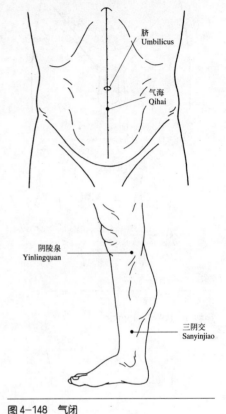

图4-148　气闭
Fig. 4-148　Qibi

通尿
Tongniao

组成　本穴组由中极、三阴交、合谷、阴陵泉四穴组合而成。

位置　中极：脐下4寸。

三阴交：内踝高点上3寸，胫骨内侧面后缘。

阴陵泉：胫骨内侧髁下缘凹陷中。

合谷：手背，第一、第二掌骨之间，约平第二掌骨中点处。

主治　尿闭。

操作　合谷直刺0.5～1寸。中极斜刺。阴陵泉、三阴交直刺1～1.5寸，得气为度。

Composition　This group of acupoints is composed of Zhongji(CV3), Sanyinjiao(SP6), Hegu(L24) and Yinlingquan (SP9).

Location　Zhongji：4 cun below the centre of the umbilicus.

Sanyinjiao：3 cun above the tip of the medial malleolus, on the posterior border of the medial side of the tibia.

Yinlingquan：in the depression below the medial condyle of the tibia.

Hegu：on the dorsum of the hand, between the 1st and 2nd metacarpal bones, and near the midpoint of the 2nd metacarpal bone.

Indication　Anuria.

Method　Hegu is needled 0.5—1 cun perpendicularly. Zhongji is needled obliquely, Yinlingquan and Sanyinjiao is needled 1—1.5 cun perpendicularly till the acu-esthesia is obtained.

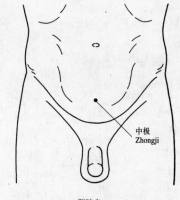
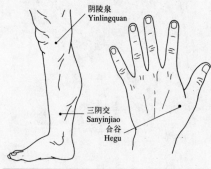

图4-149　通尿
Fig. 4-149　Tongniao

 气里

Qili

组成　本穴组由气海、足三里二穴组合而成。

位置　气海：脐下1.5寸。

足三里：犊鼻穴下3寸，胫骨前嵴外一横指处。

主治　五淋，气短。

操作　刺法：气海、足三里直刺0.8～1.2寸，得气为度，留针30分钟，留针期间可反复行针数次。

灸法：艾炷灸5～9壮，艾条温灸10～30分钟。

Composition　This group of acupoints is composed of Qihai(CV6) and Zusanli(ST36).

Location　Qihai：1.5 cun below the centre of the umbilicus.

Zusanli：3 cun below Dubi, one finger breadth from the anterior crest of the tibia.

Indication　Stranguria, shortness of breath.

Methods　Acupuncture：the needle is inserted 0.8—1.2 cun perpendicularly till the acu-esthesia is obtained.

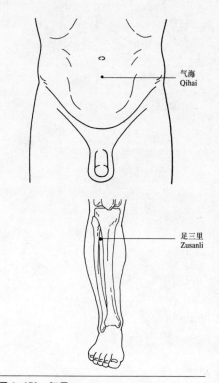

图4-150　气里
Fig. 4-150　Qili

Retain the needles for 30 minutes. Manipulations of the needles may be applied several times during the retention of the needles.

Moxibustion：moxibustion with 5-9 moxa cones, or warm moxibustion with moxa roll for 10-30 minutes is applied.

狐疝
Hushan

组成　本穴组由照海、阴交、曲泉三穴组合而成。

位置　照海：内踝下缘凹陷中。

阴交：脐下1寸。

曲泉：屈膝，当膝内侧横纹头上方凹陷中。

主治　狐疝。

操作　先针阴交，使针感沿任脉向下放散至外生殖器；然后针曲泉，使针感沿肝经向阴器放射；照海针0.3～0.4寸。诸穴留针均30分钟，三穴可加灸。

Composition　This group of acupoints is composed of Zhaohai(KI6), Yinjiao(CV7) and Ququan(LR8).

Location　Zhaohai：in the depression on the lower border of the medial malleolus.

Yinjiao：1 cun below the centre of the umbilicus.

Ququan：when the knee is flexed, in the depression above the medial end of the popliteal crease.

Indication　Hu-hernia.

Method　Yinjiao is needled first to make the acu-esthesia spread downwards to the genitals. Then Ququan is needled to make to acu-esthesia radiate towards the genitals along the Liver Meridian. Zhaohai is needled 0.3-0.4 cun. Retain the needles for 30 minutes. Moxibustion can be applied to above points.

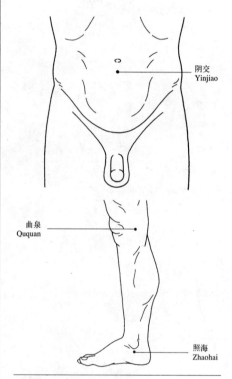

图4-151　狐疝
Fig. 4-151　Hushan

七疝
Qishan

组成　本穴组由大敦、阖门二穴组合而成。

位置　大敦：蹈趾外侧趾甲角旁约0.1寸。

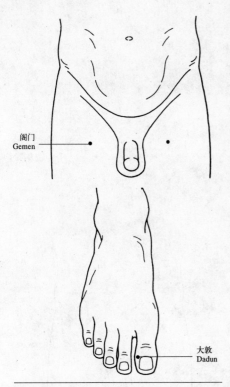

图4-152 七疝
Fig. 4-152 Qishan

阎门：阴茎根旁开3寸。

主治 七疝。

操作 大敦斜刺0.1~0.2寸。阎门针1~1.5寸，得气为度灸5~9壮。累计灸可达50壮或100壮。

Composition This group of acupoints is composed of Dadun(LR1) and Gemen.

Location Dadun：0.1 cun from the lateral corner of the toenail of the great toe.

Gemen：3 cun lateral to the root of the penis.

Indication Hernia.

Method Dadun：the needle is inserted 0.1−0.2 cun obliquely. Gemen：the needle is inserted 1−1.5 cun till the acu-esthesia is obtained. 5−9 cones of moxibustion, or a total of 50 or 100 cones can be applied.

上、中、下三才
Shangzhongxiasancai

组成 本穴组由大包(上)、天枢(中)、地机(下)三穴组成。

位置 大包：腋中线上，第六肋间隙中。

地机：阴陵泉穴下3寸。

天枢：脐旁2寸。

主治 带下痛经，胃肠疾病。

操作 刺法：大包针刺0.3~0.5寸。天枢、地机直刺1~1.5寸，局部酸胀，天枢针感可向同侧腹部扩散，地机针感可扩散至小腿部。

灸法：灸3~5壮，艾条温灸5~15分钟。

Composition This group of acupoints is composed of Dabao(SP21) (shang), Tianshu(ST25)(zhong) and Diji(SP8) (xia).

Location Dabao：on the middle axillary line, in the 6th intercostal space.

Diji：3 cun below Yinlingquan.

Tianshu：2 cun lateral to the centre of the umbilicus.

Indication Leukorrhea, dysmenorrhea, diseases of the stomach and intestine.

Method Acupuncture：Dabao is needled 0.3−0.5 cun. Tianshu and Diji are needled 1−1.5 cun perpendicularly. The acu-esthesia of soreness and dis-

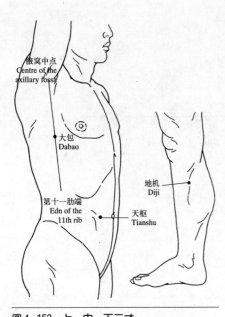

图4-153 上、中、下三才
Fig. 4-153 Shangzhongxiasancai

tension will be obtained in the part, and the feeling of Tianshu will spread to the abdomen in the same side, the feeling of Diji may spread to the leg.

Moxibustion：3–5 cones of moxibustion, or warm moxibustion with moxa roll for 5–15 minutes is applied.

梅交
Meijiao

组成　本穴组由下关梅四穴、三阴交共五穴组合而成。

位置　下关梅：以脐下 3 寸之关元穴为中点，上下左右各旁开 1 寸，共四个点。

三阴交：内踝高点上 3 寸，胫骨内侧面后缘。

主治　痛经。

操作　持壮医药线，点燃后候成珠火时，将珠火直接点按于穴上，然后分轻重按压熄灭，疼痛发作时用重按压法熄灭。在月经来潮前 1~2 日开始灸治，每日 1 次，至经净之日为止。

Composition　This group of acupoints is composed of Xiaguanmei and Sanyinjiao(SP6).

Location　Xiaguanmei：select Guanyuan which is 3 cun below the centre of the umbilicus as the centre point, the points are 1 cun respectively lateral, superior and inferior to it, 4 points in all.

Sanyinjiao：3 cun above the tip of the medial malleolus, on the posterior border of the medial side of the tibia.

Indication　Dysmenorrhea.

Method　Light the medicinal thread of the Zhuang Nationality. When the fire of the thread turns into a pearl, press the fire directly on the acupoints. Then put out the fire. During the paroxysm of pain, put out the fire with heavy press method. The treatment is given 1–2 days prior to the mens truation, treat once every day untill it's gone.

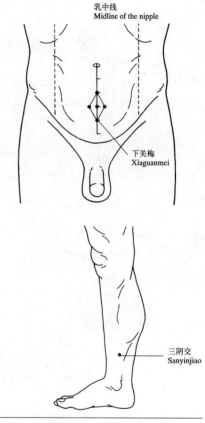

乳中线
Midline of the nipple

下关梅
Xiaguanmei

三阴交
Sanyinjiao

图 4–154　梅交
Fig. 4–154　Meijiao

痛经
Tongjing

组成　本穴组由关元、地机、三阴交、足三里四穴组合而成。

位置　关元：脐下3寸。

地机：阴陵泉穴下3寸。

三阴交：内踝高点上3寸，胫骨内侧面后缘。

足三里：犊鼻穴下3寸，胫骨前嵴外一横指处。

主治　痛经。

操作　刺法：直刺1～1.5寸，留针30分钟，留针期间可不断运针以止痛。

灸法：艾条灸10～30分钟。

Composition　This group of acupoints is composed of Guanyuan(CV4)，Diji(SP8)，Sanyinjiao(SP6) and Zusanli (ST36).

Location　Guanyuan：2 cun below the centre of the umbilicus.

Diji：3 cun below Yinlingquan.

Sanyinjiao：3 cun above the tip of the medial malleolus, on the posterior border of the medial side of the tibia.

Zusanli：3 cun below Dubi, one finger breadth from the anterior crest of the tibia.

Indication　Dysmenorrhea.

Method　Acupuncture：the needle is inserted 1−1.5 cun perpendicularly. Retain the needles for 30 minutes. The continous manipulation of needles can be applied during the retention to relieve pain.

Moxibustion：moxibustion with moxa roll for 10−30 minutes is applied.

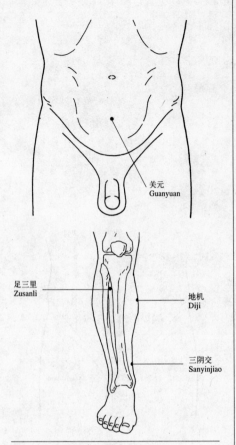

图4-155　痛经
Fig. 4-155　Tongjing

● 小腹九灵术
Xiaofujiulingshu

组成　本穴组由关元、中极、曲骨、三阴交(双)、行间、太冲、肾俞(双)共九穴组合而成。

位置　关元：脐下3寸。

中极：脐下4寸。

曲骨：耻骨联合上缘中点处。

三阴交：内踝高点上3寸，胫骨内侧面后缘。

行间：足背，第一、第二趾间缝纹端。

太冲：足背，第一、第二跖骨结合部之前凹陷中。

肾俞：第二腰椎棘突下，旁开1.5寸。

主治　痛经，月经不调，闭经，白带过多，肠痛。

操作　刺法：关元、中极、曲骨穴针 0.3~0.5 寸，针感抽至耻骨联合或外阴部。三阴交穴针 0.5~0.8 寸，针感麻、酸至内踝。行间穴进针后向上斜刺透至太冲穴，针感抽、胀至趾。肾俞穴针 0.5~0.8 寸，针感局部酸、胀。

灸法：灸 3~9 壮，艾条灸 10~20 分钟。

Composition　This group of acupoints is composed of Guanyuan(CV4), Zhongji(CV3), Qugu(CV2), Sanyinjiao(SP6), Xingjian(LR2) penetrating to Taichong(LR3) and Shenshu(BL23).

Location　Guanyuan：3 cun below the centre of the umbilicus.

Zhongji：4 cun below the centre of the umbilicus.

Qugu：at the midpoint of the upper border of the pubic symphysis.

Sanyinjiao：3 cun above the tip of the medial malleolus, on the posterior border of the medial side of the tibia.

Xingjian：on the instep of the foot, on the end of the margin of the web between the 1st and 2nd toes.

Taichong：on the instep of the foot, in the depression anterior to the commissure of the 1st and 2nd metatarsal bones.

Shenshu：1.5 cun lateral to the point below the spinous process of the 2nd lumbar vertebra.

Indication　Dysmenorrhea, irregular menstruation, amenorrhea, enteritis.

Method　Acupuncture：Guanyuan, Zhongji and Qugu are needled 0.3—0.5 cun, the acu-esthesia will spread to the pubic symphysis or the pubes. Sanyinjiao is needled 0.5—0.8 cun, the acu-esthesia will spread to the medial malleolus. Xingjian is penetrated upwards to Taichong, the acu-esthesia of twitching and distension will spread to the toes. Shenshu is needled 0.5—0.8 cun, the acu-esthesia is the feeling of soreness and distension in the part.

Moxibustion：3—9 cones of moxibustion, or moxibustion with moxa roll for 10—20 minutes is applied.

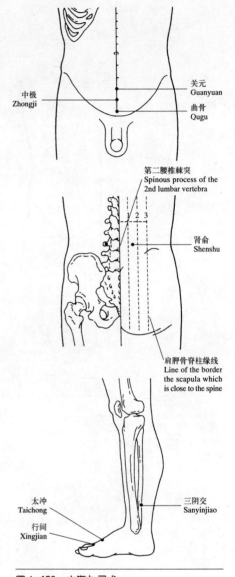

图 4-156　小腹九灵术
Fig. 4-156　Xiaofujiulingshu

调经
Tiaojing

组成　本穴组由气海、中极、照海三穴组合而成。

位置　气海：脐下1.5寸。

中极：脐下4寸。

照海：内踝下缘凹陷中。

主治　经来先后无定期，经量或多或少，经色或紫或淡。

操作　先刺气海、中极，使产生的酸胀感沿任脉向下放射至外阴部及生殖器，并可在此两穴加灸；后针照海，使酸、麻感向小腿及踝部发散。

Composition　This group of acupoints is composed of Qihai(CV6), Zhongji(CV3) and Zhaohai(KI6).

Location　Qihai：1.5 cun below the centre of the umbilicus.

Zhongji：4 cun below the centre of the umbilicus.

Zhaohai：in the depression on the lower border of the medial malleolus.

Indication　Irregular menstruation in menstrual cycle, quantity and color.

Method　Qihai and Zhongji is needled first to make the acu-esthesia of the soreness and distension transmit downwards to the pubes and genitals along the Conception Vessel. The two points can be treated with moxibustion. Then Zhaohai is needled, and the acu-esthesia of soreness and numbness will transmit to the leg and ankle.

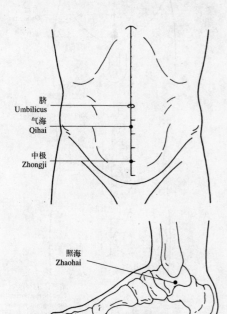

图4-157　调经
Fig. 4-157　Tiaojing

阴三针
Yinsanzhen

组成　本穴组由关元、归来、三阴交三穴组合而成。

位置　关元：脐下3寸。

归来：脐下4寸，前正中线旁开2寸。

三阴交：内踝高点上3寸，胫骨内侧面后缘。

主治　月经不调，不孕症。

操作　关元、三阴交直刺1~1.5寸，得气为度。

Composition　This group of acupoints is composed of

汉 英 对 照

Guanyuan(CV4), Guilai(ST29) and Sanyinjiao(SP6).

Location Guanyuan：3 cun below the centre of the umbilicus.

Guilai：4 cun below the centre of the umbilicus, 2 cun lateral to the anterior midline.

Sanyinjiao：3 cun above the tip of the medial malleolus, on the posterior border of the medial side of the tibia.

Indications Irregualr menstruation and sterility.

Method Guanyuan and Sanyinjiao are needled 1—1.5 cun perpendicularly till the acu-esthesia is obtained.

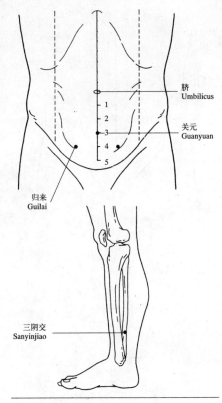

图4-158 阴三针
Fig. 4-158 Yinsanzhen

● 枢泉
Shuquan

组成　本穴组由天枢、水泉二穴组合而成。

位置　天枢：脐旁2寸。

水泉：太溪直下1寸。

主治　月经失调。

操作　刺法：天枢直刺0.8~1.2寸。水泉针0.5~0.8寸，得气为度。

灸法：艾炷灸3~5壮，艾条温灸5~15分钟。

Composition This group of acupoints is composed of Tianshu(ST25) and Shuiquan(KI5).

Location Tianshu：2 cun lateral to the centre of the umbilicus.

Shuiquan：1 cun directly below Taixi.

Indication Irregular menstruation.

Method Acupuncture：Tianshu is needled 0.8—1.2 cun perpendicularly. Shuiquan is needled 0.5—0.8 cun till the acu-esthesia is obtained.

Moxibustion：moxibustion with 3—5 moxa cones, or warm moxibustion with moxa roll for 5—15 minutes is applied.

● 下胎
Xiatai

组成　本穴组由阴交、合谷二穴组合而成。

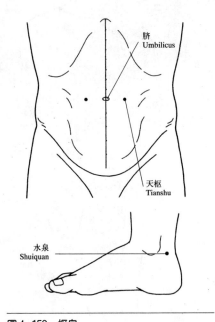

图4-159 枢泉
Fig. 4-159 Shuquan

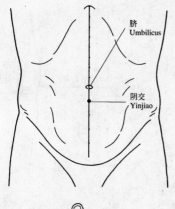

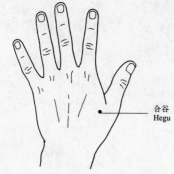

图 4-160 下胎
Fig. 4-160 Xiatai

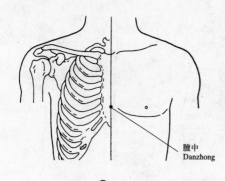

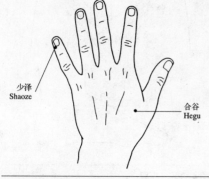

图 4-161 通乳
Fig. 4-161 Tongru

位置 阴交：脐下1寸。

合谷：手背，第一、第二掌骨之间，约平第二掌骨中点处。

主治 死胎不下。

操作 直刺0.5~1.2寸，得气为度，可用较强手法以促使胎下。

Composition This group of acupoints is composed of Yinjiao(CV7) and Hegu(LI4).

Location Yinjiao：1 cun below the centre of the umbilicus.

Hegu：on the dorsum of the hand, between the 1st and 2nd metacarpal bones, and near the midpoint of the 2nd metacarpal bone.

Indication Failure to deliver dead fetus.

Method The needle is inserted 0.5—1.2 cun perpendicularly till the acu-esthesia is obtained. Strong stimulating intensity can be applied in order to help the dilivery of the fetus.

● 通乳
Tongru

组成 本穴组由少泽、合谷、膻中三穴组合而成。

位置 少泽：小指尺侧指甲角旁约0.1寸。

合谷：手背，第一、第二掌骨之间，约平第二掌骨中点处。

膻中：前正中线，平第四肋间隙。

主治 产后乳汁不行或甚少。

操作 膻中针0.3~0.5寸，针尖向下沿皮刺，以局部胀为主，轻轻捻转针柄使两乳房发胀。少泽针0.1~0.2寸，针感多为疼痛。合谷针0.5~1寸，针感以胀、麻居多，向手指或肘、肩部放射。上诸穴均留针20~30分钟。

Composition This group of acupoints is composed of Shaoze(SI1), Hegu(LI4) and Danzhong(CV17).

Location Shaoze：0.1 cun lateral to the ulnar corner of the fingernail of the little finger.

Hegu：on the dorsum of the hand, between the 1st and 2nd metacarpal bones, and near the midpoint of the 2nd metacarpal bone.

Danzhong：on the anterior midline, at the horizonal level of the 4th intercostal space.

Indication   No or insufficient lactation after delivery.

Method   Danzhong is needled 0.3−0.5 cun under the skin with the tip of the needle downwards. The acu-esthesia is mainly distension in the part. Rotate the handle of the needle to induce distension in the breasts. Shaoze is needled 0.1−0.2 cun, the acu-esthesia is usually the pain. Hegu is needled 0.5−1 cun, the acu-esthesia of mainly distension and numbness will transmit to the fingers or to the elbow and shoulder. Retain the needles for 20−30 minutes.

● 二中
Erzhong

组成   本穴组由人中、委中二穴组合而成。

位置   人中：在人中沟的上 1/3 与中 1/3 交界处。

委中：腘横纹中央。

主治   腰背闪痛。

操作   人中向上斜刺 0.3~0.5 寸，针感酸痛。委中直刺 1~1.5 寸，或用三棱针点刺出血。

Composition   This group of acupoints is composed of Renzong(GV26) and Weizhong(BL40).

Location   Renzhong：at the junction of the upper one-third and middle one-third of the philtrum.

Weizhong：at the midpoint of the popliteal crease.

Indication   Pain due to the sprain in the lumbus and back.

Method   Renzhong is needled 0.3−0.5 cun upwards, the acu-esthesia is pain. Weizhong is needled 1−1.5 cun perpendicularly, or it can be pricked to bleed with a three-edged needle.

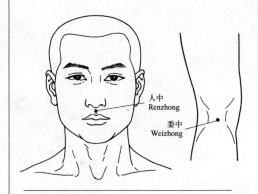

人中 Renzhong

委中 Weizhong

图 4−162 二中
Fig. 4−162 Erzhong

● 腰三针
Yaosanzhen

组成   本穴组由肾俞、大肠俞、委中三穴组合而成。

位置   肾俞：第二腰椎棘突下，旁开 1.5 寸。

大肠俞：第四腰椎棘突下，旁开 1.5 寸。

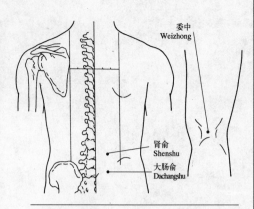

图4-163 腰三针
Fig.4-163 Yaosanzhen

委中：腘横纹中央。

主治　急慢性腰痛，性功能障碍，遗精，阳痿，月经不调。

操作　针法：肾俞穴、大肠穴直刺1～1.5寸。委中穴采用相对较浅的刺法，使之易于得气，务必使针感向腰部或下肢传导。常采用疾徐补泻和捻转补泻手法。若急性腰扭伤等痛甚者，针后加用电针，以患者能耐受为度，每次20分钟。

灸法：以艾条悬灸，时间为15分钟或涂以万花油以艾绒麦炷灸5～7壮。

Composition　This group of acupoints is composed of Shenshu(BL23), Dachangshu(BL25) and Weizhong(BL40).

Location　Shenshu：1.5 cun lateral to the point below the spinous process of the 2nd lumbar vertebra.

Dachangshu：1.5 cun lateral to the spinous process of the 4th lumbar vertebra.

Weizhong：at the midpoint of the popliteal crease.

Indications　Acute and chronic pain in the lower back, sexual disorders, seminal emission, impotence, irregular menstruation.

Method　Acupuncture：Shenshu and Dachangshu are needled 1－1.5 cun perpendicularly. Weizhong is needled with a relatively shallow puncturing method so as to induce the acu-esthesia easily, and the feeling should be made to spread to the lower back or lower limbs. Reinforcing and reducing techniques by slow and rapid puncturing or rotation are often applied. For the patient of severe pain due to acute lumbar sprain, electroacupuncture can be applied after the insertion on the basis of the patients toleran. Electrify the needles for 20 minutes every time.

Moxibustion：suspended moxibustion with moxa roll for 15 minutes, or 5－7 cones of moxibustion with the Wanhua oil　on the skin is applied.

 伛偻
Yulü

组成　本穴组由风池、悬钟二穴组合而成。

位置　风池：胸锁乳突肌与斜方肌之间凹陷中，平风府穴处。

悬钟：外踝高点上3寸，腓骨后缘。

主治　伛偻驼背。

操作　刺法：直刺0.5~1.2寸，得气为度。

灸法：悬钟用麦粒灸5~9壮。风池用艾条灸10~20分钟。

Composition　This group of acupoints is composed of Fengchi(GB20) and Xuanzhong(GB39).

Location　Fengchi：in the depression between the sternocleidomastoid and trapezius muscles, at the horizontal level of Fengfu.

Juegu：3 cun above the tip of the external malleolus, on the posterior border of the fibula.

Indication　Kyphosis.

Method　Acupuncture：the needle is inserted 0.5—1.2 cun perpendicularly till the acu-esthesia is obtained.

Moxibustion：Xuanzhong is treated with 5—9 cones of moxibustion. Fengchi is treated with 10—20 minutes' moxibustion with moxa roll.

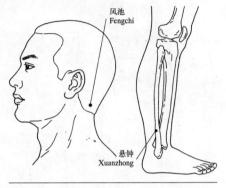

图4-164　伛偻
Fig. 4-164　Yulü

 海溜
Hailiu

组成　本穴组由气海、复溜二穴组合而成。

位置　气海：脐下1.5寸。

复溜：太溪穴上2寸。

主治　多汗。

操作　气海直刺0.8~1.5寸。复溜直刺0.5~1寸，得气为度。

Composition　This group of acupoints is composed of Qihai(CV6) and Fuliu(K27).

Location　Qihai：1.5 cun below the centre of the umbilicus.

Fuliu：2 cun above Taixi.

Indication　Excessive sweating.

Method　Qihai is needled 0.8—1.5 cun perpendicularly. Fuliu is needled 0.5—1 cun perpendicularly till the acu-esthesia is obtained.

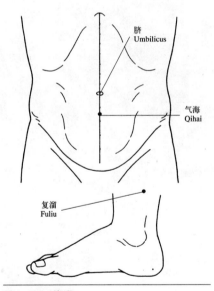

图4-165　海溜
Fig. 4-165　Hailiu

肿瘘
Zhonglou

组成　本穴组由渊液、章门、支沟三穴组合而成。

位置　渊液：举臂，腋中线上，第四肋间隙。

章门：第十一肋端。

支沟：腕背横纹上3寸，桡骨与尺骨之间。

主治　结核生于腋下，累累如贯珠之状，排列状如马刀者。

操作　先取渊液、顺肋间方向斜刺0.5～0.8寸；后刺章门、斜刺0.5～1寸；支沟直刺0.5～1寸。针刺用提插捻转泻法，行针2～3次，均留针30分钟。留针时若见溃破流水的部位，可于出针后另加艾炷灸5～7壮。

Composition　This group of acupoints is composed of Yuanye(GB22), Zhangmen(LR13) and Zhigou(TE6).

Location　Yuanye：on the midaxillary line when the arm is raised, in the 4th intercostal space.

Zhangmen：on the end of the 11th rib.

Zhigou：2 cun above the dorsal crease of the wrist, between the radius and ulna.

Indication　Scrofula in the armpit.

Method　First, Yuanye is needled 0.5−0.8 cun obliquely along the intercostal space. Then Zhangmen is needled 0.5−1 cun obliquely, Zhigou 0.5−1 cun perpendicularly. Reducing techniques by lifting, inserting and rotating are applied. Manipulate the needles for 2−3 times. Retain the needles for 30 minutes. 5−7 cones of moxibustion can be applied to the points from which the fluid flows out during the retention.

 身八邪
Shenbaxie

组成　本穴组由肺俞、风门、肩井、曲泽左右八穴组成。

位置　肺俞：第三胸椎棘突下，旁开1.5寸。

风门：第二胸椎棘突下，旁开1.5寸。

肩井：大椎穴(督脉)与肩峰连线的中点。

曲泽：肘横纹中，肱二头肌腱尺侧。

主治　风疾。

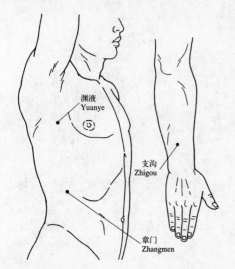

图4-166　肿瘘
Fig. 4-166　Zhonglou

操作　刺法：针0.3～0.5寸，局部酸胀感。

灸法：灸5～9壮，艾条温灸5～15分钟。

Composition　This group of acupoints is composed of Feishu(BL13), Fengmen(BL12), Jianjing(GB21) and Quze (PC3), 8 points in both sides.

Location　Feishu：1.5 cun lateral to the point below the 3rd spinous process of the thoracic vertebra.

Fengmen：1.5 cun lateral to the point below the 2nd spinous process of the thoracic vertebra.

Jianjing：at the midpoint of Dazhui and the acromion.

Indication　Diseases due to wind.

Methods　Acupuncture：the needle is inserted 0.3－0.5 cun, the acu-esthesia of soreness and distension will be　obtained in the part.

Moxibustion：5－9 cones of moxibustion, or warm moxibustion with moxa roll for 5－15 minutes is applied.

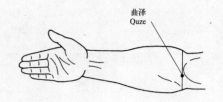

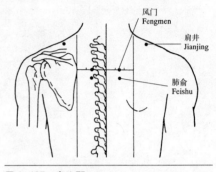

图4-167　身八邪
Fig. 4-167　Shenbaxie

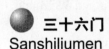

三十六门
Sanshiliumen

组成　本穴组由十四经之金门、魂门、殷门、箕门、冲门、液门、风门、肓门、哑门、命门、幽门、梁门、关门、滑肉门、章门、京门、神门、郄门、云门左右三十六穴组合而成。

位置　金门：申脉前下方的凹陷中。

魂门：第九胸椎棘突下，旁开3寸。

殷门：承扶穴与委中穴连线上，承扶穴下6寸处。

箕门：血海穴与冲门穴的连线上，血海穴直上6寸。

冲门：耻骨联合上缘中点旁开3.5寸。

液门：握拳，第四、五指之间，指掌关节前凹陷中。

风门：第二胸椎棘突下，旁开1.5寸。

肓门：第一腰椎棘突下，旁开3寸。

哑门：后发际正中直上0.5寸。

命门：第二腰椎棘突下。

幽门：脐上6寸，前正中线旁开0.5寸。

梁门：脐上4寸，前正中线旁开2寸。

关门：脐上3寸，前正中线旁开2寸。

滑肉门：脐上1寸，前正中线旁开2寸。

章门：第十一肋端。

京门：第十二肋端。

神门：腕横纹尺侧端，尺侧腕屈肌腱的桡侧凹陷中。

郄门：腕横纹上5寸，掌长肌腱与桡侧腕屈肌腱之间。

云门：胸前壁外上方，距前正中线旁开6寸，当锁骨外端下缘凹陷中取穴。

主治　风邪。

操作　灸1～3壮。

Composition　This group of acupoints is composed of Jinmen(BL63), Hunmen(BL47), Yinmen(BL37),Jimen(SR14), Chongmen(SP12), Yemen(TE2), Fengmen(BL12), Huangmen(BL51), Yamen(GV15), Mingmen(GV4), Youmen (KI21), Liangmen(ST21), Guanmen(ST22), Huaroumen (ST24), Zhangmen(LR14), Shenmen(HT7), Ximen(PC4) and Yunmen(LV2) of the 14 meridians.

Location　Jinmen：in the depression anterior and inferior to Shenmai.

Hunmen：3 cun lateral to the point below the spinous process of the 9th thoracic vertebra.

Yinmen：on the line connecting Chengfu and Weizhong, 6 cun below Chengfu.

Qimen：on the line connecting Xuehai and Chongmen, 6 cun directly above Xuehai.

Chongmen：3.5 cun lateral to the midpoint of the symphysis pubis.

Yemen：between the 4th and 5th fingers, in the front depression near the metacarpophalangeal joint when the fist is made.

Fengmen：1.5 cun lateral to the point below the 2nd spinous process of the thoracic vertebra.

Huangmen：3 cun lateral to the point below the spinous process of the 1st lumbar vertebra.

Yamen：0.5 cun directly above the midpoint of the posterior hairline.

Mingmen：below the spinous process of the 2nd lumbar vertebra.

Youmen：6 cun above the centre of the umbilicus, 0.5 cun lateral to the anterior midline.

Liangmen：4 cun above the centre of the umbilicus, 2 cun lateral to the anterior midline.

Guanmen：3 cun above the centre of the umbilicus, 2 cun lateral to the anterior midline.

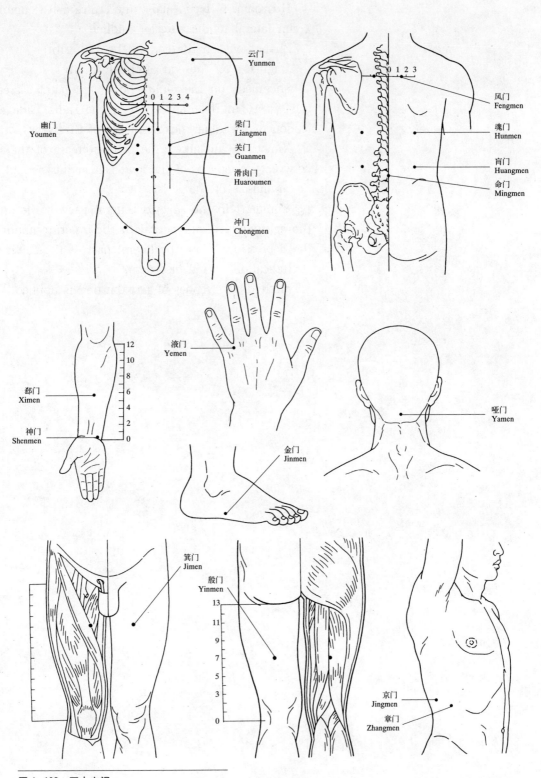

云门
Yunmen

幽门
Youmen

梁门
Liangmen

关门
Guanmen

滑肉门
Huaroumen

冲门
Chongmen

风门
Fengmen

魂门
Hunmen

肓门
Huangmen

命门
Mingmen

液门
Yemen

郄门
Ximen

神门
Shenmen

金门
Jinmen

哑门
Yamen

箕门
Jimen

殷门
Yinmen

京门
Jingmen

章门
Zhangmen

图 4-168 三十六门

Fig. 4-168 Sanshiliumen

Huaroumen: 1 cun above the centre of the umbilicus, 2 cun lateral to the anterior midline.

Zhangmen: on the end of the 11th rib.

Jingmen: on the end of the 12th rib.

Shenmen: on the ulnar end of the palmar crease of the wrist, in the depression of the radial side of the tendon of the ulnar flexor muscle of the wrist.

Ximen: 5 cun above the palmar crease of the wrist, between the tendons of the long palmar muscle and radial flexor muscle of the wrist.

Yunmen: in the superior lateral part of the anterior thoracic wall, 6 cun lateral to the anterior midline, in the depression below the lateral part of the clavicle.

Indication Wind disorders.

Method 1—3 cones of moxibustion is applied.